ATI NurseNotes

Pediatrics
Core Content At-A-Glance

WITHDRAWN

Includes "Study and Memory Aids"

Edited by:
Sally Lambert Lagerquist, RN, MS

Author:
Kathleen E. Snider, RN, MSN, CNS

ATI NurseNotes
Pediatrics
Core Content At-A-Glance

Edited by:
Sally Lambert Lagerquist, RN, MS

Former Instructor in Undergraduate and Graduate Programs
    and Continuing Education in Nursing
University of California, San Francisco, School of Nursing
President, Review for Nurses, Inc., and RN Tapes Company
San Francisco, California

Author:
Kathleen E. Snider, RN, MSN, CNS
Professor of Nursing
Los Angeles Valley College
Valley Glen, California

ATI Assessment Technologies Institute™ LLC

Acquisitions Editor: Bob Cole
Assistant Editor: Melissa Wells
Project Editor: Sally Volkoff
Production Manager: Don Walde
Programmer: Trevor Gunter
Art Director: Hara Allison
Graphic Design-Illustrators: Allen Croswhite and Eric Osterback
Design Production: Hara Allison
Indexer: Laura Steen and Melissa Wells

Library of Congress Cataloging in Publications Data

NurseNotes: Pediatric/Kathleen E. Snider; edited by Sally Lambert Lagerquist.
p.cm.
Includes bibliographical references and index.
ISBN 0-9760063-2-4
1. Pediatric nursing—Outlines, syllabi, etc. 2. Pediatric nursing—Examinations, questions, etc. I. Lagerquist, Sally L.
[DNLM: 1. Pediatric Nursing—examination questions. 2. Pediatric Nursing—outlines.
3. Child Development—examination questions. 4. Child Development—outlines. WY 18.2 C718n 2007]
RJ245.C625   1997-2007
610.73'62'076—dc20
DNLM/DLC
for Library of Congress   96-20788
                                                                                                                         CIP

Care has been taken to confirm the accuracy of the information presented and to describe generally accepted practices. However, the authors, editors, and publisher are not responsible for errors or omissions or for any consequences from application of the information in this book and make no warranty, express or implied, with respect to the contents of the publication.

The authors, editors and publisher have exerted every effort to ensure that drug selection and dosage set forth in this text are in accordance with current recommendations and practice at the time of publication. However, in view of ongoing research, changes in government regulations, and the constant flow of information relating to drug therapy and drug reactions, the reader is urged to check the package insert for each drug for any change in indications and dosage and for added warnings and precautions. This is particularly important when the recommended agent is a new or infrequently employed drug.

Some drugs and medical devices presented in this publication have Food and Drug Administration (FDA) clearance for limited use in restricted research settings. It is the responsibility of the health care provider to ascertain the FDA status of each drug or device planned for use in their clinical practice.

Last digit indicates print number   9   8   7   6   5   4   3   2   1

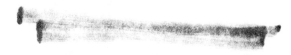

Dedications

I dedicate this book to my family. You have all given me such special "gifts."

To my husband, **Tom** –
Who always gives so much, with a generous loving touch...
...when there's another book for me to write, by many a dawn's early light.
With time rushing by so fast, let's make memories to last.
Let's toast the life we share,
...then life could be ours beyond compare.

Here's to celebrating a life "AB" (After Books!)

To our daughter, **Elana** –
Your gentle, sensitive, insightful ways
Your quiet strength and strong commitment to all that you are (a wife, parent, family member, teacher, friend.)
Your incredible artistic abilities are part of the many ways that make you such a source of joy for us.

To our son, **Kalen** –
We do so appreciate your "gifts." Thank you for sharing with us your:

Knowledge (of so many topics, so many hands-on skills.)
Achievements (your ambition and confidence has led you to see choices in opportunities)
Laughter (your wit and humor is a hallmark)
Enthusiasm (for and enjoyment of your many ventures in leisure-land)
Nostalgia (for warm memories of yesteryear with you as part of the 4LAGIES)

You have the zeal to steam ahead...may you find satisfaction and pleasure in all that you have, and in all that you do.

To our granddaughter, **Kaya Marina** –
May you always be like your first 3 years –
Laughing a lot...
Dancing as a free spirit...
Singing all day...
Talking away...

You have so many "gifts"; may you continue to find joy in dancing and singing Hawaiian songs and all your other favorites.

Sally

This book is gratefully dedicated to three very important people in my life: Edward "Pappy" Weathersbee, Martha Weathersbee Curry and Hyman Kosman. Without their guidance and direction I would still be wondering what do I want to be and have when I "grow up." My everlasting thanks.

Kathy

Author of Previous Edition

Geraldine C. Colombraro, RN, MA, PhD
Assistant Dean
Lienhard School of Nursing
Pace University
Pleasantville, New York

Dr. Colombraro was the original author of the content and questions in the first edition of this book and its accompanying disk when it was published by Lippincott. This second edition is an updated, modified version written by Ms. Snider and published by ATI.

Reviewer of Questions/Answers in Current Book and Disk & Contributing Author of Updated Questions/Answers

Janet Baatz Darrow, MS RN, CPN
Lecturer
San Jose State University
San Jose, California

Acknowledgements

A special tribute to Sally Volkoff, who was a special project coordinator for the development of this book and five other exam prep books for publication – all at the same time from start to finish, and kept an upbeat and determined it-will-be-done attitude that spanned two years of weekends and holidays. She put in inordinate effort to work with the different contributors and their styles, all in various stages of productions. Her enviable resiliency, with a smile, truly makes this "our" book.

A thank you to Don Walde for perceiving and responding to the need for that extra effort to make this Pediatric review book stand out from all the rest in this subject area.

A big word of appreciation to Hara Allison, Cheryl Appel, Molly Obetz, Laura Steen, and Melissa Wells for accepting the challenge of working with me step-by-step, detail-by-detail to shepherd the growth and development of this book, until the end result was one that reflects and continues to merit what three outstanding educators, Drs. Higgins, Lantz and Walsh, have said about this book in their Foreword.

Sally L. Lagerquist

Foreword

It is a pleasure to endorse resources for students and faculty that really work!

Faculty now has an important role in assisting the student in condensing and organizing the essential knowledge that can be translated into competent and safe nursing practice. With the exploding amount of knowledge in nursing and health care, students are often frustrated because they need to know so much. They ask questions from faculty like, "what is on the test?" and "what do I need to know?" The *ATI NurseNotes* are an incredibly easy synthesis of critical material that students need to master. Using the *NurseNotes* series along with the major nursing textbooks enhances students' comprehension of complex concepts and their application to clinical practice. The feedback from students themselves has been very positive. They comment that the *NurseNotes* save them time as they learn and review core content because concepts are graphically presented, chapters are short (yet comprehensive), with summaries and test questions at the end of each chapter to identify their problem areas.

The faculty finds that the *NurseNotes* series helps to organize their own presentations of material to students in a way that helps elevate the students' mastery of core content.

John M. Lantz, RN, PhD
Dean and Professor
School of Nursing
University of San Francisco
2130 Fulton Street
San Francisco, CA 94117

Sally Higgins, RN, PhD, FAAN
Professor and Chair of the Department of
 Family Health
University of San Francisco
2130 Fulton Street
San Francisco, CA 94117

I have found the Maternal-Newborn text to be extremely useful in the undergraduate family health course that I teach. Its concise review of all of the essential content makes it an extremely user-friendly text, particularly for students who struggle as they try to take in a tremendous amount of material during the 14 week semester. Many of my previous students have sworn that they never would have successfully completed all of the course objectives without this volume.

Linda Walsh CNM, MPH, Ph.D.
Faculty
University of San Francisco
2130 Fulton Street
San Francisco, CA 94117

x

Preface

The purpose of this book is to provide a focused overview of pediatric nursing. It covers the *most common* disorders and conditions that the nurse is likely to encounter while working with children and their families. It is our hope that the reader of this book will be better informed about the health care needs of the majority of children with whom they will work.

Intended Audience

NurseNotes: Pediatrics is intended for use by two primary audiences. *First*, it is intended for busy nursing students who currently are taking a course in pediatric nursing and need to cover the **most important information in the shortest time**. It will help students focus on the most relevant material for study, rather than having to sort through highly detailed and specialized textbooks that may be a thousand pages or longer, trying fervently to "study" for pediatric nursing quizzes, exams, midterms, and finals. It may also be helpful to students who are taking other achievement exams in pediatric nursing.

Second, it is intended for graduate nurses who are preparing to take their NCLEX-RN® licensure or certification exam. This group should include not only first-time takers but also those graduates who find they need to *repeat* their exam if they are not successful on their initial attempt. It would also be appropriate for *international nurses* who need to become more familiar with nursing care of children in the United States as they too prepare to take either the CGFNS exam or the NCLEX-RN® licensure exam.

To get the most out of this book, students are encouraged to attend all of their classes in nursing school and, of course, to use the course text first. After a lecture or reading assignment, students can use *NurseNotes: Pediatrics* for a *quick* review of *essential* content. The questions at the end of each chapter should prove helpful in preparing for quizzes or tests. In addition, the questions on the accompanying disk should be invaluable for reviewing for a midterm or final exam or an achievement test.

New graduate nurses can use this book as an organized outline review of the most common pediatric content needed to successfully prepare for the NCLEX-RN® and certification exams. For some graduates, their course in pediatric nursing may have taken place two or more years before graduation! Candidates for the NCLEX-RN® should then take, or retake, all of the questions at the end of each chapter and on the disk. By the time candidates have finished this book, they will have done 525 multiple-choice questions in *pediatric nursing*!

Features That Make This Book Stand-out From All Other Pediatric Nursing Content Review Books

1. **Time-savers:** Numerous charts (**39**), illustrations (**18**), and pharmacology tables outline a great deal of information in a few pages. Save valuable study time with *quick-access index* to instantly locate pages that cover key content, such as **36** *diets*, **58** *diagnostic tests*, **15** *tubes*, **26** *positioning*, **20** *pediatric emergencies*, **53** *hands-on care* (nursing skills, activities, procedures), **27** conditions related to *home health care/teaching*.

2. **Visual**: Unique use of icons throughout the content review sections helps important content to stand out:

Diagnostic tests	Hand washing	Memory aid
Diets	Hazard, danger	Standard precautions
Drugs	Home health care/teaching	Steps of nursing process
Hands-on care	Lab values	Summary of key points

There is also a purposeful use of **bold face** and *italics* within the text to identify content related to *diets, positions, tubes*, what to *avoid*, and *drugs*. These visual methods have proven to be particularly beneficial in boosting retention.

3. The most up-to-date, comprehensive (yet succinct!) coverage of a variety of topics, for *beginning* and *advanced* nurses already in practice, as well as for *repeat* test-takers.

4. **Self-assessment**: Questions and answers at the end of *each* chapter include *fact-packed* rationale for *each* option. Learn more from the most complete explanations!

5. **Free disk**: An integrated exam covers all essential areas in pediatric care.

6. **One-of-a-kind sections** in each chapter: *summary of key points, key words*, and *study and memory aids*.

7. **Extensive appendices** that include over **200** need-to-know *acronyms and abbreviations*; a *quick guide* to **25** *common clinical signs*; indices to help locate *test questions* covering each step of the nursing process, client needs and subneeds, and categories of human functions; and a list of addresses for *health care agencies and resources*.

8. A list of **21** *mnemonics* (↑ memory!) for various conditions.

9. A *crossword puzzle on pediatric cardiopulmonary* failure.

How to Benefit From This Book

1. Use the *key words* and *key points* sections at the beginning of each chapter to *anticipate* the content that will be covered in the chapter.

2. Take the questions at the end of each chapter, not only to test yourself on the content covered in the chapter but also to review added information.

3. Use the various *indices* in the appendices to quickly locate and pull out for study and review *separate* key topics, such as **58** *diagnostic tests and medical procedures*; **20** pediatric *emergencies*; *lab values*; **53** *nursing skills, activities* and *procedures* (*hands-on care*) necessary for beginning nursing students to master; hands-on care related to **26** *positions* of choice and *tubes* (**15** different ones!); **36** *diets*; and **27** conditions related to *home health care/health teaching*.

We wish you much success as you prepare for nursing exams with the aid of *NurseNotes: Pediatrics*.

Sally Lambert Lagerquist, RN, MS
Editor, *ATI NurseNotes* series
Kathleen E. Snider, RN, MSN, CNS
Author of *ATI NurseNotes: Pediatrics*

How to Use the ATI NurseNotes Series

The *ATI NurseNotes* series was written to lower students' stress while increasing mastery of essential subjects (i.e. core content), by presenting concise information in a visual way to enable an at-a-glance approach to increasing understanding and retention.

Students can use this series as a basis for doing care plans (care maps) at the *beginning* of and *throughout* a course, as well as an *end–point* review for the course exam or for *NCLEX-RN® review*. This is the only nursing review series with content and practice questions that *directly relate to the NCLEX-RN® test plan blue print.*

Step–By–Step Approach To the Most Effective Use of This Book By Students

❖ Quickly glance at the *outline* at the start of each chapter to see what topics/conditions will be covered.

❖ Go over the *key words* that are basic and *need-to-know.*

❖ Carefully read the **summaries** of key points 🔑 at the start of each chapter to be aware of what you need to understand and retain as the key points when you read through the chapter.

❖ Look over the outline format that is used, noting that there is a brief *introduction,* followed by concisely worded description of *physiology* and a relevant *risk factors/causes,* and incidence.

❖ Spend significant time going over the *assessment* section, especially the diagnostic tests/procedures and any related lab data. Note that the symbol in the margins 〰, quickly identifies diagnostic tests.

❖ Briefly glance at the *nursing diagnosis,* which can relate to pathophysiology, with implications for nursing interventions.

❖ Spend the most concentrated time in the section: *nursing plan* (i.e., the general goals)/ *implementation* (i.e., specific interventions). Pay special attention to *diets* 🍎, *positioning, hands-on care aspects* ☞, *medications* ▭, *infection control situations* ⚠, hazards ⚡, and *home health care/teaching* 🏠.

❖ Next, study all the information in table format, the words and phrases that are in **boldface** (very important) and *italic* type, as well as boxed content and shaded areas. These visual cues are time-savers for the reader because they serve the same purpose as when students spend time doing their own highlighting and underlining for emphasis. These visual cues allow for faster learning!

❖ Look at the end of each chapter for a synthesis of need-to-remember points about the condition(s), diets, drugs and diagnostic tests/procedures.

❖ Now take the *test questions* at the end of *each* chapter. Read the rationale not only for the best answer, but also the rationale for all the other options. Determine your percentage correct; if it was less than 85% correct (this is a higher benchmark than you'd expect to find on the licensure exam), then we suggest that you re-read that chapter.

❖ When you have completed all the chapters in the book for an end-point review, be sure to go through the content-packed **appendices**. The indices there can also lead you to pages where specific content (e.g. diets) and specific questions (e.g. safety and infection control) are located in the book. For example, this means that you can go through the book and only review all the diets; then you can go through the book and do a review of all the tubes or positioning etc.

❖ Follow this approach before you use the 275 questions on the *CD* in this book as your final "test and assess."

Suggestions for Instructor's Use of the Books in the ATI NurseNotes Series

While these books offer a <u>synthesis</u> of essential content in a condensed format, the instructor can then use lecture time to focus on <u>expansion</u> of content, to illustrate key concepts with <u>clinical scenarios</u> (to use in conjunction with *ATI Nursing Q&A: Critical Thinking Exercises* and the 75 case scenarios).

❖ These books can increase time for the focus of the instructor's lecture to be on a re-emphasis of more <u>complex</u> concepts (e.g. acid-base).

❖ If any clinical experience in the nursing program is reduced in scope, the instructor can select from these books certain chapters for special supplemental coverage to fill in those gaps. In that way, their lectures can be <u>tailored</u> to the particular needs of the nursing program.

❖ Instructors can use these books to point out <u>major</u> nursing care problems, to <u>separate</u> them from secondary ones; and to provide a *hands-on care skills assessment checklist* (see ☞ throughout the chapters), with an opportunity to learn and fill in gaps in the how-to aspects of nursing care.

❖ A focus on sections in these books that cover **assessment** data is another way the instructor can point out patterns, relationships and make appropriate inferences based on assessment data.

❖ The instructor should also call students' attention to the many appendices that provide **multiple ways** that students can use these books for self-assessment in addition to the usual end-of-chapter questions and questions on the *CD*. For example, show students how they can do a focused review of <u>special topics</u> (e.g. use the index in an Appendix to locate throughout the book a review of diets, diagnostic studies/procedures, common tubes, positioning of the client.) They can also review by <u>questions</u> throughout the book which directly relate to the NCLEX-RN® Test Plan (e.g. by client needs/subneeds), by nursing process steps; and by level of complexity of questions (from basic knowledge/comprehension to application and analysis.)

❖ These books can help *new* instructors to zero-in on core content, and can give *experienced* lecturers more time to focus on clinically-based anecdotal illustrations.

Contents

Appendixes

List Of Illustrations

xx

List of Tables

Clinical Assessment of the Child

1

Chapter Outline

- Key Words
- Summary of Key Points
- Mortality Rates in the Pediatric Population
- Selected Principles of Growth and Development
- Family and Cultural Influences

- Physical Assessment of the Child
- Developmental Assessment of the Child
- Study and Memory Aids
- Questions
- Answers/Rationale

Key Words

cephalocaudal pattern of development that proceeds from the head, down the spinal column, to the toes.

culture all mores, traditions, and beliefs about people's functioning; encompasses products of human works and thoughts specific to members of an intergenerational group, community, or population.

development progressive increase in the ability to function; includes physiological, psychosocial and cognitive changes over the lifespan.

ethnicity heritage of shared race, culture, society, and language.

growth progressive increase in physical size.

habituation the ability to decrease responses to disturbing stimuli; protects newborn from over stimulation and frees energy to meet physiologic demands.

maturation changes that are due to genetic inheritance rather than life experience, illness or injury; allows children to function at increasingly higher and more sophisticated levels as they get older.

morbidity prevalence of a specific illness in the population at a particular time.

mortality incidence/number of individuals who have died over a specific period of time.

proximodistal pattern of development that proceeds from the midline of the body to the extremities.

race group of people who share similar physical characteristics, such as skin color, that are transmitted genetically and are sufficient to characterize the group as a distinct human type.

🔑 Summary of Key Points

1. The leading cause of death from birth through 28 days is *congenital anomalies*.

2. The leading cause of death from age 1–12 mo is disorders relating to: short gestation, unspecified low birth weight, sudden infant death syndrome (SIDS).

3. The leading cause of death from age 1–19 yr is unintentional injuries (*accidents*); motor vehicle accidents are the most common type of accident.

4. The growth and development of children are affected by a wide variety of factors.

5. There are predictable stages of growth and development.

6. There are standard parameters for various aspects of growth and development.

7. Growth and development occur in a uniform sequence of predictable patterns.

8. The exact time at which a child exhibits a specific behavior related to growth and development varies.

9. There are *three main theories of personality development*: Erikson, Freud, and Piaget.

10. Play is the work of children and is one way children learn about their world.

11. A family can be defined in many different ways.

12. The nurse must understand the influence of culture, race, and ethnicity on the child and family.

13. The ability to have culturally sensitive interactions is an important skill for the nurse.

14. When examining a child, the nurse should remember that children generally cooperate best when a parent is allowed to remain with them.

15. Growth measurements such as height, weight, and head circumference should be compared with those on standard growth charts with national percentiles.

16. Physiologic measurements, or vital signs, should be done carefully to provide accurate data, and should be compared with standard norms.

17. The assessment of developmental functioning is a vital component of a child's complete health assessment.

18. The *Denver Developmental Screening Test* (DDST) is the best known and most widely used developmental assessment tool.

TABLE 1.1 GENERAL TRENDS IN HEIGHT AND WEIGHT GAIN DURING CHILDHOOD

Age	Weight*	Height*
Infant Birth–6 months	Weekly gain: 140–200 g (5–7 oz) Birth weight **doubles** by end of first 4–7 mo	Monthly gain: 2.5 cm (1 in.)
6–12 months	Weight gain: 85–140 g (3–5 oz) Birth weight **triples** by end of first yr	Monthly gain: 1.25 cm ($1/2$ in.) Birth length increases by approximately **50%** by end of first yr
Toddler	Birth weight **triples** by 14–17 mo Birth weight **quadruples** by age $2^1/_2$ yr Yearly gain: 2–3 kg ($4^1/_2$-$6^1/_2$ lb)	Height at age 2 yr is approximately **50% of eventual adult height** Gain during second yr: about 12 cm ($4^3/_4$ in.) Gain during third yr: about 6-8 cm ($2^3/_8$-$3^1/_4$ in.)
Preschool	Yearly gain: 2–3 kg ($4^1/_2$–$6^1/_2$ lb)	Birth length **doubles** by age 4 yr Yearly gain: 5.0–7.5 cm (2–3 in.)
School-age	Yearly gain: 2–3 kg ($4^1/_2$–$6^1/_2$ lb)	Yearly gain after age 7 yr: 5 cm (2 in.) Birth length **triples** by about age 13 yr
Pubertal growth spurt *Girls* 10–14 yr	Weight gain: 7–25 kg (15–55 lb) Mean: 17.5 kg ($38^1/_8$ lb)	Height gain: 5–25 cm (2–10 in.); approximately **95%** of mature height achieved by onset of menarche or skeletal age of 13 yr Mean: 20.5 cm ($8^1/_4$ in.)
Boys 11–16 yr	Weight gain: 7–30 kg (15–65 lb) Mean: 23.7 kg ($52^1/_8$ lb)	Height gain: 10–30 cm (4–12 in.); approximately **95%** of mature height achieved by skeletal age of 15 yr Mean: 27.5 cm (11 in.)

*Yearly weight and height gains for each age group represent averaged estimates from a variety of sources.

Source: Adapted from Wong D. *Wong's Nursing Care of Infants and Children* (7th ed). St. Louis, Mosby.

Mortality Rates in the Pediatric Population

I. *Congenital* anomalies are the leading cause of death in the *first 28 days* of an infant's life.

II. Disorders relating to: short gestation; unspecified low birth weight; sudden infant death syndrome (SIDS) are leading causes of death from age 1–12 mo.

III. Unintentional injuries (*accidents*) are the leading cause of death in children from age 1–19 yr.
  A. The most common accident during the first year of life is *aspiration*.
  B. The most common accident in all other pediatric age groups is *motor vehicle accidents*, as either a passenger, pedestrian, or driver. Motor vehicle accidents are responsible for nearly 50% of all accidental deaths in children.

IV. *Homicides* are the *second* leading cause of death in children.

V. *Suicide* is the *third* leading cause of death in children.

Selected Principles of Growth and Development

I. Growth and development are the totality of all changes that take place during a person's life.
  A. Growth: progressive increase in physical size.
  B. Development: progressive increase in the ability to function.

II. *Stages* of growth and development
  A. *Prenatal* period: from conception through birth.
  B. *Infancy* period: from birth–12 mo.
    1. Neonatal: 1–28 days.
    2. Infancy: 1–12 mo.
  C. *Toddler*: 1–3 yr.
  D. *Preschool*: 3–5, 6 yr.
  E. *School-aged*: 6–11, 12 yr.
  F. *Prepubertal*: 10–13 yr.
  G. *Adolescence*: 13–18 yr.

III. Standards (norms) define the average age for selected parameters to appear, e.g., height, weight, motor skills.

(*continued on p. 4*)

TABLE 1.2 ERIKSON'S EIGHT STAGES IN THE HUMAN LIFE CYCLE

Task and Subtasks*	Task's Negative Counterpart	Significant Persons	Significant Supporting Experiences
Infancy (Oral) (0–1 yr) Sense of *trust*: realization of hope Tolerating frustration in small doses Recognizing mother as distinct from others and self	*Mistrust*	Primary caregiver	Consistency and quality in the care received
Toddler (Anal) (1–3 yr) Sense of *autonomy*: realization of will Child will try out new powers of speech Beginning acceptance of reality vs. pleasure principle	*Shame and doubt*	Parent(s)	Opportunity to attain some self-control based on a feeling of self-esteem rather than fear
Preschool (Oedipal) (3–6 yr) Sense of *initiative*: realization of purpose Questioning Exploring own body and environment Differentiation of sexes	*Guilt*	Basic family	Opportunity to do for self with a balance between imaginative exploration and set limits
School-Age (Latent) (6–12 yr) Sense of *industry*: realization of competence Learning to win recognition by producing things Exploring, collecting Learning to relate to own sex	*Inferiority*	Neighborhood; school; same-sex peers; adult, non-parent idols	Opportunity to achieve success and recognition by engaging in manageable tasks in the child's social world so he or she can learn responsibility, social and work skills, cooperation, and fair play
Adolescence (Mature) (12–? yr) Sense of *identity*: realization of fidelity Moving toward heterosexuality Selecting vocation Beginning separation from family Integrating personality (e.g., altruism)	*Identity diffusion*	Peer groups and out groups; models of leadership	Opportunity to establish who the child is and what her or his purpose in society is to be through both private and social experiences that build self-esteem, foster increased need for independence, and cushion periods of feeling of not belonging
Late Adolescence and Young Adulthood Sense of *intimacy* and *solidarity*: realization of love Becoming capable of establishing a lasting relationship with a member of the opposite sex Learning to be creative and productive	*Isolation*	Partner in friendship, sex, competition, cooperation	Opportunity to experience close, shared relationships with individuals of own and opposite sex in which the child's identity is verified and accepted and he or she accepts the identity of others
Adulthood Sense of *generativity*: realization of care Learning effective skills in communicating with and managing children Developing active interest in the next generation	*Self-absorption* and *stagnation*	Spouse; children; friends and work associates	Opportunity for involvement in activities that arouse concern for and advocacy for the next generation
Late Adulthood Sense of *integrity*: realization of wisdom Reconciling life accomplishments Learning to accept death Putting life in order Accepting retirement without quitting life	*Despair*	Spouse; children and grandchildren; friends	Opportunity to be acknowledged for life accomplishments by self, children, peers in a manner that emphasizes what was achieved, rather than what was not, so that end of life can be dealt with gracefully and peaceably

*The corresponding stage in Freud's theory of development is listed in parentheses.

Source: Betz, et al. *Family Centered Nursing Care of Children*. Philadelphia, WB Saunders, (out of print).

IV. *Patterns* of growth and development
  A. Growth and development occur in a uniform sequence of predictable patterns. Each child's growth and development is unique; the exact time at which a child exhibits a specific behavior related to growth and development varies.
  B. Growth and development have two major patterns:
    1. *Cephalocaudal*: Development proceeds from the head, down the spinal column, to the toes. Infants achieve control of the head before they can control the trunk or extremities.
    2. *Proximodistal*: Development proceeds from the midline of the body to the extremities. Infants achieve control of their torso before their shoulders or arms.

V. *Physical* growth and development—height and weight: see **Table 1.1, p. 2** for general trends in height and weight gain during childhood.

VI. *Personality* development—Erikson, Freud, Piaget: see **Table 1.2, p. 3** for a summary of Erikson's theory.

VII. *Play*
  A. Play is vitally important to children's growth and development.
  B. Role of play in the growth and development of children: play teaches children about the world in which they live and how they can or should function there. Sometimes referred to as the "work" of children, play allows children to practice how to communicate with others and establish satisfactory relationships with others.
  C. Types of play:
    1. *Solitary* play: infants usually do not seek out the company of other infants to "play." This does not mean that the infant should be left alone with toys; however, social stimulation from parents, older siblings, and children is still critical to the infant's development.
    2. *Parallel* play: two toddlers play next to, but not necessarily with, each other. They are engaged in separate activities, do not have shared rules, and have no apparent organization.
    3. *Associative* play: preschoolers play in a group in activities that may be the same or similar, but there are few, if any, rules and little organization to the group.
    4. *Cooperative* play: slightly more advanced than associative play. The preschooler or school-aged child plays in a group with other children in an organized activity that has rules and goals, generally led by one or two group members.

VIII. *Factors that can influence growth and development:*
  A. *Genetics*: sex, physical characteristics, certain diseases.
  B. *Prenatal* influences: smoking, drinking, drugs used by the mother during pregnancy.
  C. *Gender*: cultural expectations regarding the sex of the child.
  D. *Family structure*: birth order, family size, and family characteristics.
  E. *Socioeconomic level*: children from lower socioeconomic levels generally have poorer nutrition and health than do children from middle or upper classes.
  F. *Culture*: customs, mores, and norms related to food, health care practices, and social interactions.
  G. *Environment*: media, school, community/neighborhood.
  H. *Environmental hazards*: water, air, food contaminants.
  I. *Nutrition*: single most important factor that affects growth at all ages and stages.

Family and Cultural Influences

I. *Definitions* of "family" are many and varied and depend on the definer's frame of reference, discipline, and values. In *Whaley and Wong*, family is defined as "the relationships between dependent children and one or more protective adults. It also implies relationships among siblings. Family members share a sense of belonging to their own family that deeply affects their lives."[a] Betz, et al define family as "a complex organization of one or more persons with a pattern of interrelationships that have a past, present and future."[b]

II. The *traditional* family structure has been conceptualized as the nuclear (or extended) family; however, in recent years, *contemporary* families include many different types of families such as the single-parent family, the blended family, or the gay/lesbian family.

III. In addition to understanding families, the nurse must also understand the influence of culture, race, and ethnicity on the child and the family.
  A. *Culture* is all mores, traditions, and beliefs about people's functioning and encompasses products of human works and thoughts specific to members of an intergenerational group, community, or population.[c]
  B. *Race* refers to a group of people who share similar physical characteristics, such as skin color, that are transmitted genetically and are sufficient to characterize the group as a distinct human type.[d]

[a]Wong D. L. *Wong's Nursing Care of Infants and Children*, (7th. Ed) St. Louis, Mosby.
[b]Betz C, Hunsberger M, and Wright S. *Family-Centered Nursing Care of Children* (2nd ed.) Philadelphia W. B. Saunders, (out of print).
[c]Wong D. L. *Wong's Nursing Care of Infants and Children*, (7th ed.) St. Louis, Mosby.
[d]Wong D. L. *Wong's Nursing Care of Infants and Children*, (7th ed.) St. Louis., Mosby.
[e]Wong D. L. *Wong's Nursing Care of Infants and Children*, (7th ed.) St. Louis, Mosby.

TABLE 1.3 GUIDELINES FOR CULTURALLY SENSITIVE INTERACTIONS

Nonverbal Strategies

Invite family members to choose where they would like to sit or stand, allowing them to select a comfortable distance.

Observe interactions with others to determine which body gestures (e.g., shaking hands) are acceptable and appropriate. Ask when in doubt.

Avoid appearing rushed.

Be an active listener.

Observe for cues regarding appropriate eye contact.

Learn appropriate use of pauses or interruptions for different cultures.

Ask for clarification if nonverbal meaning is unclear.

Verbal Strategies

Learn proper terms of address.

Use a positive tone of voice to convey interest.

Speak slowly and carefully, not loudly, when families have poor language comprehension.

Encourage questions.

Learn basic words and sentences of family's language, if possible.

Avoid professional terms.

When asking questions, tell family why the questions are being asked, the way in which the information they provide will be used, and how it might benefit their child.

Repeat important information more than once.

Always give the reason or purpose for a treatment or prescription.

Use information written in family's language.

Offer the services of an interpreter when necessary.

Learn from families and representatives of their culture methods of communicating information without creating discomfort.

Address intergenerational needs (e.g., family's need to consult with others).

Be sincere, open, and honest and, when appropriate, share personal experiences, beliefs, and practices to establish rapport and trust.

Source: Wong D. *Wong's Nursing Care of Infants and Children* (7th ed). St. Louis, Mosby.

    C. *Ethnicity* refers to a shared racial, cultural, social, and linguistic heritage[e]. Ethnic differences include family structure, language, food preferences, moral codes, and how emotion is expressed.

  IV. Communication skills of the nurse must include culturally sensitive interactions (see **Table 1.3**). For effective therapeutic interactions to occur, the nurse must acknowledge and respect the patient's culture.

◄ Physical Assessment of the Child

Author's Note: Physical assessment can be presented in any one of three ways: *body systems, head-to-toe,* or *focused*. For this review book, the author has elected to present the head-to-toe order; however, a body systems approach or a focused assessment might also be appropriate for the nurse to select.

I. When examining a child, the nurse should remember that children generally cooperate best when a parent is allowed to remain with them; see **Table 1.4, p. 6** for *age-specific approaches to physical examination* during childhood.

II. *Growth measurements* should include length or height, weight, and head circumference. Growth charts are available from the National Center for Health Statistics for boys and girls of three age groups: birth–36 mo, 2–18 yr, and prepubescence. The child's measurements should be compared with NCHS percentiles.

III. *Vital signs* should include: temperature, pulse, respiration, and blood pressure.

    A. See **Table 1.5, p. 7** for *normal* measurements of *vital signs* and *variations* with age.

    B. The most common cause of inaccurate blood pressure readings in children is use of the wrong size cuff. When measuring blood pressure in a child, the nurse should select a cuff that covers $^2/_3$ to $^3/_4$ of the child's upper arm. (If the correct size cuff is not available, the use of an oversize cuff rather than an undersized one is recommended.)

IV. *General appearance* should document the nurse's impression of the child, including overall physical appearance, hygiene, nutritional status, and behavior.

☞ V. *Skin, hair, and nails*

    A. Examination primarily involves *inspection* and *palpation*.

    B. Skin should be evaluated for variations in: color, texture, temperature, moistness, and resilience (turgor). *Skin turgor* is best assessed on the infant/child's abdomen or thigh.

    C. Hair should be evaluated for: color, distribution, and cleanliness.

    D. Nails should be evaluated for: size, shape, and color. Capillary refill should also be checked.

☞ VI. *Lymph nodes* should be *palpated* in the cervical, axillary, and inguinal areas. The nurse should note their size, mobility, any tenderness, and any enlargement.

VII. *Head* should be observed for: shape, symmetry, head control and posture, and range of motion.

  ☞ A. The *skull* should be *palpated* for suture lines and fontanels. The anterior fontanel remains open until *12–18 mo*. of age while the posterior fontanel closes at *2 mo*. of age. Palpation of the anterior fontanel should be conducted in the *supine* postion.

    B. The *face* should be observed for: shape, mobility, and symmetry.

  ☞ C. The *sinuses* should be percussed for any evidence of pain, indicative of infection.

(*continued on p. 7*)

TABLE 1.4 AGE-SPECIFIC APPROACHES TO PHYSICAL EXAMINATION DURING CHILDHOOD

Position	Sequence	Preparation
INFANT		
Before sits alone: *supine* or *prone*, preferably in parent's lap; before 4–6 mo: can place on examining table	If quiet, auscultate heart, lungs, abdomen Record heart and respiratory rates Palpate and percuss same areas	Completely undress if room temperature permits Leave diaper on boy Gain cooperation with distraction, bright objects, rattles, talking
After sits alone: use sitting in parent's lap whenever possible	Proceed in usual head-to-toe direction	Have older infants hold a small block in each hand; until voluntary release develops toward end of the first yr, infants will be unable to grasp other objects (e.g., stethoscope, otoscope)
If on table, place with parent in full view	Perform traumatic procedures last (eyes, ears, mouth [while crying]) Elicit reflexes as body part examined Elicit *Moro* reflex last	Smile at infant; use soft, gentle voice Soothe with bottle or pacifier Enlist parent's aid for restraining to examine ears, mouth *Avoid* abrupt, jerky movements
TODDLER		
Sitting or standing on/ by parent *Prone* or *supine* in parent's lap	Inspect body area through play: "count fingers," "tickle toes" Use minimal physical contact initially Introduce equipment slowly Auscultate, percuss, palpate whenever quiet Perform traumatic procedures last (same as for infant)	Have parent remove outer clothing Remove underwear as body part examined Allow to inspect equipment; demonstrating use of equipment is usually ineffective If uncooperative, perform procedures quickly Use restraint when appropriate; request parent's assistance Talk about examination if cooperative; use short phrases Praise for cooperative behavior
PRESCHOOL		
Prefer standing or sitting Usually cooperative prone/supine Prefer parent's closeness	If cooperative, proceed in head-to-toe direction If uncooperative, proceed as with toddler	Request self-undressing Allow to wear underpants if shy Offer equipment for inspection; briefly demonstrate use Make up "story" about procedure: "I'm seeing how strong your muscles are" (blood pressure) Use paper-doll technique Give choices when possible Expect cooperation; use positive statements: "Open your mouth"
SCHOOL-AGE		
Prefer sitting Cooperative in most positions Younger child prefers parent's presence Older child may prefer privacy	Proceed in head-to-toe direction May examine genitalia last in older child Respect need for privacy	Request self-undressing Allow to wear underpants Give gown to wear Explain purpose of equipment and significance of procedure, such as otoscope to see eardrum, which is necessary for hearing Teach about body functioning and care
ADOLESCENT		
Same as for school-aged child Offer option of parent's presence	Same as for older school-aged child	Allow to undress in private Give gown Expose only area to be examined Respect need for privacy Explain findings during examining: "Your muscles are firm and strong" Matter-of-factly comment about sexual development: "Your breasts are developing as they should be" Emphasize normalcy of development Examine genitalia as any other body part; may leave to end

Source: Wong D. *Wong's Nursing Care of Infants and Children* (7th ed). St. Louis, Mosby.

TABLE 1.5 NORMAL MEASUREMENTS OF VITAL SIGNS AND VARIATIONS WITH AGE

Age	Heart Rate (beats/min)	Respiratory Rate (breaths/min)	Blood Pressure (mm Hg)
Newborn	120–160	30–40	70/55
1 yr	100–140	25–35	90/55
2 yr	80–120	20–30	90/56
5 yr	70–100	18–24	95/56
10 yr	60–90	18–22	102/62
14 yr	55–90	16–20	110/65
18 yr	55–90	16–18	116/68

Source: Adapted from Wong D. Wong's *Nursing Care of Infants and Children* (7th ed. St. Louis: Mosby.

TABLE 1.6 NEUROLOGIC "SOFT" SIGNS

Short attention span
Unusual body movement, such as mirroring
Poor coordination and sense of position
Excessive, sustained, and purposeless movement (hyperactivity)
Hypoactivity
Impulsiveness
Labile emotions
Distractibility
No established handedness
Language and articulation problems
Perceptual deficits (space, form, movement, time)
Problems with learning, especially reading, writing, and arithmetic

Source: Wong D. *Wong's Nursing Care of Infants and Children* (7th ed). St. Louis, Mosby.

VIII. The *neck* should be assessed for: size, edema, pulses, and neck veins. The thyroid gland and trachea should also be *palpated*.

IX. The *eyes* should be inspected for: size, symmetry, color, and motility. The retina should be examined by using an ophthalmoscope. Vision testing should also be done when appropriate.

   A. The *Snellen symbol* (E) chart should be used to test the vision of *preschoolers*.

   B. The *Snellen letter* chart should be used to test the vision of *school-aged* children and *adolescents*.

   C. Color vision should be checked by using *Ishihara Plates*.

X. The *ears* should be inspected externally and internally.

   A. External ears should be inspected for shape, position, placement, and cleanliness. Remember: The *top* of the pinna of the ear should be at the *same* level as the outer canthus of the eye.

   B. The otoscope should be used to inspect the internal structures of the ear.

   C. Auditory testing should be done when appropriate.

XI. The *nose* should be inspected externally and internally by using an otoscope with a nasal speculum.

XII. The *mouth* and *throat* should be inspected in three main areas:

   A. The oral cavity.

   B. The oropharynx.

   C. The nasopharynx.

XIII. The *chest* should be inspected for: size, shape, symmetry, and movement.

   ☞ A. The *lungs* should be inspected through observation of respiration and by *palpation* by placing each hand flat against the child's back or chest while the child takes several deep breaths. The lungs should also be *auscultated* by using the diaphragm side of the stethoscope.

   ☞ B. *Cardiac sounds* should also be *auscultated* for: quality, intensity, rate, and rhythm. Murmurs should be referred for further evaluation. Heart sounds should be auscultated by using the *bell* side of the diaphragm.

☞ XIV. The *abdomen* should be *inspected first, then auscultated, percussed*, and *palpated* in all four quadrants: right upper quadrant (RUQ), right lower quadrant (RLQ), left upper quadrant (LUQ), left lower quadrant (LLQ). The stethoscope must be pressed firmly against the abdominal surface to hear bowel sounds.

XV. The *genitalia* should be assessed next:

   A. In *boys*, the nurse should assess the penis including the glans (head) and the shaft, the prepuce or foreskin, the meatal opening, the scrotum and testes, and hair distribution.

   B. In *girls*, assessment should be limited to inspection and palpation of external structures including: the vulva, mons pubis, the clitoris, the urethral meatus, and the vaginal orifice.

XVI. The *anus* should be inspected for: patency, muscle tone of anal sphincter, and any deviations from the norm such as prolapse or hemorrhoids.

XVII. The *back and spine* should be inspected for any curvature or dimpling. Mobility should also be assessed.

XVIII. *Extremities* should be inspected for: symmetry of length and size, temperature, and color. The shape of the bones and any deviations should be noted.

   ☞ Range of motion (ROM) should also be checked.

XIX. *Cerebral functioning* should be evaluated by a careful history as well as physical exam.

   A. *Behavior* is not assessed via any one particular test or exam; assessment is based on overall sense of the child's personality, posture, activity level, speech, and attention span.

   B. *Cognitive-perceptual* development is assessed via standard screening tests.

TABLE 1.7 FACTS ABOUT THE DENVER DEVELOPMENTAL SCREENING TEST (DDST)

Parents' Questions	Nurse's Best Response
"Will this be used as a measure of my child's IQ?"	"No, it is a screening test for your child's development."
"What ages can be tested?"	"Infants through preschoolers, or from birth to 6 years."
"What will they test?"	"There are four areas: personal-social, fine motor-adaptive, language, gross motor."
"Can I stay with my child?"	"Yes, in fact it is preferred that you be there."
"If my child fails, does it mean he is retarded?"	"No, this is not a diagnostic tool, but rather a screening test."
"If he fails, what do we do?"	"Repeat the test in a week or two to rule out temporary factors."
"Why didn't my child accomplish everything?"	"He is not expected to."
"Why did my child score so poorly?"	"Perhaps it's a bad day for the child; he isn't feeling up to par, etc."

C. *Motor* functioning is assessed via voluntary muscle control and age-specific developmental milestones such as head control or handedness.

D. *Sensory* functioning is assessed in relation to the cranial nerves (vision and hearing) as well as peripheral sensation.

E. *Cerebellar* functioning is assessed in terms of balance and coordination.

☞ F. The *reflexes* should be elicited and graded from 4+ (extremely brisk, hyperactive reflex) to 0+ (absent).

G. "Soft" signs are neurologic signs that fall into a gray area between normal and abnormal findings. Although soft signs may be normal in a younger child, their appearance in an older child in whom such behavior would not normally be expected can indicate problems Refer to **Table 1.6** for neurologic soft signs.

Developmental Assessment of the Child

I. The assessment of developmental functioning is a vital component of a child's complete health assessment.

II. The *Denver Developmental Screening Test* (DDST) is the best known and most widely used developmental assessment tool. It was first published in 1967 as the DDST but was revised in 1981 as the DDST-R; a newer, standardized version is called the Denver-II. The Screening Manual provides complete directions for the administration of this important screening test.

III. If an infant was born prematurely, the nurse should adjust the age of the child until the child is age 24 mo; after that, no adjustment should be made.

IV. The nurse should explain to the parents (and child, if appropriate) that this is a *screening* test of development, *not* an intelligence test. In addition, the nurse should stress that the child is not expected to perform each item on the test. For additional information about the DDST, refer to **Table 1.7**.

A. The DDST screens infants and children to age 6 yr in four categories:
1. Personal-social.
2. Fine motor-adaptive.
3. Language.
4. Gross motor.

💡 Study and Memory Aids

Mortality Rates

Accidents are the most common cause of death in children aged 1-19 yr.

Patterns of Growth and Development

All children follow the same order of growth and development; however, the exact age at which an individual child learns to sit or walk, for example, varies.

Role of Play in Growth and Development

Play is the work of children; through play children learn about their world.

Cultural Influences

The nurse must understand the effect that culture, race, and ethnicity have on the child and family.

Approach to Physical Examination of Child

Allowing parents to remain with the child during physical examination maximizes the child's cooperation.

Physical Assessment Must Include:

Capillary refill: normal < 2 sec

The Denver Developmental Screening Test—The best known and most widely used; it screens four developmental areas:

1. PERSONAL-SOCIAL.
2. FINE MOTOR-ADAPTIVE.
3. LANGUAGE.
4. GROSS MOTOR.

Questions

1. When preparing to teach a class about safety to parents of children aged 1 yr and older, the nurse should focus on preventing the most common type of accidental death, which is:
   1. Poisoning.
   2. Aspiration.
   3. Drowning.
   4. Motor vehicle accidents.

2. The nurse should recognize which item as an example of cephalocaudal development in an infant?
   1. The infant's head gradually enlarges in proportion to body growth.
   2. The infant plays with the hands before playing with the toes.
   3. The infant develops a palmar grasp before a pincer grasp.
   4. The infant smiles in response to the smile of an adult.

3. While the nurse is administering the Denver Developmental Screening Test to an infant, a mother expresses concern that her baby is not doing well. Which response is most appropriate for the nurse to make?
   1. "Why are you so worried? Have you been having problems at home too?"
   2. "Please let me finish this test before you start worrying. Maybe the baby will do better on the rest of the test."
   3. "You really sound worried. Please keep in mind that no baby is expected to do all the things on this test."
   4. "Unfortunately, your concerns seem to be valid. I will write up a consult with the child developmental specialist to follow up on this."

4. The nurse must perform an admitting assessment on a preschooler who is very upset and crying. The most appropriate action for the nurse to take initially is:
   1. Avoid any physical contact with the child, but remain in the room and speak with the parents.
   2. Give the child a brief explanation of what the nurse needs to do during the admission.
   3. Ask the parents to hold the child so the nurse can complete the assessment.
   4. Show the child a video about another child entering the hospital.

5. The RN observes a nursing student entering a toddler's room to check vital signs and begins to take the child's temperature first. The RN should:
   1. Suggest the student start with the pulse.
   2. Suggest the student start with the blood pressure.
   3. Suggest the student start with the respirations.
   4. Say nothing; this action is appropriate.

6. When examining an infant's abdomen, which assessment should be done first?
   1. Inspection.
   2. Auscultation.
   3. Percussion.
   4. Palpation.

7. The nurse's note reads "Vesicular breath sounds noted." The nurse heard:
   1. Normal breathing.
   2. Crackles.
   3. Wheezing.
   4. Rhonchi.

8. When checking capillary refill, the nurse should normally expect to see refill in:
   1. Less than 1 sec.
   2. 2 secs.
   3. 5 secs.
   4. 8-10 secs.

Answers/Rationale

1. **(4)** The leading cause of death by accidents for children aged 1 yr and older is motor vehicle accidents. The type of motor vehicle accident may vary with age: the *toddler* may be killed when not wearing a seat belt; the *preschooler* may be killed when struck by a car after running out into the street to chase a ball; the *school-aged* child may be struck by a car when riding a bike in the street; the *adolescent* may be killed when driving or riding as a passenger in the car with other teens. Poisoning **(1)** is most common in toddlers and young preschoolers; aspiration **(2)** is common in infants, and drowning **(3)** is common in toddlers and older children. None of these answers represent the most common type of accidental death *across all age groups.* **AN, COM, 1, HPM, Health promotion and maintenance**

2. **(2)** Cephalocaudal development means that the infant learns to control the body in an orderly fashion from the head, down the torso, to the legs; therefore, the infant is able to control and manipulate hands before achieving control over lower extremities. The growth of the head in proportion to the body **(1)** is normal physical development. The development of a palmar grasp before a pincer grasp **(3)** is an example of *proximodistal* development. A social smile **(4)** represents *psychosocial* development. **EV, COM, 5, HPM, Health promotion and maintenance**

3. **(3)** In performing the Denver Developmental Screening Test, the examiner should ask about items that are slightly *above* the infant's expected performance to get a true range of the infant's capabilities; however, the examiner should assure the parents that the infant is not expected to do everything. The nurse should not need to

discuss other problems (1) or refer the child for a consultation (4) at this time. Simply proceeding with the exam (2) without reassuring her that the infant is not expected to do everything will further alarm the mother and is inappropriate. **IMP, APP, 7, PsI, Psychosocial integrity**

4. (1) No. 1 is correct because a quiet, nonthreatening presence helps establish trust and calm the child. Attempting to explain procedures (2) or showing a video (4) to a child who is visibly upset and crying will not be effective because the child is incapable of attending to the material being presented. Starting off with a show of force, even if the parents are holding the child (3), can further frighten the child and prolong crying. **IMP, APP, 7, PsI, Psychosocial integrity**

5. (3) The nurse should perform the *least* intrusive procedure first; the nurse can observe the character of the respirations and count the respiratory rate without disturbing the toddler in any way. When the infant is disturbed, crying, or upset, the heart and respiratory rates can be affected as well as blood pressure, which can cause inaccurate readings. Starting with the pulse (1) or blood pressure (2) would disturb the toddler and should *not* be done first. Starting with the temperature is also *not* appropriate (4) because it would disturb the toddler. **IMP, ANL, 5, SECE, Management of care**

6. (1) Before the nurse touches the abdomen, the nurse should *first* visually inspect it for any unusual findings such as redness, bulging, or distention. Inspection does not affect other findings that follow from percussion, palpation, or auscultation. Auscultating first (2) could stimulate peristalsis, which would affect later findings. Percussing or palpating first (3 and 4) could increase bowel sounds, which again, may affect later findings. **IMP, ANL, 8, HPM, Health promotion and maintenance**

7. (1) "Vesicular breath sounds" reflect normal inspiration and exhalation, without any pathology. Vesicular breath sounds do *not* mean crackles (2), wheezing (3), or rhonchi (4). Crackles (rales) are interrupted sounds that are fairly loud but low pitched; they are caused by air passing through fluid-filled airways. A wheeze is a continuous, high pitched, hissing sound caused by a narrowing of the airway. Rhonchi are continuous, low pitched sounds, similar to snoring, that are caused by partial airway obstruction. **EV, APP, 6, PhI, Physiological adaptation**

8. (2) Normally, capillary refill should be quite brisk, less than 2 sec. A refill of less than 1 sec (1) is *quicker* than normal; a longer refill time (3 and 4) is *prolonged* beyond the norm. Prolonged or delayed refill may indicate poor systemic perfusion. **EV, COM, 6, PhI, Reduction of risk potential**

Key to Codes

Nursing process: AS, assessment; **AN**, analysis; **PL**, planning; **IMP**, implementation; **EV**, evaluation. (See **Appendix L** for explanation of nursing process steps.)

Cognitive level: RE/KN, recall/knowledge; **COM**, comprehension; **APP**, application; **ANL**, analysis; **EVL**, evaluation; **SYN**, synthesis. (See **Appendix L** for explanation.)

Category of human function: 1, protective; **2**, sensory-perceptual; **3**, comfort, rest, activity, and mobility; **4**, nutrition; **5**, growth and development; **6**, fluid-gas transport; **7**, psychosocial-cultural; **8**, elimination. (See **Appendix N** for explanation.)

Client need: SECE, safe, effective care environment; **HPM**, health promotion and maintenance; **PsI**, psychosocial integrity; **PhI**, physiological integrity. (See **Appendix O** for explanation.)

Client subneed: See **Appendix O** for explanation.

Growth and Development of the Infant

2

Chapter Outline

- Key Words
- Summary of Key Points
- Infant (28 days–1 yr)
  - Erikson's Theory of Personality Development
  - Physical Growth
  - Denver Developmental Screening Test Norms
  - Nursing Interventions/Parental Guidance
    - Play/Toys
    - Safety
    - Immunizations
  - Hospitalization of Infants
- Study and Memory Aids
- Questions
- Answers/Rationale

Key Words

deciduous teeth   the first teeth, or "baby" teeth, that an infant has; referred to as "deciduous" because they fall out and are replaced with adult or permanent teeth.

fontanel   an unossified soft spot lying between the bones of the head of a fetus or infant.

immunization   the process of rendering a client immune to a specific communicable disease by the administration of a vaccine that protects the client from developing that disease.

kinetic stimulation   sensory stimulation that consists of movement or motion.

palmar grasp   the process whereby the infant reaches for an object using the palm of the hand, hits the object with the palm, and rakes the object in with the fingertips.

pincer grasp   the process whereby the infant reaches for an object using the thumb and forefinger in neat opposition, closes on the object, and neatly picks the object up with two fingers.

reflex   an involuntary response to a stimulus.

solitary play   infants usually do not seek out the company of other infants to "play."

weaning   switching an infant from breast feeding to bottle feeding, or getting an infant to give up the bottle and drink from a cup.

Summary of Key Points

1. The period of infancy extends from *28 days* to *1 yr*.

2. According to Erikson, the central task for the infant is to develop basic *trust*.

3. The infant's height increases by 50% by the first birthday.

4. The infant's weight *doubles* by age 4–7 mo, and *triples* by 1 yr.

5. The *posterior* fontanel closes by 6–8 wk; the *anterior* fontanel remains open, or patent, through 12–18 mo of age.

6. Teething generally begins about age *6 mo*.

7. The Denver Developmental Screening Test is used to screen the development of infants; the average infant learns to:
   a. Roll over from stomach to back by *3 mo*.
   b. Sit with support by *6 mo*.
   c. Crawl by *9 mo*.
   d. Stand alone by *12 mo*.

8. Play during the first year of life is considered "solitary" play.

9. The most common accident during the first year of life is the *aspiration* of foreign bodies.

10. Routine immunizations for hepatitis B, diphtheria, tetanus, pertussis, haemophilus influenzae type b, polio, measles, mumps, rubella, varicella, pneumococcal, and influenza should be given per MD order.

11. For a hospitalized infant, the nurse should encourage rooming in by the primary caretaker and should observe behavioral cues in the nonverbal infant.

Infant (28 days–1 yr)

Erikson's Theory of Personality Development

I. *Central task*: basic trust vs. mistrust; central person: primary caretaker.

II. *Behavioral indicators*
  A. Crying is only means of communicating needs.
  B. Quieting usually means needs are met.
  C. *Fear* of strangers at 6–8 mo.

III. *Parental guidance/teaching*
  A. Must meet infant's needs consistently–cannot "spoil" infant by holding, comforting.
  B. Neonatal *reflexes* fade at 4–6 mo; replaced with increase in purposeful behavior, e.g., babbling, reaching.
  C. *Fear of strangers* is normal–indicates attachment between infant and primary caretaker.
  D. Infant may repeat over and over newly learned behaviors, e.g., sitting or standing.
  E. *Weaning* can begin around the time child begins walking.

IV. Additional information about behavioral concerns for each age group may be found in **Tables 2.1** and **2.2**.

Physical Growth

I. *Height* (length): *50% increase by first birthday.*

II. *Weight*
  A. *Doubles* by 4–7 mo, *triples* by 1 yr.
  B. Gains 5–7 oz/wk in first 6 mo.
  C. Gains 3–5 oz/wk in second 6 mo.

III. *Vital signs*: see **Chapter 1, Table 1.5, p. 7.**

IV. *Fontanels*
  A. *Posterior*–closed by 6–8 wk.
  B. *Anterior*–remains open through first 12 mo.

V. *Teething*
  A. Generally begins around *6 mo.*
  B. "Baby" teeth are deciduous (primary) teeth.
  C. First two teeth: lower central incisors.
  D. By 1 yr: 6–8 teeth.

Denver Developmental Screening Test (DDST) Norms: see **Chapter 1, Table 1.7, p. 8**

I. **Birth–3 mo**
  A. *Personal–social*:
    1. Smiles responsively, then spontaneously.
  B. *Fine motor–adaptive*:
    1. Follows 180 degrees, past midline.
    2. Grasps rattle.
    3. Holds hands together.
  C. *Language*:
    1. Laughs/squeals.
    2. Vocalizes without crying.
  D. *Gross motor*:
    1. While on stomach, lifts head 45-90 degrees.
    2. Able to hold head steady and erect.
    3. Rolls over from stomach to back.

II. **4–6 mo**
  A. *Personal–social*:
    1. Works for toy.
    2. Feeds self (bottle).
  B. *Fine motor-adaptive*:
    1. Palmar grasp.
    2. Reaches for objects.
  C. *Language*:
    1. Turns toward voice.
    2. Imitates speech.
  D. *Gross motor*:
    1. Some weight-bearing on legs.
    2. No head lag when pulled to sitting.
    3. Sits with support.

III. **7–9 mo**
  A. *Personal–social*:
    1. Indicates wants.
    2. Plays pat-a-cake.
    3. Waves bye-bye.
  B. *Fine motor–adaptive*:
    1. Takes two cubes in hands and bangs them together.
    2. Passes cube hand to hand.
    3. Makes crude pincer grasp.
  C. *Language*:
    1. Says "dada" and "mama."
    2. Non specific jabbers.
  D. *Gross motor*:
    1. Creeps on hands and knees.
    2. Gets self to sitting position.
    3. Pulls self to standing position.
    4. Stands holding on.

IV. **10–12 mo**
  A. *Personal–social*:
    1. Plays ball.
    2. Imitates activities.
    3. Drinks from cup.
  B. *Fine motor-adaptive*:
    1. Neat pincer grasp.
  C. *Language*:
    1. Says "dada" and "mama" (specific).
  D. *Gross motor*:
    1. Stands alone well.
    2. Walks holding on.
    3. Stoops and recovers.

TABLE 2.1 PEDIATRIC BEHAVIORAL CONCERNS: NURSING IMPLICATIONS AND PARENTAL GUIDANCE

Behavioral Concern	◄ Nursing Implications/Parental Guidance	Behavioral Concern	◄ Nursing Implications/Parental Guidance
"Accidents" (enuresis)	*Occasional*—common and normal through preschool *If frequent*—need complete physical exam to rule out pathology "Training": after dinner—*avoid* fluids; before bed—toilet (perhaps awaken once during night) *Never* put back into diapers or attempt to shame	Smoking/ drinking	May begin in *older school-aged* child or adolescent Serve as role model with own habits
Cursing	*Avoid* overreacting Defuse use of a word by simply stating "not here, not now" Distract, change subject, substitute activity Serve as role model by own language	Teething	Begins around age 4 mo—infant may seem unusually fussy and irritable but should *not* run a fever Provide relief with teething rings, acetaminophen, topical preparations
Discipline	*Not* for infant Can begin with *toddler*, within limits Be consistent and clear *Avoid* excessively strict measures	Temper tantrums	Normal in the *toddler*—occurs in response to frustration *Avoid* abrupt end to play or making excessive demands Offer only allowable choices Once a decision is verbalized, *avoid* sudden changes of mind Provide diversion to achieve cooperation If tantrum occurs, best means to handle is to *ignore* the outburst
Lying	*In preschool child*: not deliberate; child often unable to differentiate between "real" and "lie." By saying something that the child often feels, it makes it real *In older child*: may indicate problems and need for professional attention if persists Serve as role model—no "white lies"	Thumb sucking	Need to suck varies: may be caused by hunger, frustration, loneliness Do *not stop infant* from doing this—usually stops by preschool years. If behavior persists, evaluate need for attention, peer play
Masturbation	Normal, common in *preschooler* Set firm limits *Avoid* overreacting	Toilet training	Assess child for readiness: awareness of body functions, form of mutual communication, physical control over sphincters Use child-size seat No distractions (food, toys, books) Offer praise for success or efforts (*never* shame accidents)
Sibling rivalry	Fairly common, normal Allow older child to "help" Give each child "special" time, with individual attention		

◄ Nursing Interventions/Parental Guidance

I. **Play/Toys**
  A. First year—generally solitary.
  B. *Visual stimulation*:
    1. Best color: red.
    2. *Toys*: mirrors, brightly colored pictures.
  C. *Auditory stimulation*:
    1. Talk and sing to infant.
    2. *Toys*: musical mobiles, rattles, bells.
  D. *Tactile stimulation*:
    1. Hold, pat, touch, cuddle, swaddle/keep warm; rub body with lotion.
    2. *Toys*: various textures; nesting and stacking; plastic milk bottle with blocks to dump in, out.

TABLE 2.2 PEDIATRIC SLEEP AND REST NORMS: NURSING IMPLICATIONS AND PARENTAL GUIDANCE

Pediatric Sleep and Rest Norms	◄ *Nursing Implications/Parental Guidance*
Infant: 16–20 h/day	No set schedule can be predetermined
3 mo: nocturnal pattern	If waking at night after age 3 mo, investigate hunger as probable cause
6 mo: 1–2 naps, with 12 h at night	Monitor behavior to determine sleep needs: alert and active? growing, developing?
12 mo: 1 nap, with 12 h at night	Routine fairly well established
Toddler: 12–14 h/night	
"Dawdles" at bedtime	Set firm, realistic limits
Dependency on security object	Place favorite blanket or toy in crib/bed
May ask to sleep with bottle	*Avoid* "bottle mouth syndrome" (caries)
May rebel against going to sleep	Establish bedtime "ritual"
Preschool: 10–12 h/night	May regress in behavior when tired
Gives up afternoon nap	Provide "quiet time" in place of nap
Difficulty falling asleep/nighttime waking	*Avoid* overstimulation in evening
Fear of dark	Leave nightlight on, door open
Enuresis	Occasional accidents are normal
May begin to have nightmares	Comfort child but leave in own bed
School-age: 8–12 h/night	
Nightmares common	Comfort child but leave in own bed
Awakens early in morning	Important that child play/relax before school
May not be aware he/she is tired	Remind about bedtime
Likes to stay up late	"Privilege" of later bedtime can be "awarded" as child gets older
Slumber parties	Permit—good opportunity to socialize
Adolescent: 10–14 h/night	Needs vary greatly among individuals
Need for sleep increases greatly	Rapid growth rate
May complain of excessive fatigue	Related to rapid growth and overall increased activity

E. *Kinetic stimulation*:
  1. Cradle, stroller, carriage, infant seat, car rides, wind-up infant swing, jumper seat, furniture strategically placed for walking.
  2. *Toys*: cradle gym, push-pull.

⚡ **II. Safety**
  A. *Note*: Most common accident during first twelve months is the *aspiration of foreign bodies*.
    1. Keep small objects out of reach.
    2. Use one-piece pacifier only.
    3. *No* nuts, raisins, hot dogs, popcorn, *avoid* "coin-cut" slices of vegetables.
    4. *No* toys with small, removable parts.
    5. *No* balloons or plastic bags.
  B. *Falls*
    1. Raise crib rails.
    2. *Never* place child on high surface unsupervised.
    3. Use restraining straps in seats, swings, highchairs, etc.
  C. *Poisoning*
    1. Check that paint on toys/furniture is *lead-free*.
    2. Treat all medications as drugs, *never* as "candy."
    3. Store all poisonous substances in locked cabinet, closet.

  4. Have phone number of poison control center on hand.
  5. Instruct in use of *syrup of ipecac*; controversial (consult with pediatrician first for children under 1 yr of age).

D. *Burns*
  1. Use microwave oven to heat refrigerated formula only; heat at least 4 oz. or more for about 30 sec. Test formula on *top* of hand, *not* inside wrist.
  2. Check temperature of bath water; *never* leave infant alone in bath; reduce temperature of hot water heater.
  3. Take special care with cigarettes, hot liquids.
  4. Do *not* leave infant in sun.
  5. Cover all electrical sockets.
  6. Keep electrical wires out of sight/reach.
  7. *Avoid* tablecloths with overhang.
  8. Put guards around heating devices.

E. *Motor vehicles*
  1. Use only federally approved car seat for all car rides.
  2. *Never* leave stroller behind parked car.
  3. Do *not* allow infant to crawl near parked cars or in driveway.

(*continued on p. 17*)

TABLE 2.3 A RECOMMENDED CHILDHOOD & ADOLESCENT (SAMPLE) IMMUNIZATION SCHEDULE* (U.S.)

Vaccine ▼ Age ►	Birth	1 month	2 months	4 months	6 months	12 months	15 months	18 months	24 months	4–6 years	11–12 years	13–14 years	15 years	16–18 years
Hepatitis B[1]	HepB	HepB		HepB[1]		HepB					HepB Series			
Diphtheria, Tetanus, Pertussis[2]			DTaP	DTaP	DTaP		DTaP			DTaP	Tdap		Tdap	
Haemophilus influenzae type b[3]			Hib	Hib	Hib[3]	Hib								
Inactivated Poliovirus			IPV	IPV		IPV				IPV				
Measles, Mumps, Rubella[4]						MMR				MMR		MMR		
Varicella[5]						Varicella				Varicella				
Meningococcal[6]										MPSV4	MCV4		MCV4 / MCV4	
Pneumococcal[7]			PCV	PCV	PCV	PCV				PCV	PPV			
Influenza[8]						Influenza (Yearly)				Influenza (Yearly)				
Hepatitis A[9]										HepA Series				

Vaccines within broken line are for selected populations

This schedule indicates the recommended ages for routine administration of currently licensed childhood vaccines, for children through age 18 years. Any dose not administered at the recommended age should be administered at any subsequent visit when indicated and feasible.

▒ Indicates age groups that warrant special effort to administer those vaccines not previously administered. Additional vaccines may be licensed and recommended during the year. Licensed combination vaccines may be used whenever any components of the combination are indicated and other components of the vaccine are not contraindicated and if approved by the Food and Drug Administration for that dose of the series. Providers should consult the respective ACIP statement for detailed recommendations. Clinically significant adverse events that follow immunization should be reported to the Vaccine Adverse Event Reporting System (VAERS). Guidance about how to obtain and complete a VAERS form is available at www.vaers.hhs.gov or by telephone, 800-822-7967

▒ Range of recommended ages   ▒ Catch-up immunization   ▒ 11–12 year old assessment

1. **Hepatitis B vaccine (HepB).** *AT BIRTH:* **All newborns** should receive monovalent HepB soon after birth and before hospital discharge. **Infants born to mothers who are HBsAg-positive** should receive HepB and 0.5 mL of hepatitis B immune globulin (HBIG) within 12 hours of birth. **Infants born to mothers whose HBsAg status is unknown** should receive HepB within 12 hours of birth. The mother should have blood drawn as soon as possible to determine her HBsAg status; if HBsAg-positive, the infant should receive HBIG as soon as possible (no later than age 1 week). **For infants born to HBsAg-negative mothers,** the birth dose can be delayed in rare circumstances but only if a physician's order to withhold the vaccine and a copy of the mother's original HBsAg-negative laboratory report are documented in the infant's medical record. *FOLLOWING THE BIRTHDOSE:* The HepB series should be completed with either monovalent HepB or a combination vaccine containing HepB. The second dose should be administered at age 1–2 months. The final dose should be administered at age ≥24 weeks. It is permissible to administer 4 doses of HepB (e.g., when combination vaccines are given after the birth dose); however, if monovalent HepB is used, a dose at age 4 months is not needed. **Infants born to HBsAg-positive mothers** should be tested for HBsAg and antibody to HBsAg after completion of the HepB series, at age 9–18 months (generally at the next well-child visit after completion of the vaccine series).

2. **Diphtheria and tetanus toxoids and acellular pertussis vaccine (DTaP).** The fourth dose of DTaP may be administered as early as age 12 months, provided 6 months have elapsed since the third dose and the child is unlikely to return at age 15–18 months. The final dose in the series should be given at age ≥4 years.

   Tetanus and diphtheria toxoids and acellular pertussis vaccine (Tdap – adolescent preparation) is recommended at age 11–12 years for those who have completed the recommended childhood DTP/DTaP vaccination series and have not received a Td booster dose. Adolescents 13–18 years who missed the 11–12-year Td/Tdap booster dose should also receive a single dose of Tdap if they have completed the recommended childhood DTP/DTaP vaccination series. Subsequent **tetanus and diphtheria toxoids (Td)** are recommended every 10 years.

3. *Haemophilus influenzae* **type b conjugate vaccine (Hib).** Three Hib conjugate vaccines are licensed for infant use. If PRP-OMP (PedvaxHIB® or ComVax® [Merck]) is administered at ages 2 and 4 months, a dose at age 6 months is not required. DTaP/Hib combination products should not be used for primary immunization in infants at ages 2, 4 or 6 months but can be used as boosters after any Hib vaccine. The final dose in the series should be administered at age ≥12 months.

4. **Measles, mumps, and rubella vaccine (MMR).** The second dose of MMR is recommended routinely at age 4–6 years but may be administered during any visit, provided at least 4 weeks have elapsed since the first dose and both doses are administered beginning at or after age 12 months. Those who have not previously received the second dose should complete the schedule by age 11–12 years.

5. **Varicella vaccine.** Varicella vaccine is recommended at any visit at or after age 12 months for susceptible children (i.e., those who lack a reliable history of chickenpox). Susceptible persons aged ≥13 years should receive 2 doses administered at least 4 weeks apart.

6. **Meningococcal vaccine (MCV4).** Meningococcal conjugate vaccine (MCV4) should be given to all children at the 11–12 year old visit as well as to unvaccinated adolescents at high school entry (15 years of age). Other adolescents who wish to decrease their risk for meningococcal disease may also be vaccinated. All college freshmen living in dormitories should also be vaccinated, preferably with MCV4, although **meningococcal polysaccharide vaccine (MPSV4)** is an acceptable alternative. Vaccination against invasive meningococcal disease is recommended for children and adolescents aged ≥2 years with terminal complement deficiencies or anatomic or functional asplenia and certain other high risk groups (see *MMWR* 2005;54 [RR-7]:1-21); use MPSV4 for children aged 2–10 years and MCV4 for older children, although MPSV4 is an acceptable alternative.

7. **Pneumococcal vaccine.** The heptavalent **pneumococcal conjugate vaccine (PCV)** is recommended for all children aged 2–23 months and for certain children aged 24–59 months. The final dose in the series should be given at age ≥12 months. **Pneumococcal polysaccharide vaccine (PPV)** is recommended in addition to PCV for certain high-risk groups. See *MMWR* 2000; 49(RR-9):1-35.

8. **Influenza vaccine.** Influenza vaccine is recommended annually for children aged ≥6 months with certain risk factors (including, but not limited to, asthma, cardiac disease, sickle cell disease, human immunodeficiency virus [HIV], diabetes, and conditions that can compromise respiratory function or handling of respiratory secretions or that can increase the risk for aspiration), healthcare workers, and other persons (including household members) in close contact with persons in groups at high risk (see *MMWR* 2005;54[RR-8]:1-55). In addition, healthy children aged 6–23 months and close contacts of healthy children aged 0–5 months are recommended to receive influenza vaccine because children in this age group are at substantially increased risk for influenza-related hospitalizations. For healthy persons aged 5–49 years, the intranasally administered, live, attenuated influenza vaccine (LAIV) is an acceptable alternative to the intramuscular trivalent inactivated influenza vaccine (TIV). See *MMWR* 2005;54(RR-8):1-55. Children receiving TIV should be administered a dosage appropriate for their age (0.25 mL if aged 6–35 months or 0.5 mL if aged ≥3 years). Children aged ≤8 years who are receiving influenza vaccine for the first time should receive 2 doses (separated by at least 4 weeks for TIV and at least 6 weeks for LAIV).

9. **Hepatitis A vaccine (HepA).** HepA is recommended for all children at 1 year of age (i.e., 12–23 months). The 2 doses in the series should be administered at least 6 months apart. States, counties, and communities with existing HepA vaccination programs for children 2–18 years of age are encouraged to maintain these programs. In these areas, new efforts focused on routine vaccination of 1-year-old children should enhance, not replace, ongoing programs directed at a broader population of children. HepA is also recommended for certain high risk groups (see *MMWR* 1999; 48[RR-12]1-37).

*Schedule is approved by American Academy of Pediatrics (http://www.aap.org), Advisory Commitee on Immunization Pediatrics (http://www.cdc.gov/nip/acip)

TABLE 2.3 B RECOMMENDED (SAMPLE) IMMUNIZATION SCHEDULE FOR CHILDREN AND ADOLESCENTS WHO START LATE OR WHO ARE MORE THAN 1 MONTH BEHIND (UNITED STATES)

The tables below give catch-up schedules and minimum intervals between doses for children who have delayed immunizations. There is no need to restart a vaccine series regardless of the time that has elapsed between doses. Use the chart appropriate for the child's age.

CATCH-UP SCHEDULE FOR CHILDREN AGED 4 MONTHS THROUGH 6 YEARS

Vaccine	Minimum Age for Dose 1	Minimum Interval Between Doses			
		Dose 1 to Dose 2	Dose 2 to Dose 3	Dose 3 to Dose 4	Dose 4 to Dose 5
Diphtheria, Tetanus, Pertussis	6 wks	**4 weeks**	**4 weeks**	**6 months**	**6 months**[1]
Inactivated Poliovirus	6 wks	**4 weeks**	**4 weeks**	**4 weeks**[2]	
Hepatitis B[3]	Birth	**4 weeks**	**8 weeks** (and 16 weeks after first dose)		
Measles, Mumps, Rubella	12 mo	**4 weeks**[4]			
Varicella	12 mo				
Haemophilus influenzae type b[5]	6 wks	**4 weeks** if first dose given at age <12 months **8 weeks (as final dose)** if first dose given at age 12–14 months **No further doses needed** if first dose given at age ≥15 months	**4 weeks**[6] if current age <12 months **8 weeks (as final dose)**[6] if current age ≥ 12 months and second dose given at age <15 months **No further doses needed** if previous dose given at age ≥15 mo	**8 weeks (as final dose)** This dose only necessary for children aged 12 months–5 years who received 3 doses before age 12 months	
Pneumococcal[7]	6 wks	**4 weeks** if first dose given at age <12 months and current age <24 months **8 weeks (as final dose)** if first dose given at age ≥12 months or current age 24–59 months **No further doses needed** for healthy children if first dose given at age ≥24 months	**4 weeks** if current age <12 months **8 weeks (as final dose)** if current age ≥ 12 months **No further doses needed** for healthy children if previous dose given at age ≥24 months	**8 weeks (as final dose)** This dose only necessary for children aged 12 months–5 years who received 3 doses before age 12 months	

CATCH-UP SCHEDULE FOR CHILDREN AGED 7 YEARS THROUGH 18 YEARS

Vaccine	Minimum Interval Between Doses		
	Dose 1 to Dose 2	Dose 2 to Dose 3	Dose 3 to Booster Dose
Tetanus, Diphtheria[8]	**4 weeks**	**6 months**	**6 months** if first dose given at age <12 months and current age <11 years; otherwise **5 years**
Inactivated Poliovirus[9]	**4 weeks**	**4 weeks**	IPV[2,9]
Hepatitis B	**4 weeks**	**8 weeks** (and 16 weeks after first dose)	
Measles, Mumps, Rubella	**4 weeks**		
Varicella[10]	**4 weeks**		

1. **DTaP.** The fifth dose is not necessary if the fourth dose was administered after the fourth birthday.
2. **IPV.** For children who received an all-IPV or all-oral poliovirus (OPV) series, a fourth dose is not necessary if third dose was administered at age ≥4 years. If both OPV and IPV were administered as part of a series, a total of 4 doses should be given, regardless of the child's current age.
3. **HepB.** Administer the 3-dose series to all children and adolescents <19 years of age if they were not previously vaccinated.
4. **MMR.** The second dose of MMR is recommended routinely at age 4–6 years but may be administered earlier if desired.
5. **Hib.** Vaccine is not generally recommended for children aged ≥5 years.

6. **Hib.** If current age <12 months and the first 2 doses were PRP-OMP (PedvaxHIB® or ComVax® [Merck]), the third (and final) dose should be administered at age 12–15 months and at least 8 weeks after the second dose.
7. **PCV.** Vaccine is not generally recommended for children aged ≥5 years.
8. **Td.** Adolescent tetanus, diphtheria, and pertussis vaccine (Tdap) may be substituted for any dose in a primary catch-up series or as a booster if age appropriate for Tdap. A five-year interval from the last Td dose is encouraged when Tdap is used as a booster dose. See ACIP recommendations for further information.
9. **IPV.** Vaccine is not generally recommended for persons aged ≥18 years.
10. **Varicella.** Administer the 2-dose series to all susceptible adolescents aged ≥13 years.

TABLE 2.4 ⊂⊃ IMMUNIZATIONS: ASSESSMENT OF SIDE EFFECTS AND NURSING CARE

Immunization	▶ Assessment: Side Effects	▶ Nursing Care
Diphtheria	Crankiness, irritability Moderate fever within 24–48 h Soreness, redness, swelling at injection site	General teaching for DTP: ⊂⊃ Prophylactic use of acetaminophen Apply ice/cool soak to injection site
Tetanus	Lump at injection site	Extra "TLC"
Pertussis	Seizures or changes in level of consciousness	Notify physician promptly of any other side effects/severe side effects (seizures, temperature >101.5°F)
Polio	Essentially none	Explain to parent that benefit of being protected by immunization outweighs risk associated with vaccine or disease
Measles	Reaction is delayed until 7–10 d after immunization: fever, rash, coryza	Teach parents about delay in side effects
Mumps	Essentially none	Explain to parent that benefit of being protected by immunization out weighs risk associated with vaccine or disease
Rubella	Mild rash for 24–48 h Arthralgia, arthritis—more common in older children and adults; may last weeks	⊂⊃ Teach parents about side effects; use mild *analgesics*; reassure that symptoms will subside Women of childbearing age should *not* become pregnant for 3 mo after immunization
Hepatitis B	Pain or redness at injection site	⊂⊃ Teach parents about side effects; use mild *analgesics*; reassure that symptoms will subside
H. influenzae (Hib)	Pain, redness, swelling at injection site Low-grade fever	⊂⊃ Teach parents about side effects; use mild *analgesics*; reassure that symptoms will subside
Varicella	Pain or redness at injection site	⊂⊃ Teach parents about side effects; use mild *analgesics*
Pneumococcal	Fever, fussiness	Explain to parents benefits/rationale for immunization in children younger than 2 yr or in older "high-risk" category children
Influenza	Pain or redness at injection site	Teach parents importance of immunization in healthy children aged 0–23 mo as well as in children aged 6 mo and older with certain risk factors (e.g. asthma, cardiac disease, sickle cell disease, etc.)

⊂⊃ **III. Immunizations**

    A. *Recommended* schedule for active immunization of normal infants and children: see **Table 2.3 A-B, p. 15-16.**

    B. *Side effects* of immunizations and nursing care: see **Table 2.4.**

    C. *Contraindications/precautions* to immunizations:

        1. Child who has a severe *febrile* illness (e.g., upper respiratory infection (URI), gastroenteritis, or any fever).

        2. Child with alteration in *skin* integrity: rash, eczema.

        3. Child with alteration in *immune system;* on: *steroids, chemotherapy, radiation therapy;* HIV/AIDS (no live virus vaccine).

        4. Child with a known *allergic* reaction to previous immunization or substance in the immunization vaccine.

Hospitalization of Infants

See **Table 2.5, p. 18** for information on the nursing care of hospitalized infants as it relates to key developmental differences.

TABLE 2.5 NURSING CARE OF HOSPITALIZED INFANTS AND CHILDREN: KEY DEVELOPMENTAL DIFFERENCES

Age	▸ Assessment: Reaction to Hospitalization	▸ Nursing Plan/Implementation: Key Nursing Behaviors
Infant	Difficult to assess needs, pain Wants primary caretaker	Close observation, need to look at behavioral cues Rooming-in
Toddler	Separation anxiety Frustration, loss of autonomy Regression Fears intrusive procedures	Rooming-in Punching bag, pounding board, clay Behavior modification Axillary temperatures
Preschool	Fearful Fantasy about illness/hospitalization (may feel punished, abandoned) Peak of body mutilation fear Behavior problems: aggressive, manipulative Regression	Therapeutic play with puppets, dolls Therapeutic play with puppets, dolls Care with dressings, casts, IMs Clear, consistent limits Behavior modification
School-age	Cooperative Quiet, may withdraw May complain of being bored Fears loss of control Competitive—afraid of "failing"	Use diagrams, models to teach Indirect interview: tell story, draw picture Involve in competitive game with peer Encourage peers to call, send get well cards, and visit Provide privacy; allow to make some decisions Provide tutor prn, get books and homework
Adolescent	Difficulty with body image Does not want to be separated from peers Rebellious behavior	Provide own clothes; give realistic feedback Phone in room; liberal visiting; teen lounge Set clear rules; form teen "rap groups"

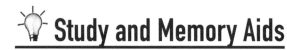

Study and Memory Aids

Personality Development

Major task for infant: trust vs. mistrust.

Physical Development

Birth weight should *double* by 4–7 mo, *triple* by 1 yr. (This period of rapid growth is unparalleled; never again should an individual triple weight in a 1-yr period!)
Deciduous (primary) teeth: first tooth at 6 mo; 6–8 teeth at 1 yr.

Gross Motor Development

No. of Mo	Normal Infant Activity
3	Roll Over
6	Sit (with support)
9	Crawl
12	Walk

Fine Motor–Adaptive Development

Palmar grasp, 4-6 mo: infant uses fingertips to touch object, then rakes object in against palm of hand.
Pincer grasp, 7-9 mo: infant uses thumb and forefinger in neat opposition to pick up object.

Play—Parental Guidance

Best color for toys:
Neonate (birth–28 d):   black and white
Infant (1–12 mo):   red
Infants develop a sense of object permanence or a sense that objects that leave one's visual field still exist at 9–10 mo.

Safety—Accidents

The most common accident during the first 12 mo is *aspiration* of foreign bodies.

⚡ Safety—Burns

Microwave ovens can be used to heat formula *with caution*. 4 oz. or more should be heated for 30 sec; *never* heat amounts of less than 4 oz. Test temperature of formula on the top of hand, **not** inside wrist.

Safety—Car Seats

Use *rear*-facing infant seat placed in the middle of the backseat for first year;
After 20 pounds: use *front*-facing infant/toddler seat until child is *4 yr/40 lb*, then use booster seat;
Use specially designed car restraints until *8 yr or 60 lb*, then "graduate" to factory installed manual shoulder belts in the rear seat.

Questions

1. The nurse should suggest to parents of an infant that the best way for them to assist their child to complete the core developmental task of the first year is to:
   1. Be consistent in their responses.
   2. Provide as many sensory experiences as possible.
   3. Avoid leaving their infant with professional care givers.
   4. Include the infant in their planned activities.

2. The grandparents of a 3-month-old infant ask the nurse what kind of toys they should purchase to have in their home when their infant grandchild comes to visit. Which should the nurse **not** recommend for purchase at this time?
   1. A mobile for the crib.
   2. Brightly colored blocks.
   3. Unbreakable mirrors.
   4. A stuffed animal.

3. Anticipatory gross motor guidance for the parents of a 5-month-old infant should include instructions:
   1. Not to leave the infant unattended on a changing table.
   2. To cover all electrical outlets with "finger-proof" caps.
   3. To continue supporting the infant's head when the infant is pulled into a sitting position.
   4. To remove small items from coffee and end tables.

4. What type of response should the nurse anticipate from an 8-month-old infant when the nurse gets physically close to and smiles at the infant?
   1. Smiles at the nurse.
   2. Reaches out to be picked up.
   3. Turns away from the nurse.
   4. Makes no response to the nurse.

5. In terms of fine motor development, which behavior would be most characteristic of a 9-month-old infant?
   1. Grasping a rattle.
   2. Demonstrating evidence of palmar grasp.
   3. Passing a block from hand to hand.
   4. Showing a pincer grasp.

6. The concerned parent of a 10-month-old infant tells the nurse, "I take all the toys out of the crib when I put the baby down for a nap, but my baby keeps looking under the blanket for the toys. Is this normal?" The best response by the nurse is:
   1. "This is an example of solitary play and it is normal."
   2. "Apparently, the baby prefers to have toys to cuddle with when napping."
   3. "This is an example of object permanence and is perfectly normal for a 10-month-old infant."
   4. "Why don't you rock the baby to sleep so that this behavior stops?"

7. Which physical finding on a 12-month-old infant warrants further investigation?
   1. Posterior fontanel is closed.
   2. A total of six teeth are present.
   3. Birth weight has doubled.
   4. Infant has regular pattern of bowel elimination.

8. Using the Denver Development Screening Test (DDST-II) to assess an infant with chronic heart failure, the nurse should anticipate a developmental lag in which area?
   1. Language.
   2. Personal-social.
   3. Fine motor-adaptive.
   4. Gross motor.

Answers/Rationale

1. **(1)** According to Erikson, the infant's core developmental task is acquiring a sense of trust while overcoming a sense of mistrust. The trust that develops is a trust of self, of others, and of the world; consistency of care is essential for the development of trust. Providing an appropriate number and type of sensory experiences **(2)** is also important during the first year of life; however, experiences in themselves do not replace the more essential trust bond that must develop between parent and infant. The provision of competent, loving infant care by someone other than the parents **(3)** is not detrimental to the child's future development. The nurse plays an important role in providing guidance to parents in selecting well-qualified facilities or individuals to care for their infant. Infants should be included, within reason, in the parent's activities **(4)**; however, parents also need occasional respite activities from 24-hour-a-day parenting. Grandparents and extended family members can assist in this area with offers of babysitting. **IMP, APP, 5, HPM, Health promotion and maintenance**

2. **(2)** Playing with blocks requires the fine motor skills of a 12-month-old infant. Mobiles **(1)**, unbreakable mirrors **(3)** and stuffed animals **(4)** *are* all *age-appropriate* toys for a 1–6-month-old infant. Infants in the 1–12-mo age group are especially attracted

to red objects and toys. **IMP, ANL, 5, HPM, Health promotion and maintenance**

3. **(1)** By 5 mo, the infant can turn from back to side as well as from abdomen to back. If left unattended on a changing table, the infant is capable of rolling off the table and falling to the floor. It is wise to "childproof" the house before bringing the infant home from the hospital; however, covering electrical outlets **(2)** is not necessary until the infant is 9 mo or can creep on hands and knees to such structures. Head lag **(3)** begins to fade at 4–5 mo; parents should be informed of this, but preventing possible injury via a fall is *more critical* than knowing when to expect discontinuance of head lag. Items on low tables **(4)** pose no risk until the 8-month-old infant can stand holding onto furniture. **IMP, ANL, 5, HPM, Health promotion and maintenance**

4. **(3)** "Stranger anxiety" begins at approximately 7 mo and peaks at 8 mo. This is demonstrated by a preference for "mother" as evidenced by clinging to the parent and crying and turning away from the stranger. Smiling back **(1)** is evidenced at 2 mo; reaching out to be held **(2)** occurs at 6 mo. Making no response **(4)** is *inappropriate* for *any* age group; its cause should be determined as soon as possible. **EV, APP, 5, PsI, Psychosocial integrity**

5. **(4)** Pincer grasp (use of thumb and index finger simultaneously) is usually evidenced at 9 mo. Care must be taken with this age group that infants do not pick up small objects, place them in their mouths, and possibly aspirate the objects. Grasping a rattle **(1)** should be evidenced by 4 mo. A palmar grasp **(2)** is demonstrated by 5 mo. Transferring objects from one hand to another **(3)** should be seen by 7 mo. **EV, APP, 5, HPM, Health promotion and maintenance**

6. **(3)** Realizing that objects that leave one's visual field still exist is known as object permanence. It is normal developmental milestone for a 9-10-month-old infant. During the first year of life, infant play practices are solitary or one-sided **(1)**, in that the infant is the center of play, but this does *not* specifically answer the parent's question regarding the infant's behavior. Suggesting the parent place toys in the crib **(2)** does *not* demonstrate a knowledge of infant play practices; the crib should be used for sleeping only—not as a playpen—so that

the infant associates the crib with sleep, not activity. When infants are accustomed to falling asleep in the parent's arms **(4)** and are then transferred to the crib, they awaken in unfamiliar surroundings and are unable to fall asleep until the routine is repeated. One constructive way to prevent sleep problems is to place the infant in the crib while he or she is awake. **IMP, APP, 5, HPM, Health promotion and maintenance**

7. **(3)** Birth weight should be doubled by 4–7 mo and *tripled* by 12 mo. The cause of delay in weight gain requires immediate investigation. The posterior fontanel should close **(1)** at approximately 2 mo. At 12 mo 6-8 deciduous teeth **(2)** should be present. A regular pattern of bowel and bladder elimination **(4)** *should* be evidenced about 8 mo. **EV, ANL, 5, HPM, Health promotion and maintenance**

8. **(4)** Heart failure is a clinical syndrome that reflects the inability of the heart to meet the metabolic needs of the body. Infants with heart failure may sleep much of the time; may fall asleep during feedings; and may be delayed in gross motor activities such as turning over, crawling, and sitting. The older child with heart failure may show fatigue and inability to keep up with peers during physical activities because of decreased perfusion to peripheral tissues and the energy required by the heart in failure. Language **(1)**, personal-social **(2)**, and fine motor-adaptive **(3)** development might also lag because of the infant's poor health, but not to the same extent as gross motor development. **EV, APP, 6, HPM, Health promotion and maintenance**

Key to Codes

Nursing process: AS, assessment; **AN**, analysis; **PL**, planning; **IMP**, implementation; **EV**, evaluation. (See **Appendix L** for explanation of nursing process steps.)

Cognitive level: RE/KN, recall/knowledge; **COM**, comprehension; **APP**, application; **ANL**, analysis; **EVL**, evaluation; **SYN**, synthesis. (See **Appendix L** for explanation.)

Category of human function: 1, protective; **2**, sensory-perceptual; **3**, comfort, rest, activity, and mobility; **4**, nutrition; **5**, growth and development; **6**, fluid-gas transport; **7**, psychosocial-cultural; **8**, elimination. (See **Appendix N** for explanation.)

Client need: SECE, safe, effective care environment; **HPM**, health promotion and maintenance; **PsI**, psychosocial integrity; **PhI**, physiological integrity. (See **Appendix O** for explanation.)

Client subneed: See **Appendix O** for explanation.

Growth and Development of the Toddler

Chapter Outline

- Key Words
- Summary of Key Points
- Toddler (1–3 yrs)
  - Erikson's Theory of Personality Development
  - Physical Growth
  - Denver Developmental Screening Test Norms
  - Nursing Interventions/Parental Guidance
    Play

- Toys
- Safety
- Immunizations
  - Hospitalization of Toddlers
- Study and Memory Aids
- Questions
- Answers/Rationale

Key Words

lordosis   an anterior convexity of the spine; normal in the toddler, who walks with a broadbased gait, but should be outgrown in the preschooler and older child.

parallel play   toddlers play next to, but not necessarily with, one another; engage in separate activities and generally do not share rules, goals, purposes.

physiologic anorexia   decreased appetite because the toddler's growth is much *slower* than that of the infant. Parents may perceive decreased appetite as abnormal when it usually is quite normal during the toddler years.

ritual   a routine that toddlers come to feel is essential to their sense of security and well-being; must be carried out regularly and exactingly.

security object   something a toddler becomes strongly attached to (doll, stuffed animal, or blanket); if separated from the security object, the toddler usually reacts with extreme frustration and anxiety.

temper tantrum   the reaction a toddler has when unable to do what he or she wants, and the toddler feels frustrated and angry; toddler explodes into action with kicking, screaming, hitting, biting, and other gross motor activity instead of verbally expressing these feelings.

🔑 Summary of Key Points

1. The toddler period extends from age 1–3 yr.
2. According to Erikson, the central task for the toddler is *autonomy vs. shame and doubt.*
3. The two words that are most commonly associated with the toddler period are "No!" and "Mine!" Toddlers are very *negativistic* and do not understand the concept of sharing.
4. Toddlers prefer *rituals*, which give them a sense of security.
5. The best method to handle temper tantrums is to *ignore* the behavior.
6. The toddler's growth is slow and steady.
7. Birth weight should *quadruple* by $2^1/_2$ yr.
8. By age 30 mo, *all* 20 "baby" teeth (primary teeth) should be present. The first dental check-up should be between 12 and 18 mo.

9. The Denver Developmental Screening Test is used to screen the development of toddlers. Most toddlers can remove their own clothes between *12 and 18 mo* and put their own clothes on between *19 and 24 mo.*
10. Play during the toddler years is considered "*parallel*" play.
11. Accidents are the chief cause of death in toddlers; most accidental deaths in children under age 3 yr are related to *motor vehicle accidents.*
12. Routine immunizations should continue as recommended for toddlers.
13. When caring for a toddler in the hospital, the nurse should prevent *separation anxiety* by encouraging rooming-in. To help the toddler deal with frustration and loss of autonomy, the nurse should provide the toddler with a *pounding board* or *punching bag.*

Toddler (1–3 yrs)

Erikson's Theory of Personality Development

I. *Central task: autonomy vs. shame and doubt*; central person(s): parent(s).

II. *Behavioral indicators*
   A. Does not separate easily from parents.
   B. Negativistic.
   C. Prefers rituals and routine activities.
   D. Active physical explorer of environment.
   E. Begins attempts at self-assertion.
   F. Easily frustrated by limits.
   G. Temper tantrums.
   H. May have favorite "security object."
   I. Uses "mine" for everything—does not understand concept of sharing.

III. **Parental guidance/teaching**
   A. *Avoid* periods of prolonged separation if possible.
   B. *Avoid* constantly saying "no" to toddler.
   C. *Avoid* "yes"/"no" questions.
   D. Stress that child may use "no" even when he or she means "yes."
   E. Establish and maintain rituals, e.g., toilet training, going to sleep.
   F. Offer opportunities for play, *with* supervision.
   G. Allow child to feed self.
   H. Offer only allowable choices.
   I. Best method to handle temper tantrums: ignore them.
   J. Keep security object with child, if so desired.
   K. Do *not* force toddler "to share."

IV. Additional information about behavioral concerns for each age group may be found in **Chapter 2, Tables 2.1, p. 13** and **Table 2.2, p. 14**.

Physical Growth

I. *Height*
   A. Slow, steady growth at 2–4 in./yr, mainly in *legs* rather than trunk.
   B. Adult height is roughly *twice* child's height at 2 yr.

II. *Weight*
   A. Slow, steady growth, 4–6 pounds/yr.
   B. Birth weight *quadruples* by $2^{1}/_{2}$ yr.

III. *Vital signs*: refer to **Chapter 1, Table 1.5, p. 7**.

IV. *Anterior fontanel*—closes between 12 and *18 mo.*

V. *Teething*
   A. Introduce tooth brushing as a "ritual."
   B. By 30 mos: *all* 20 primary teeth present.
   C. First dental check-up should be between 12 and 18 mo.

VI. *Vision*
   A. Full binocular vision well developed.
   B. Visual acuity of toddler: 20/40.

VII. *Posture and gait*
   A. Lordosis: abdomen protrudes.
   B. Walks like a duck: wide-based gait, side-to-side.

Denver Developmental Screening Test (DDST) Norms

I. **12–18 mo**
   A. *Personal-social*
      1. Imitates housework.
      2. Uses spoon, spills little.
      3. Removes own clothes.
      4. Drinks from cup.
      5. Feeds doll.
   B. *Fine motor-adaptive*
      1. Scribbles spontaneously.
      2. Builds tower with 2–4 cubes.
   C. *Language*
      1. Says 3–6 words other than "mama," "dada."
      2. Points to at least one named body part.
   D. *Gross motor*
      1. Kicks ball forward.
      2. Walks up steps.

II. **19–24 mo**
   A. *Personal-social*
      1. Puts on clothing.
      2. Washes and dries hands.
      3. Brushes teeth with help.
   B. *Fine motor-adaptive*
      1. Builds tower with 4–6 cubes.
      2. Imitates vertical line.
   C. *Language*
      1. Combines 2–3 words.
      2. Names one picture.
      3. Speech is half-understandable.
   D. *Gross motor*
      1. Throws ball overhand.
      2. Jumps in place.

III. **2–3 yr**
   A. *Personal-social*
      1. Puts on T-shirt.
      2. Can name a friend.
   B. *Fine motor-adaptive*
      1. Wiggles thumbs.
      2. Builds tower of 8 cubes.
   C. *Language*
      1. Knows two actions (verbs) and two adjectives.
      2. Names one color.
   D. *Gross motor*
      1. Balances on one foot briefly.
      2. Pedals tricycle.

⋈ Nursing Interventions/Parental Guidance

I. **Play**: toddler years—generally *parallel*.

II. **Toys**—stimulate multiple senses simultaneously:
A. Push-pull.
B. Riding toys, e.g., straddle horse or car.
C. Small, low slide or gym.
D. Balls, in various sizes.
E. Blocks—multiple shapes, sizes, colors.
F. Dolls, trucks, dress-up clothes.
G. Drums, horns, cymbals, xylophones, toy piano.
H. Pounding board and hammer, clay.
I. Finger paints, chalk and board, thick crayons.
J. Wooden puzzles with large pieces.
K. Toy record player with kiddie records.
L. Talking toys—dolls, "see 'n say," phones.
M. Sand, water, soap bubbles.
N. Picture books, photo albums.
O. Nursery rhymes, songs, music.

⚡ III. **Safety**
A. *Accidents* are the leading cause of death among toddlers.
B. *Motor vehicles*: most accidental deaths in children under age 3 yr are related to motor vehicles.
1. Use only federally approved car seat for all car rides (see **Chapter 2, Memory Aids, Safety—Car Seats**).
2. Follow manufacturer directions carefully.
3. Make car seat part of routine for toddler.
C. *Drowning*
1. Always supervise child near water—tub, pool, Jacuzzi, lake, ocean.
2. Keep bathroom locked to prevent drowning in toilet.
D. *Burns*
1. Turn pot handles *in* when on stove top.
2. Do *not* allow child to play with electrical appliances.
3. Decrease water temperature in house to avoid scald burns.
E. *Poisonings*: most common in 2-year-olds.
1. Consider every nonfood substance a hazard and place out of child's sight/reach.
2. Keep all medications, cleaning materials, etc. in clearly marked containers in locked cabinets.
⊂⊃ 3. Instruct caregivers in use of *syrup of ipecac*; (controversial; consult with pediatrician).
F. *Falls*
1. Provide barriers on open windows.
2. *Avoid* gates on stairs—child can strangle on gate.
3. Move from crib to bed.
🍎 G. *Choking*: *avoid* foods on which child might choke:
1. Fish with bones.
2. Fruit with seeds or pits.
3. Nuts, raisins.
4. Hot dogs.
5. Chewing gum.
6. Hard candy.

⊂⊃ IV. **Immunizations**
A. Recommended schedule for active immunization of normal infants and children: see **Chapter 2, Table 2.3 A-B, p. 15-16**.
B. Side effects of immunizations and nursing care: see **Chapter 2, Table 2.4, p. 17**.

Hospitalization of Toddlers

⋈ Refer to **Chapter 2, Table 2.5, p. 18** for information on the nursing care of hospitalized toddlers as it relates to key developmental differences.

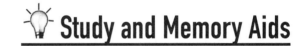

💡 Study and Memory Aids

Personality Development

Major task for toddler: *autonomy* vs. *shame* and *doubt*.
Toddler's most common words: "No!" and "Mine!"
Ignore temper tantrums.

Physical Growth

Toddler growth: slow and steady.
Toddler weight: *quadruples by* age 2½ yr.
Teeth: first dental screening at 12–18 months; all deciduous teeth (20) present at *2½ yr*.

Personal–Social

The toddler feeds self with spoon at 12–18 mo.

Play

Play for a toddler is *parallel*: two toddlers play next to, but not with, each other.

Safety

Number one cause of death in toddler years: *accidents*.
Most common accident: *motor vehicle* accidents.

Questions

1. The parents of an infant ask the nurse when the child should be seen by the dentist for the first time. The nurse would be most correct in advising the parents that ideally a child should see the dentist:
1. Before teeth erupt.
2. Soon after the first teeth erupt, usually by age 1.
3. Between 12 and 18 mo.
4. Around the second birthday.

2. A toddler who is to be hospitalized brings a dirty, ragged Barney stuffed animal with him. The nurse's most appropriate action is:
    1. Ask the toddler's parents to find an identical, new Barney stuffed animal.
    2. Remove Barney while the child is sleeping and when the child wakes up, say Barney is "lost."
    3. Allow the toddler to keep the Barney stuffed animal.
    4. Distract the toddler by taking him to the playroom and letting him select another stuffed animal.

3. Knowing that toddlers can be very negative and often use the word "no!," the nurse who is working with a toddler should:
    1. Offer the toddler only choices that are acceptable.
    2. Offer the toddler no choices at all.
    3. Involve the toddler in choices about his care.
    4. Read the toddler a book about making the right choices.

4. The nurse should suggest that the best way for a toddler's parents to assist their child to complete the core developmental task of the toddler years is to:
    1. Allow the toddler to make simple decisions.
    2. Allow the toddler to "help."
    3. Assign the toddler simple tasks or errands.
    4. Teach the toddler car- and street-safety rules.

5. A toddler repeatedly says "no" to everything the nurse offers to the child. The nurse realizes that the best way to deal with this situation is to:
    1. Reduce the opportunities for a "no" answer.
    2. Keep offering the toddler choices until the toddler accepts one.
    3. Say "no" to the toddler in return.
    4. Discipline the toddler to curb negative behavior.

6. Parents ask the nurse how to toilet-train their toddler. Which is not an appropriate statement by the nurse?
    1. Wanting to please the parent helps motivate the toddler to use the toilet.
    2. Awareness of the urge to defecate must be developed.
    3. Practice sessions should be limited to once or twice a day.
    4. Free-standing potty chairs help to make the toddler feel more secure.

7. In assessing a toddler, the nurse should know that the toddler may best demonstrate the achievement of gross motor skills by:
    1. Stacking two blocks.
    2. Pushing and pulling toys.
    3. Turning the pages in a book two or three at a time.
    4. Dumping a raisin from a bottle.

8. If observed in a home with a 2-year-old child, which action would the nurse identify as an ineffective safety measure?
    1. Keeping the poison control number by the phone.
    2. Installing safety latches on kitchen and bathroom cabinets.
    3. Keeping poisonous items in a locked cabinet.
    4. Keeping all substances in their original containers.

Answers/Rationale

1. **(2)** The American Academy of Pediatric Dentistry recommends that children see a dentist soon after their first teeth erupt, no later than one year of age. Seeing a dentist before teeth erupt **(1)** is *too early* to have value. The second birthday **(4)** and 12-18 mo **(3)** is now considered *too late* for the initial visit. **IMP, COM, 5, HPM, Health promotion and maintenance**

2. **(3)** Toddlers often have security objects, such as a stuffed animal, that help them feel safe and secure. Since the child has been living with the stuffed animal for some time, there is no harm in allowing the toy; in fact, real psychological harm could be done by attempting to separate the child from his beloved Barney at this stressful time. The parents should *not* attempt to replace Barney **(1)**, nor should the nurse attempt to distract the child and suggest he pick another animal **(4)** as these actions could prove frightening and even threatening for the child and disrupt his sense of trust and security. In addition, the nurse should not remove the stuffed animal while the child is asleep **(2)** because this could also prove frightening, disrupt his sense of trust, and cause a period of sleep disturbances and nightmares for the toddler. **IMP, APP, 5, PsI, Psychosocial integrity**

3. **(1)** The nurse and parents should offer the toddler only choices that are allowable and be prepared to live with the choice the toddler selects. For example, the nurse could offer the toddler a choice about which adhesive bandage he would like after he has an IM injection, but should not offer a choice about having the injection. Because the toddler asserts autonomy through excessive use of the word "no," it is *not* appropriate to offer no choices **(2)**. Unlike an older school-aged child or adolescent, the toddler does *not* have the ability to participate meaningfully in choices about his care **(3)**. Toddlers like being read to and generally like simple stories; a book with a moral to it, such as a book about making choices **(4)**, is beyond a toddler's comprehension. **PL, APP, 5, PsI, Psychosocial integrity**

4. **(1)** According to Erikson, the toddler is concerned with acquiring a sense of autonomy while overcoming a sense of doubt and shame. Toddlers must learn that their behavior is their own and must begin to trust their judgments. Allowing the toddler to make simple decisions from allowable choices is one way of assisting the toddler in developing autonomy. "Helping" **(2)**, errands **(3)**, and learning rules **(4)** are beyond the cognitive scope of a toddler. These skills are appropriate for a *preschooler* rather than a toddler. **PL, APP, 5, PsI, Psychosocial integrity**

5. **(1)** Negativism is an acknowledged part of toddlerhood and occurs because children attempt to express their will in their quest for autonomy. Reduce opportunities for a "no" answer—offer the toddler two appropriate choices. For example, "You may have milk or apple juice," *not* "Do you want milk?" or "Do you want apple juice?" Offering additional choices **(2)** only further frustrates the toddler. Parents (or nurses), in their own frustration in dealing with a toddler, should *not* resort to toddler-like behaviors themselves **(3)**. Setting simple rules and applying them consistently are of greater value in reducing negativism than is disciplining the toddler **(4)**. **PL, APP, 5, PsI, Psychosocial integrity**

6. **(3)** Practice sessions should be limited to 5–10 min/session, *frequent* sessions need to be scheduled throughout the day to reinforce what the toddler is being asked to do. Wanting to please parents **(1)**, awareness of the urge to defecate **(2)**, and small, child-sized equipment **(4)** *are* some essential elements in a successful potty-training regime for a toddler. **IMP, APP, 5, HPM, Health promotion and maintenance**

7. **(2)** Pushing and pulling toys demonstrates gross motor development on the toddler's part. Stacking blocks **(1)**, turning the pages of a book **(3)**, and dumping a raisin from a bottle **(4)** are *fine motor* skills acquired during the toddler years. **AS, ANL, 5, HPM, Health promotion and maintenance**

8. **(2)** Unlike the infant, the toddler, by trial and error, can manage to undo safety latches and childproof medicine caps. For this age group, only a *locked* cabinet is safe. Keeping the poison control number **(1)** handy, having locked cabinets **(3)**, and keeping poisonous items in their original containers **(4)** are *all appropriate* safety measures in a home with a toddler. **EV, APP, 5, SECE, Safety and infection control**

Key to Codes

Nursing process: AS, assessment; **AN**, analysis; **PL**, planning; **IMP**, implementation; **EV**, evaluation. (See **Appendix L** for explanation of nursing process steps.)

Cognitive level: RE/KN, recall/knowledge; **COM**, comprehension; **APP**, application; **ANL**, analysis; **EVL**, evaluation; **SYN**, synthesis. (See **Appendix L** for explanation.)

Category of human function: 1, protective; **2**, sensory-perceptual; **3**, comfort, rest, activity, and mobility; **4**, nutrition; **5**, growth and development; **6**, fluid-gas transport; **7**, psychosocial-cultural; **8**, elimination. (See **Appendix N** for explanation.)

Client need: SECE, safe, effective care environment; **HPM**, health promotion and maintenance; **PsI**, psychosocial integrity; **PhI**, physiological integrity. (See **Appendix O** for explanation.)

Client subneed: See **Appendix O** for explanation.

Growth and Development of the Preschooler

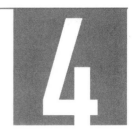

Chapter Outline

- Key Words
- Summary of Key Points
- Preschooler (3–5 yrs)
  - Erikson's Theory of Personality Development
  - Physical Growth
  - Denver Developmental Screening Test Norms
  - Nursing Interventions/Parental Guidance
    Play

        Toys/Games
        Safety
        Immunizations
-    Hospitalization of Preschoolers
- Study and Memory Aids
- Questions
- Answers/Rationale

Key Words

associative play   preschoolers will play in a group with other preschool children doing the same or similar activities, but there are few—if any—rules and little organization to the group.

cooperative play   slightly more advanced than associative play; preschoolers will play in a group with other preschool children in one, organized activity that has rules and goals.

enuresis   bedwetting, involuntary urination, most often during sleep.

🔑 Summary of Key Points

1. The preschool period extends from age 3–5 yr.
2. According to Erikson, the central task for the preschooler is *initiative vs. guilt*.
3. The word most frequently associated with the preschooler is *"Why?"*
4. The preschool period is characterized by *fantasy, magical thinking,* and many *fears.*
5. The preschool period is one of continued slow and steady growth.
6. Preschoolers should be screened annually for dental, vision, and hearing health.
7. The Denver Developmental Screening Test is used to screen the development of preschoolers; normal developmental steps are:

   a. a *3-year-old* can pedal a tricycle.
   b. a *4-year-old* can tie own shoes.
   c. a *5-year-old* can verbalize number sequences, i.e., telephone numbers.
8. Play during the preschool years is considered *"associative"* and *"cooperative"* play.
9. Accidents are the leading cause of death in the preschool years; *motor vehicle accidents* are the most common accident for preschoolers.
10. Routine immunizations should continue as recommended for preschoolers.
11. When caring for a preschooler in the hospital, the nurse should incorporate *therapeutic play* to help the child cope with fears and fantasies.

Preschooler (3–5 yrs)

Erikson's Theory of Personality Development

I. *Central task: initiative vs. guilt*; central person(s): basic family unit.

II. *Behavioral indicators*
  A. Attempts to perform activities of daily living (ADL) independently.
  B. Attempts to make things for self/others.
  C. Tries to "help."
  D. Talks constantly: verbal exploration of the world ("Why?").
  E. Extremely active, highly creative imagination: *fantasy* and *magical thinking.*
  F. May demonstrate *fears*: "monsters," dark rooms, etc.
  G. Able to tolerate short periods of separation.

III. *Parental guidance/teaching*
  A. Encourage child to dress self by providing simple clothing.
  B. Remind to go to bathroom (tends to "forget").
  C. Assign small, simple tasks or errands.

D. Answer questions patiently, simply; do *not* offer child more information than he or she is asking for.
E. Normal to have "imaginary playmates."
F. Offer realistic support and reassurance with regard to fears.
G. Expose to a variety of experiences: zoo, train ride, shopping, sleigh riding, etc.
H. Enroll in preschool/nursery school program; kindergarten at 5 yr.
IV. Additional information about behavioral concerns for each age group may be found in **Chapter 2, Tables 2.1, p. 13** and Table 2.2, p. 14.

Physical Growth

I. *Height and weight*
   A. Continued slow, steady growth.
   B. Generally grows more in *height* than weight.
   C. Posture: appears taller and thinner; lordosis of toddler gradually *disappears*.
II. *Vital signs*: see **Chapter 1, Table 1.5, p. 7.**
III. *Teeth*
   A. *All* 20 "baby teeth" present.
   B. Annual dental check-ups, daily brushing.
IV. *Vision*
   A. Visual acuity: 20/30 at 3–5 yr.
   B. Do vision/hearing screening prekindergarten.

Denver Developmental Screening Test (DDST) Norms

I. **3 yr**
   A. *Personal-social*
      1. Dresses without help.
      2. Plays board/card games.
   B. *Fine motor-adaptive*
      1. Picks longer of two lines.
      2. Copies circle, intersecting lines.
      3. Draws person with three parts.
   C. *Language*
      1. Comprehends "cold," "tired," "hungry."
      2. Comprehends prepositions: "over," "under."
      3. Names four colors.
   D. *Gross motor*
      1. Pedals tricycle; hops, skips on alternating feet.
      2. Broad jumps, jumps in place.
      3. Balances on one foot.
II. **4 yr**
   A. *Personal-social*
      1. Brushes own teeth, combs own hair.
      2. Dresses without supervision.
      3. Knows own age and birthday.
      4. Ties own shoes.
   B. *Fine motor-adaptive*
      1. Draws person with six body parts.
      2. Copies a square.
   C. *Language*
      1. Knows opposite analogies (2 of 3).
      2. Defines seven words.
   D. *Gross motor*
      1. Balances on each foot for 5 sec.
      2. Can walk heel-to-toe.
III. **5 yr**
   A. *Personal-social*
      1. Interested in money.
      2. Knows days of week, seasons.
   B. *Fine motor-adaptive*
      1. Prints name.
   C. *Language*
      1. Counts to 10.
      2. Verbalizes number sequences (e.g., telephone number).
   D. *Gross motor*
      1. Attempts to ride bike.
      2. Rollerskates, jumps rope, bounces ball.
      3. Backward heel-toe walk.

Nursing Interventions/Parental Guidance

I. **Play**: preschool years—associative and cooperative.
II. **Toys/Games:**
   A. Likes to play house, "work," school, firehouse.
   B. "Arts and crafts": color, draw, paint, dot-to-dot, color by number, cut and paste, simple sewing kits.
   C. Ball, roller skates, jump rope, jacks.
   D. Swimming.
   E. Puzzles, blocks (e.g., Lego blocks).
   F. Tricycle, then bike (with/without training wheels).
   G. Simple card games and board games.
   H. Costumes and dress-up: "make-believe."
III. **Safety**: Emphasis shifts from protective supervision to teaching simple safety rules. Preschoolers are "the great imitators" of parents, who now serve as role models.
   A. Teach child car/*street* safety rules.
   B. Change to "booster seat" in car at age 4 yr, 40 pounds. (see **page 18, Chapter 2, Memory Aids**)
   C. Teach child not to go with strangers or accept gifts or candy from strangers.
   D. Teach child danger of *fire*, matches, flame: "drop and roll."
   E. Teach child rules of *water* safety; provide swimming lessons.
   F. Provide adult supervision, frequent checks on activity/location. Despite safety teaching, preschooler is still a child and may be unreliable.

⊂▭ IV. **Immunizations**
  A. Recommended schedule for active immunization of normal infants and children: see **Chapter 2, Table 2.3 A-B, p. 15-16.**
  B. Side effects of immunizations and nursing care: see **Chapter 2, Table 2.4, p. 17.**

Hospitalization of Preschoolers

Refer to **Chapter 2, Table 2.5, p. 18** for information on ⋈ the nursing care of hospitalized preschoolers as it relates to key developmental differences.

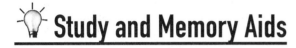 **Study and Memory Aids**

Personality Development

Major task for preschooler: *initiative vs. guilt.*
Preschoolers' most common word: "Why?"
Fears, fantasies, magical thinking characterize preschool period.

Physical Growth

Growth during preschool years continues to be slow and steady.

Developmental Norms

3 years—3 wheels. Once the preschooler learns the alternate foot pedaling needed for the tricycle, the child can go down stairs using alternating feet, skip on alternating feet, or hop on alternating feet.
Four-year-olds: tie their own shoes.
Five-year-olds: can repeat their telephone numbers.

Play

Play for a preschooler is *associative* and *cooperative*: preschoolers play in a group with other children.

Safety

Leading cause of death in preschool years: *accidents.*
Most common accident: *motor vehicle* accidents.

Questions

1. The nurse should counsel parents of a preschooler that the best way for them to assist their child to complete the core developmental task of the preschooler is to:
   1. Have the preschooler watch the parents do chores.
   2. Answer their preschooler's questions simply but truthfully.
   3. Minimize the preschooler's fear of the dark and monsters.
   4. Insist on clear, fluent speech.

2. A nutritional teaching goal for a preschooler would be to:
   1. Decrease the number of mealtime spills.
   2. Introduce new food gradually.
   3. Enforce table manners.
   4. Encourage the child to eat a specific amount of food each day.

3. The nurse should anticipate, that in terms of fine motor development, a 4-year-old is unable to:
   1. Copy a circle.
   2. Use safety scissors.
   3. Tie shoes.
   4. Print own name.

4. The nurse should advise parents that injury prevention for a preschooler can best be enforced by:
   1. Constant vigilance on the part of the parent.
   2. Role modeling and teaching safety rules.
   3. A small teacher-child ratio in the child's nursery school.
   4. Discipline for unsafe behaviors.

5. A preschooler hospitalized on the pediatrics unit asks the nurse, "Where do babies come from?" Before answering this question, the nurse should:
   1. Determine exactly what the child is asking.
   2. Tell the child that babies come from the stork.
   3. Discuss the question with the child's parents.
   4. Tell the child to ask his parents because the nurse is not sure.

6. The nurse should advise parents that normally a child learns to tie shoes at what age?
   1. 3 yr.
   2. 4 yr.
   3. 5 yr.
   4. 6 yr.

7. The nurse should expect a 4-year-old child to be capable of three of the behaviors listed. Which behavior is more advanced than the nurse should expect in a 4-year-old?
   1. Uses scissors to cut out pictures by following an outline.
   2. Names coins, e.g., penny, nickel, dime, quarter.
   3. Throws a ball overhand and catches a ball reliably.
   4. Knows simple songs and names one or more colors.

8. The mother of a preschooler expresses disappointment when her child's weight has increased only 4 pounds since the child's physical 1 year ago. The nurse should advise this mother that:
   1. A weight gain of 4–6 pounds/yr is normal for a preschooler.
   2. The poor weight gain may be a result of poor nutrition; the mother should meet with the dietician.
   3. The poor weight gain may indicate a more serious problem; the child should be seen by the MD.
   4. The weight gain is not ideal but may be nothing to worry about; the child should be checked again in 3 mo.

Answers/Rationale

1. **(2)** According to Erikson, the preschooler's core developmental task is initiative vs. guilt. Preschoolers are in a stage of energetic learning and feel a sense of satisfaction in their abilities. For these reasons, parents can best aid the preschooler's development by answering the many questions simply but truthfully. Preschoolers want to "help," *not* just watch **(1)**. Parents should offer realistic support and reassurance regarding their child's fears **(3)**, *not* minimize the fears. Age 2–4 yr is the most critical period for speech development; however, lack of fluency in speech **(4)**, such as stuttering or stammering while trying to say a word, is a normal characteristic of language development in a preschooler. **IMP, APP, 5, HPM, Health promotion and maintenance**

2. **(2)** Preschoolers have so much curiosity about what is happening around them that they may have little interest in eating; therefore, it is best to introduce new food gradually and include a variety of tastes, colors, and consistencies. An adult's likes and dislikes greatly influence preschoolers. Mealtime spills **(1)** are unavoidable for the preschooler and should be accepted, cleaned up, and forgotten. Table manners at this age are best learned by observation and should *not* be stressed **(3)**. It is normal for the child to want more food on some days than others **(4)**. **PL, APP, 4, HPM, Health promotion and maintenance**

3. **(4)** Printing, a fine motor skill, is the task of a *5-year-old* child. By 5 yr, preschoolers can print a few letters, numbers, or words, such as a first name. Copying a circle **(1)**, a fine motor skill, is usually achieved during the *third* year. Using scissors **(2)** and tying shoes **(3)** *are* fine-motor skills achieved in the *fourth* year. **AS, APP, 5, HPM, Health Promotion and Maintenance**

4. **(2)** By appealing to the preschooler's sense of initiative, safety rules are usually readily learned. Poor judgment and lack of experience may cause the preschooler to forget the rules, so repetition, modeling and reinforcement are needed by the parent. Constant vigilance by the parent **(1)** can interfere with the child's sense of initiative. Adequate supervision in the child's nursery school **(3)** is essential, but it is *not* a substitute for teaching the child about safety. Limit setting is always more effective than discipline **(4)**; this is especially true in gaining the child's cooperation with safety rules. **IMP, APP, 5, HPM, Health promotion and maintenance**

5. **(1)** The nurse needs to find out what the child is really asking by a question like this. One child might be asking about sex; another might be thinking "Johnny came from California, and Mary came from Texas. How can that be?" A good response to elicit more information from the preschooler would be, "You sound really interested in learning more about babies. Tell me what you'd like to know and I'll try to help you." It would *not* be appropriate to lie to a preschooler **(2)** by telling him a story about the stork. Depending on what the child wants to know, there may be no need to involve the parents at this time **(3)**. The nurse should *not* close off communication with the preschooler who has asked a question by redirecting the child to talk with parents **(4)**. **AS, ANL, 5, PsI, Psychosocial integrity**

6. **(2)** The normal 4-year-old child is expected to have the skills necessary to tie shoes. Children younger than 5 **(1)** may mimic parts of the process but are generally too young to complete the skill. A child normally learns to tie shoes before turning 5 or 6 **(3 and 4)**. **IMP, COM, 5, HPM, Health promotion and maintenance**

7. **(2)** A 5-year-old, *not* a 4-year-old, is capable of naming coins. A 4-year-old *should be capable* of using scissors and following an outline **(1)**, playing ball **(3)**, knowing simple songs, and naming colors **(4)**. **EV, ANL, 5, HPM, Health promotion and maintenance**

8. **(1)** A preschooler normally gains only 4–6 pounds/yr. The nurse should reassure the mother that the weight gain is well within normal limits. It is *not* appropriate to call the weight "poor weight gain" since it is within normal limits; a referral to the dietician **(2)** or the MD **(3)** is *not* necessary. Because the weight gain *is* within normal limits, there is no need to recheck the child in 3 mo **(4)**. **EV, COM, 5, HPM, Health promotion and maintenance**

Key to Codes

Nursing process: AS, assessment; **AN**, analysis; **PL**, planning; **IMP**, implementation; **EV**, evaluation. (See **Appendix L** for explanation of nursing process steps.)

Cognitive level: RE/KN, recall/knowledge; **COM**, comprehension; **APP**, application; **ANL**, analysis; **EVL**, evaluation; **SYN**, synthesis. (See **Appendix L** for explanation.)

Category of human function: 1, protective; **2**, sensory-perceptual; **3**, comfort, rest, activity, and mobility; **4**, nutrition; **5**, growth and development; **6**, fluid-gas transport; **7**, psychosocial-cultural; **8**, elimination. (See **Appendix N** for explanation.)

Client need: SECE, safe, effective care environment; **HPM**, health promotion and maintenance; **PsI**, psychosocial integrity; **PhI**, physiological integrity. (See **Appendix O** for explanation.)

Client subneed: See **Appendix O** for explanation.

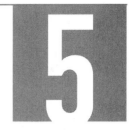

Growth and Development of the School-Aged Child

Chapter Outline

- Key Word
- Summary of Key Points
- School-Aged (6–12 yrs)
  - Erikson's Theory of Personality Development
  - Physical Growth
  - Developmental Norms
  - Nursing Interventions/Parental Guidance
    Play

    Toys/Games
    Safety
    Immunizations
  - Hospitalization of School-Aged Children
- Study and Memory Aids
- Questions
- Answers/Rationale

Key Word

pubescence   preadolescent physical changes that usually occur at age 10 yr in *girls* and age 12 yr in *boys*.

🔑 Summary of Key Points

1. The school-aged years extend from age 6–12 yr.
2. According to Erikson, the central task for the school-aged child is *industry vs. inferiority*.
3. The school-aged child is highly *competitive*.
4. Growth during these years continues to be slow and steady. Height almost *doubles* between ages 6–12 yr; boys and girls differ little in size.
5. The school-aged child begins to lose primary teeth around the *sixth* birthday and permanent teeth begin to erupt. There should be 28 *permanent* teeth present by the *twelfth* birthday.
6. Pubescence, the preliminary physical changes of adolescence, begins at *10 yr* in *girls* and at *12 yr* in *boys*.
7. The Denver Developmental Screening Test is *not used* to screen the development of school-aged children.
8. Children learn to tell time and read between *6 and 8 yrs*.
9. Play during the school-aged years is *cooperative* and focuses on team or group activities.
10. Accidents are the leading cause of death in the school-aged child; *motor vehicle accidents* are the most common type of *accident* for school-aged children.
11. Routine immunizations should continue as recommended for school-aged children.
12. When caring for a school-aged child in the hospital, the nurse should use *diagrams* or models to teach the child about the illness or surgery. If the school-aged child appears quiet or withdrawn, the nurse should use the *indirect interview* method (tell story, draw picture) to elicit feelings.
13. If a hospitalized school-aged child complains of feeling bored, the nurse should suggest a *competitive* board game with a *same-sex peer*.

School-Aged (6–12 yrs)

Erikson's Theory of Personality Development

I. *Central task: industry vs. inferiority;* central person(s): school, neighborhood friend(s).

II. *Behavioral indicators*
   A. Moving toward complete independence in activities of daily living (ADL).
   B. May be very competitive—wants to achieve in school, at play.
   C. Likes to be alone occasionally, may seem shy.
   D. Prefers friends and peers to siblings.

III. **Parental guidance/teaching**
   A. Be accepting of the child as he or she *is*.
   B. Offer consistent support and guidance.
   C. *Avoid* authoritative or excessive demands on child.
   D. Respect need for privacy.
   E. Assign household tasks, errands, chores.

IV. Additional information about behavioral concerns for each age group may be found in **Chapter 2, Tables 2.1, p. 13** and **Tables 2.2 p, 14.**

Physical Growth

I. *Height and weight*
   A. Period of slow, steady growth.
   B. 1–2 in./yr.
   C. 3–6 pounds/yr (Almost *double* in weight during 6–12 yr).
   D. Girls and boys differ very little in size.

II. *Vital signs*: refer to **Chapter 1, Table 1.5, p. 7.**

III. *Teeth*
   A. Begins to lose primary teeth about *sixth* birthday.
   B. Eruption of permanent teeth, including molars; *28* permanent teeth by age *12 yr.*
   C. Dental screening annually, daily brushing.

IV. *Vision and hearing*
   A. Should be screened annually—usually in school.
   B. 20/20 vision well established at 9–11 yr.

V. *Pubescence* (preliminary physical changes of adolescence)
   A. Average age of onset: girls at 10 yr, boys at 12 yr.
   B. Beginning of growth spurt.
   C. Some sexual changes may begin.

Developmental Norms

I. 6–8 yr
   A. Dramatic, exuberant, boundless energy.
   B. Alternating periods: quiet, private behavior.
   C. Conscientious, punctual.
   D. Wants to care for own needs, but needs reminders, supervision.
   E. Oriented to time and space.
   F. Learns to read, tell time, follow map.
   G. Interested in money—asks for "allowance."
   H. Eagerly anticipates upcoming events, trips.
   I. Can ride bike, swim, play ball.

II. 9–11 yr
   A. Worries over tasks; takes things seriously, but also develops sense of humor—likes to tell jokes.
   B. Keeps room, clothes, toys relatively tidy.
   C. Enjoys physical activity, has great stamina.
   D. Very enthusiastic at work and play; has lots of energy—may fidget, drum fingers, tap foot.
   E. Wants to work to earn money: mow lawn, babysit, deliver papers.
   F. Loves secrets (secret clubs).
   G. Very well behaved outside own home (or with company).
   H. Uses tools, equipment; follows directions, recipes.
   I. By *twelfth* birthday: paradoxic stormy behavior, onset of adolescent conflicts.

▶◀ Nursing Interventions/Parental Guidance

I. **Play**; school-aged years–cooperative

II. **Toys/Games:**
   A. Wants to win; likes competitive games.
   B. Prefers to play with same-sex children.
   C. Enjoys group, team play.
   D. Loves to do magic tricks and other "show-off" activities (e.g., puppet shows, plays, singing).
   E. Likes collecting: cards, records.
   F. Does simple scientific experiments; plays computer games.
   G. Has hobbies: needlework, woodwork, models.
   H. Enjoys pop music, musical instruments, radio, audio tapes, videos, posters.

III. **Safety**—motor vehicles
   A. As passenger: teach to wear safety belt, not distract driver.
   B. As pedestrian: teach bike, street safety.
   C. Teach how to swim, rules of water safety.
   D. Sports: teach safety rules.
   E. Adult supervision still necessary; serve as role model for safe activities.
   F. Suggest Red Cross courses on first aid, water safety, babysitting, etc.

IV. **Immunizations**
   A. Recommended schedule for active immunization of normal infants and children: see **Chapter 2, Table 2.3 A-B, p. 15-16.**
   B. Side effects of immunizations and nursing care: see **Chapter 2, Table 2.4, p. 17.**

Hospitalization of School-Aged Children

▶◀ Refer to **Chapter 2, Table 2.5, p. 18** for information on the nursing care of hospitalized school-aged children as it relates to key developmental differences.

💡 Study and Memory Aids

Personality Development

Major task for school-aged child: *industry* vs. *inferiority*. The school-aged child is very competitive, achievement oriented.

Physical Growth

Growth of the school-aged child continues to be slow and steady.

The school-aged child loses all 20 primary teeth, which are replaced by permanent (or adult) teeth; of 32 adult teeth, *28* are present by *12 yr.*

The growth spurt and pubescence begins *earlier* in *girls*, at about *10 yr*, than it does in boys, at 12 yr.

Developmental Norms

6– and 7–year-olds learn how to tell time and to read.

Play

The school-aged years feature *cooperative* play, focused on team or group activities.

Safety

Leading cause of death in school-aged years: *accidents*. Most common accident: *motor vehicle* accidents.

Questions

1. The nurse should counsel the parents of a school-aged child that the best way for them to assist their child to complete the core developmental task of the school-aged years is to:
   1. Give recognition and positive feedback for accomplishments.
   2. Avoid giving the child set responsibilities.
   3. Limit family outings to family members.
   4. Assist the child in selecting a vocation.

2. A school-aged child undergoing an annual physical examination has gained 5 pounds during the past year. The parents question the weight gain. The nurse should reply:
   1. "This is a little more than average, so we need to discuss some dietary restrictions."
   2. "This is expected for a school-aged child."
   3. "Weight gain is a little low this year, but it will catch-up next year."
   4. "Your child's weight will triple between ages 6–12."

3. The nurse should be aware that which description is uncharacteristic of the play practices of children in the school-aged years?
   1. Boys and girls seek each other out to play.
   2. Both sexes like to collect things.
   3. School-aged children prefer to play with same-sex children.
   4. School-age children like competitive games.

4. For the parents of a school-aged child, anticipatory guidance regarding homework should include which item?
   1. Parents should participate in their child's assignments.
   2. Parents are responsible for their child's scholastic successes and failures.
   3. Parents should withdraw privileges for poor academic performance.
   4. Parents should promptly confer with their child's teacher when problems arise.

5. A school-aged child who has just lost the first tooth comes into the school nurse's office and asks the nurse, "How many baby teeth will I lose?" The nurse would be most correct in saying the child will lose:
   1. All the baby teeth.
   2. 8 baby teeth.
   3. 12 baby teeth.
   4. 16 baby teeth.

6. A school-aged child asks the school nurse how many adult teeth she will have when they are all "in." The school nurse should tell this child that she can expect to have a total of:
   1. 20 adult teeth.
   2. 24 adult teeth.
   3. 28 adult teeth.
   4. 32 adult teeth.

7. A hospitalized school-aged boy has a large collection of comic books with him. On seeing the stacks of comics scattered in his room, which action by the nurse is most appropriate?
   1. Ask the child to select some favorite comics and send the rest home with his parents.
   2. Advise the parents to remove the comics while the child is sleeping, because they are cluttering up the child's room.
   3. Allow the child to keep the comics with him, provided they are kept reasonably neat.
   4. Tell the child that he can keep them, but that he must share his comics with the other children in his room.

8. When teaching a class about safety to 10- and 11-year-old boys and girls, on which type of accident should the school nurse focus as the primary cause of serious accidental injury and death in school-aged children?
   1. Bicycle accidents.
   2. Motor vehicle accidents.
   3. Rollerblading accidents.
   4. All-terrain vehicle accidents.

Answers/Rationale

1. **(1)** According to Erikson, industry vs. inferiority is the core developmental task of school-aged children. This period is usually the first time that the child is making truly independent judgments. Parents need to give praise and recognition for good judgments and accomplishments so that the child feels competent. School-aged children *need* and *want* set tasks, errands, and chores **(2)**, which contribute to their sense of industry. Peers are very important to school-aged children; this is an age at which children may enjoy friends more than siblings or parents—including a friend in a family outing often makes the event more enjoyable for everyone **(3)**. Selecting a vocation **(4)** is the task of an *adolescent*. **IMP, APP, 5, HPM, Health promotion and maintenance**

2. (2) 3–6 pounds/yr is an average yearly weight gain for a school-aged child. For a school-aged child, a 5-pound weight gain during 1 yr is neither excessive (1) nor deficient (3). The child's weight should almost double, *not triple*, between ages 6-12 yr (4). **IMP, COM, 5, HPM, Health promotion and maintenance**

3. (1) About age 10, children begin to show interest in the opposite sex, but do not actively seek to play with members of the opposite sex. Boys and girls tend to play with same-sex children throughout the school-aged years (3). Collecting things (2) and playing competitively (4) *are* also characteristics of the school-aged child. **AS, APP, 5, HPM, Health promotion and maintenance**

4. (4) Teachers are a vital source of support for the school-aged child. They are with the child for prolonged periods of time and can detect subtle changes in the child's behavior and performance before problems occur. It is therefore wise for parents to confer with the teacher before problems reach crisis proportions. Parents should guide the child with homework but not "help" or do the homework for the child (1); intervention deters the child's sense of industry. The child, *not* the parent, is responsible for the child's successes and failures (2). The reason for poor academic performance should be determined and corrected instead of punishing the child for the performance (3). Punishment rarely improves academic performance. **PL, APP, 5, HPM, Health promotion and maintenance**

5. (1) School-aged children lose all 20 primary ("baby") teeth—usually between 6 and 12 yr. The teeth are replaced with adult teeth, also known as permanent or secondary teeth. A school-aged child will *not* lose only 8 (2), 12 (3), or 16 (4) teeth. **IMP, COM, 5, HPM, Health promotion and maintenance**

6. (4) The normal child can expect to have a total of 32 adult or permanent (secondary) teeth. The normal child should *not* have *less* than 32 teeth; thus, 20 (1), 24 (2), or 28 (3) teeth is well *below* the norm. **IMP, COM, 5, HPM, Health promotion and maintenance**

7. (3) School-aged children are avid collectors, and this kind of behavior is perfectly normal. The comics must be kept reasonably neat so as not to interfere with any treatments or procedures the child may need. It is not necessary to limit the child to keep just a few comics (1) because thin books do not take up an inordinate amount of room. Neither the parents nor the nurse should remove the child's comics while he is sleeping (2) because, this will cause the child to become suspicious and distrustful of them. It would be unreasonable to expect the child to share a personal collection with the other children (4), just as a hospitalized adult is not asked to share personal belongings with other patients. **IMP, APP, 5, PsI, Psychosocial integrity**

8. (2) In the school-aged group, as in all other pediatric age groups, the most common cause of serious accidental injury and death is motor vehicle accidents, either as a pedestrian or as a passenger. Pedestrian deaths are two-and-a-half times more common than are passenger deaths. The school nurse should thoughtfully discuss how to prevent motor vehicle accidents and encourage older school-aged children to model appropriate behavior for younger children. Although accidents caused by bikes (1), roller blades (3) and all-terrain vehicles (4) do account for a large number of trips to an MD or to a hospital emergency department every year, they are not the *most* common cause of serious accidental injury or death in school-aged children. **AN, APP, 5, HPM, Health promotion and maintenance**

Key to Codes

Nursing process: AS, assessment; **AN,** analysis; **PL,** planning; **IMP,** implementation; **EV,** evaluation. (See **Appendix L** for explanation of nursing process steps.)

Cognitive level: RE/KN, recall/knowledge; **COM,** comprehension; **APP,** application; **ANL,** analysis; **EVL,** evaluation; **SYN,** synthesis. (See **Appendix L** for explanation.)

Category of human function: 1, protective; 2, sensory-perceptual; 3, comfort, rest, activity, and mobility; 4, nutrition; 5, growth and development; 6, fluid-gas transport; 7, psychosocial-cultural; 8, elimination. (See **Appendix N** for explanation.)

Client need: SECE, safe, effective care environment; **HPM,** health promotion and maintenance; **PsI,** psychosocial integrity; **PhI,** physiological integrity. (See **Appendix O** for explanation.)

Client subneed: See **Appendix O** for explanation.

Growth and Development of the Adolescent

Chapter Outline

- Key Words
- Summary of Key Points
- Adolescent (12–18 yrs)
  - Erikson's Theory of Personality Development
  - Physical Growth
  - Developmental Norms
  - Nursing Interventions/Parental Guidance
    Play

  - Toys/Activities
  - Safety
  - Immunizations
  - Hospitalization of Adolescents
- Study and Memory Aids
- Questions
- Answers/Rationale

Key Words

menarche   the first menstrual period a girl experiences.

menstruation   the monthly flow of blood and discharge from the uterus through the vagina that a girl/woman experiences at periodic intervals from puberty to menopause.

nocturnal emission   the involuntary discharge of semen that occurs during sleep in a boy/man.

puberty   the period of life during which an adolescent becomes functionally capable of reproduction; accompanied by the development of secondary sexual characteristics.

sebaceous glands   oil-secreting glands of the skin.

Summary of Key Points

1. Adolescence extends from age 12–18 yr.

2. According to Erikson, the central task for the adolescent is *identity vs. role diffusion*.

3. Adolescents develop a sense of identity in two ways: through *identification* with a *peer group* and through *hostility* toward *parents*, *adults*, and *family*.

4. Adolescence is marked by an *enormous* growth spurt that begins at age 10 in girls and at age 12 in boys.

5. *Thirty-two* permanent teeth should be present by age 18–21 yr.

6. In girls, changes in the *nipple* and *areola* accompanied by the development of *breast buds* are the first sexual changes noted.

7. The average age for the onset of menstruation is 12.8 yr.

8. In boys, the first sexual change noted is an enlargement of the *genitalia*.

9. Accidents are the leading cause of death in adolescence; *motor vehicle accidents* are the most common fatal accidents during adolescence.

10. Routine immunizations should continue as recommended for adolescents.

11. When caring for an adolescent in the hospital, the nurse should *promote a sense of identity* by allowing the teen to wear own clothes, use own grooming aids, and have maximum contact with *peers*.

12. To decrease rebellious behavior by hospitalized adolescents, the nurse should identify *clear rules for behavior*, e.g., "No sex, no drinking, no drugs."

Adolescent (12–18 yrs)

Erikson's Theory of Personality Development

I. *Central task: identity vs. role diffusion*; central person(s): peer group.

II. *Behavioral indicators*
   A. Changes in body image related to sexual development.
   B. Awkward and uncoordinated.
   C. Much interest in opposite sex: girls become romantic.
   D. Wants to be exactly like peers.
   E. Becomes hostile toward parents, adults, family.
   F. Concerned with vocation, life after high school.

III. **Parental guidance, teaching**
   A. Offer firm but realistic limits on behavior.
   B. Continue to offer guidance, support.
   C. Allow child to earn own money, control own finances.
   D. Assist adolescent to develop positive self-image.

IV. Additional information about behavioral concerns for each age group may be found in **Chapter 2, Tables 2.1, p. 13** and **Table 2.2, p. 14**.

Physical Growth

I. *Height and weight*
   A. Adolescent growth spurt lasts 24–36 mo.
   B. Growth in height commonly *ceases* at age 16–17 in girls, age 18–20 in boys.
   C. Boys gain *more weight* than girls, are generally *taller* and *heavier*.

II. *Vital signs* approximately those of the adult. See **Chapter 1, Table 1.5, p. 7**.

III. *Teeth*: 32 permanent teeth by 18–21 yr.

IV. *Sexual changes*
   A. *Girls*
      1. Changes in nipple and areola; development of breast buds.
      2. Growth of pubic hair.
      3. Change in vaginal secretions.
      4. Menstruation—12.8 yr (average).
      5. Growth of axillary hair.
      6. Ovulation.
   B. *Boys*
      1. Enlargement of genitalia.
      2. Growth of pubic, axillary, facial, and body hair.
      3. Lowering of voice.
      4. Production of sperm; nocturnal emission ("wetdreams").

Developmental Norms

I. **Motor development**
   A. *Early (12–15 yr)*—awkward, uncoordinated, poor posture; decrease in energy and stamina.
   B. *Later (15–18 yr)*—increased coordination, better posture; more energy and stamina.

II. **Cognitive**
   A. Academic ability and interest vary greatly.
   B. "Think about thinking"—period of introspection.

III. **Emotional**
   A. Same-sex best friend, leading to strong friendship bonds.
   B. Highly romantic period for boys and girls.
   C. May be moody, unpredictable, inconsistent.

IV. **Social**
   A. Periods of highs and lows, sociability and loneliness.
   B. Turmoil with parents—related to changing roles, desire for increased independence.
   C. Peer group is important socializing agent— *conformity* increases sense of belonging.
   D. Friendships: same-sex best friend, advances to heterosexual "relationships."

▶◀ Nursing Interventions/Parental Guidance

I. **Play:** adolescent years–cooperative

II. **Toys/Activities:**
   A. School-related group activities and sports.
   B. Develops talents, skills, and abilities.
   C. Television—watches soap operas, romantic movies, sports.
   D. Develops interest in art, writing, poetry, musical instrument.
   E. *Girls*: increased interest in makeup and clothes.
   F. *Boys*: increased interest in mechanical and electrical devices.

III. **Safety**—motor vehicles (cars and motorcycles)—as *passenger* or as *driver*
   A. Encourage driver education; serve as positive role model.
   B. Teach rules of safety for water sports.
   C. Wants to earn money but still needs guidance: advocate safe job, reasonable hours.

IV. **Immunizations**
   A. Recommended schedule for active immunization of normal infants and children: see **Chapter 2, Table 2.3 A-B, p. 15-16**.
   B. Side effects of immunizations and nursing care: see **Chapter 2, Table 2.4, p. 17**.

Hospitalization of Adolescents

Refer to **Chapter 2, Table 2.5, p. 18** for information on ▶◀ the nursing care of hospitalized adolescents as it relates to key developmental differences.

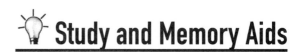

Study and Memory Aids

Personality Development

Major task for adolescent: *identity vs. role diffusion*.
Adolescents develop a sense of identity in two ways:
   They identify with a peer group.
   They become overtly hostile toward others.

Physical Growth

Adolescence is marked by a tremendous growth spurt.
All *32* adult teeth should be present by age *18–21*.

Sexual Changes

The first sexual changes noticed in girls are changes in the
   nipple and areola and the development of breast buds.
Menstruation begins, on average, at 12.8 yr.
The first sexual change noted in boys is enlargement of
   the genitalia.

Safety

Leading cause of death in adolescent years: *accidents*.
Most common accident: *motor vehicle* accidents.

Questions

1. The nurse should counsel the parents of an adolescent that the best way for them to assist their child to complete the core developmental task of the teenage years is to:
   1. Set limits and offer simple, concrete choices.
   2. Allow the adolescent to set his or her own limits.
   3. Allow participation in the decision-making process.
   4. Base limits on what the teenager's peers are allowed to do.

2. The parents of an adolescent tell the nurse, "Everything we say seems to upset our teenager." The nurse best assists the parents in understanding their adolescent's response by saying:
   1. "Perhaps a few counseling sessions would benefit you as a family."
   2. "These outbursts are hormonal in nature."
   3. "Your teenager needs to show more respect in responding to you."
   4. "Adolescence can be a difficult time for everyone. What upsets you the most about these interactions with your teenager?"

3. Which best demonstrates to the nurse that an adolescent is achieving the goal of identity vs. role diffusion?
   1. The adolescent selects a college to attend and a field to major in.
   2. The adolescent drops out of high school and gets a job.
   3. The adolescent becomes involved in a "first romance."
   4. The adolescent begins to save part of a paycheck from a part-time job.

4. When interviewing an adolescent who is ill, the nurse should ask the parents to:
   1. Wait outside the office.
   2. Remain in the office but not to participate in the interview.
   3. Remain in the office and actively participate in the interview.
   4. Answer most questions for the adolescent since the teen is ill.

5. A teenager newly diagnosed with asthma is hospitalized for further evaluation and stabilization. The teen seems to be having a hard time with the peak flow meter and medications. The nurse should be aware that the most important factor that influences compliance with the treatment regimen after discharge is:
   1. The teen's knowledge about asthma.
   2. Parental control over treatment regimen.
   3. The reaction of the teen's peer group.
   4. The extent and quality of the nurse's discharge teaching.

6. A 15-year-old boy expresses concern to the nurse about his height, saying that all his friends are growing much taller than he is and he is worried that he will always be very short. The nurse would be most correct in telling this adolescent:
   1. "The growth spurt in boys is completed at age 14."
   2. "Don't worry, you're far too young yet to be concerned."
   3. "A growth spurt normally occurs during adolescence, but it happens at different times for different people."
   4. "Boys generally grow taller than girls, so even if you're not as tall as the other boys, you'll still be just fine."

7. While reviewing the immunization history of an adolescent, the school nurse notes that the teen has received only one immunization for measles-mumps-rubella (MMR). Which action by the school nurse is most appropriate?
   1. Say nothing because this is normal.
   2. Recommend the teen be immunized against rubella only.
   3. Recommend the teen be immunized against measles only.
   4. Recommend the teen be given a second MMR.

8. An adolescent with acne asks the nurse what she can do to improve her skin. The best advice the nurse can offer her is:
   1. Wash her face three times a day with an antibacterial soap and then use an abrasive cleanser pad.
   2. Avoid wearing makeup or use only oil-free makeup.
   3. Gently squeeze any pimples to manually express the infected material.
   4. Get adequate rest with moderate exercise, eat a well-balanced diet, and try to avoid stress.

Answers/Rationale

1. (3) According to Erikson, adolescents are engaged in establishing identity and becoming their "own person," which sets the stage for conflict over independence and control. Parents need to reduce control gradually by allowing increasing participation in the decision-making process. Setting limits and offering simple, concrete choices (1) is appropriate for parents with children in younger age groups. Adolescents lack the judgment and experience to set their own limits (2); they still require guidance and support from parents. Parents must base limits on what behaviors are and are not acceptable to them, *not* on what their adolescent's peers are allowed to do (4). PL, APP, 5, HPM, **Health promotion and maintenance**

2. **(4)** Acknowledging that adolescence is a difficult time for all concerned establishes the nurse as an empathetic, supportive figure. Assisting the parents in identifying their feelings about their teenager's response is the first step in opening up parent-adolescent communication. Counseling **(1)** might prove to be of benefit, but further assessment of the depth and scope of the communication problem should be undertaken by the nurse *before* this is suggested. The adolescent is undergoing hormonal changes **(2)**, but the changes do *not* explain the basic difficulty between parent and teenager. Developmental issues are the primary reason for conflict. Suggesting that the adolescent is being disrespectful **(3)** indicates a lack of understanding as to why the teenager is having parental communication difficulties. **IMP, APP, 5, PsI, Psychosocial integrity**

3. **(1)** By selecting a career and operationalizing a plan to attain the goal through education, the adolescent moves from a present orientation to a future orientation—a major step in establishing an independent identity as an individual. Dropping out of school, **(2)** an unfortunate, frequent occurrence among adolescents, does not assist the adolescent in establishing a positive identity. A first relationship with a member of the opposite sex **(3)** demonstrates social growth; starting to save money **(4)** also shows maturation; however, neither demonstrate achievement of identity as well as planning for the future. **EV, ANL, 5, PsI, Psychosocial integrity**

4. **(1)** The nurse should interview an adolescent without parents present to ensure confidentiality and protect privacy. It is inappropriate for the nurse to interview the adolescent with the parents in the room **(2, 3, and 4)** because this does not show respect for the teen's privacy. **IMP, APP, 7, PsI, Psychosocial integrity**

5. **(3)** The peer group is the most important factor affecting the compliance of adolescents; peers are the normative group against which teens gauge their own behavior. Although the teen's knowledge about the disease **(1)** and the nurse's discharge teaching **(4)** are important, these factors are *not as important* as the teen's own peer group. The parents **(2)** should not try to control the treatment. The teen needs to have more independence and control over the treatment, although parental support is very important. **AN, ANL, 7, PsI, Psychosocial integrity**

6. **(3)** Although accelerated growth occur in all adolescents, the age of onset, duration, and extent vary greatly among individuals. This response

acknowledges the child's concern about his friends' growth and also offers factual information that may help the child to realize his own growth is still normal but may occur somewhat differently than that of his friends. The growth spurt *peaks* at about 14 yr in boys, but is far from complete **(1)** at that time. It is *not* appropriate to tell an adolescent "not to worry" **(2)**; this effectively cuts off any further communication with the teen. Nor is it appropriate to tell the child that even if he's not as tall as the other boys, he'll "be just fine" **(4)**; this is exactly the concern the adolescent is expressing, and he is saying it is *not* fine. **IMP, COM, 5, HPM, Health promotion and maintenance**

7. **(4)** All adolescents, with the exception of pregnant teens, should receive a second MMR unless they have already received two MMR vaccinations during childhood (after 12 mo). It is *not* appropriate to not say anything **(1)** because having only one MMR immunization does not meet the guidelines for immunizing children. The adolescent should not receive only rubella **(2)** or only measles **(3)** immunizations because a second complete MMR immunization is recommended. **IMP, APP, 1, HPM, Health promotion and maintenance**

8. **(4)** An improvement in the teen's overall health status is considered an important part of treatment. Antibacterial soaps **(1)** are considered ineffective and may be too drying for the skin; gentle cleansing with a mild cleanser once or twice a day is adequate. Abrasive pads are harsh and may aggravate acne and damage the skin. Contrary to popular belief, cosmetics do not cause acne **(2)**, and it does not matter whether the makeup is oil-free; however, makeup should always be removed at night. Squeezing pimples **(3)** causes damage to the skin and worsens acne. **IMP, APP, 1, HPM, Health promotion and maintenance**

Key to Codes

Nursing process: AS, assessment; **AN,** analysis; **PL,** planning; **IMP,** implementation; **EV,** evaluation. (See **Appendix L** for explanation of nursing process steps.)

Cognitive level: RE/KN, recall/knowledge; **COM,** comprehension; **APP,** application; **ANL,** analysis; **EVL,** evaluation; **SYN,** synthesis. (See **Appendix L** for explanation.)

Category of human function: 1, protective; 2, sensory-perceptual; 3, comfort, rest, activity, and mobility; 4, nutrition; 5, growth and development; 6, fluid-gas transport; 7, psychosocial-cultural; 8, elimination. (See **Appendix N** for explanation.)

Client need: SECE, safe, effective care environment; **HPM,** health promotion and maintenance; **PsI,** psychosocial integrity; **PhI,** physiological integrity. (See **Appendix O** for explanation.)

Client subneed: See **Appendix O** for explanation.

Respiratory Disorders

Chapter Outline

- Key Words
- Summary of Key Points
- Selected Respiratory Disorders
  - Cystic Fibrosis
  - Pediatric Respiratory Infections
  - Asthma
  - Disorders of Unknown Etiology:

    - Apnea of Infancy
    - SIDS
- CPR, Foreign Body Airway Obstruction
- Commonly Prescribed Medications
- Study and Memory Aids
- Questions
- Answers/Rationale

Key Words

aphonic   unable to produce speech sounds from the larynx.

dyspnea   difficulty breathing.

meconium ileus   failure of a newborn to pass meconium stool within the first twenty-four hours of life.

mucolytic   a medication that thins the mucus.

paroxysmal cough   cough that occurs suddenly, periodically, and recurrently.

postural drainage   drainage of mucus and secretions from the lungs by use of gravity to enhance the flow of mucus and secretions up so they can be expectorated by the client.

prophylactic   any medication or treatment that contributes to the prevention of illness.

steatorrhea   bulky, foul-smelling, frothy, fatty stools that are commonly found in certain malabsorption conditions such as cystic fibrosis and celiac disease.

tachycardia   abnormally rapid heart rate.

tachypnea   abnormally rapid respiratory rate.

🔑 Summary of Key Points

1. *Cystic fibrosis*, a generalized dysfunction of the exocrine glands, produces multisystem involvement; however, the child's ultimate prognosis depends on the *degree of pulmonary* involvement.

2. *Cystic fibrosis* is inherited as an *autosomal recessive* disorder.

3. Common signs and symptoms of *cystic fibrosis* include: meconium ileus, recurrent pulmonary infections, malabsorption syndrome, steatorrhea, and sweat that is excessively high in sodium and chloride.

4. The most commonly used diagnostic test for cystic fibrosis is the *sweat test*.

5. The most common respiratory tract infections are the "*croup syndromes*": croup, laryngotracheobronchitis, and epiglottitis.

6. Of all respiratory tract infections, the most acute and life-threatening is *epiglottitis*.

7. *Asthma* is a chronic lower airway disorder characterized by heightened airway reactivity with bronchospasm and obstruction.

8. Common signs and symptoms of *asthma* include: expiratory wheeze, coughing (especially at night), and dyspnea/respiratory distress.

9. Infants with *apnea* should be on an apnea monitor at home; the family should be taught how to use the monitor and effective interventions should apnea occur.

10. A leading cause of death in infants 1–12 mo is *sudden infant death syndrome* (SIDS).

11. Infants should be positioned supine, *never* prone, to prevent SIDS.

12. Nursing care for the family of an infant who died from SIDS includes providing factual information regarding SIDS in both oral and written form, and referring the family to a local perinatal bereavement group to cope with the infant's death.

13. *Home care* for all children with respiratory disorders: **NEVER** allow rapid/labored breathing for more than 1 hour before seeking medical attention.

Selected Respiratory Disorders

Cystic Fibrosis

I. *Introduction*: Cystic fibrosis is a generalized dysfunction of the exocrine glands that produces *multisystem* involvement. Although the disorder is inherited as an *autosomal recessive* defect, the basic biochemical defect is unknown. However, its probable cause is an alteration in a protein or an enzyme, e.g., *pancreatic enzyme deficiency*. The basic problem is one of *thick, sticky, tenacious mucous secretions that obstruct the ducts* of the exocrine glands, which affect their ability to function. Cystic fibrosis is found in all races and socioeconomic groups, although there is a significantly *lower* incidence in *African Americans* and *Asians*. It is a chronic disease with no known cure and *guarded* prognosis; median age at death is 31 yr.

II. **Assessment:**
   A. Newborn: *meconium ileus* (see **Chapter 9, p. 72**).
   B. Frequent, recurrent *pulmonary infections*: bronchitis, bronchopneumonia, pneumonia, and ultimately chronic obstructive pulmonary disease (COPD) caused by mechanical obstruction of respiratory tract as a result of thick, tenacious mucous gland secretions.
   C. *Malabsorption syndrome*: failure to gain weight, distended abdomen, thin arms and legs, lack of subcutaneous fat due to disturbed absorption of nutrients that results from the inability of pancreatic enzymes to reach intestinal tract.
   D. *Steatorrhea*: bulky, foul-smelling, frothy, fatty stools in increased amounts and frequency (predisposed to rectal prolapse).
   E. Parents may note that child "*tastes salty*" when kissed, caused by excessive loss of sodium and chloride in sweat.
   F. *Sweat* test reveals *high* sodium and chloride levels in child's sweat, unique to children with cystic fibrosis.
   G. Sexual development
      1. *Boys*: sterile (due to aspermia).
      2. *Girls*: difficulty conceiving and bearing children (from increased viscosity of cervical mucus, which acts as a plug and mechanically blocks the entry of sperm).

III. **Analysis/nursing diagnosis:**
   A. *Ineffective breathing patterns* related to thick, viscid secretions.
   B. *Altered nutrition, less than body requirements*, related to diarrhea and poor intestinal absorption of nutrients.
   C. *Infection* related to thick viscid secretions.
   D. *Knowledge deficit*, related to disease process, treatments, medications, genetics.
   E. *Noncompliance* (risk for), related to complicated and prolonged treatment regimen.

IV. **Nursing care plan/implementation:**
   A. Goal: *assist child to expectorate sputum.*
      1. Perform *postural drainage* as prescribed: first thing in morning, between meals, before bedtime (**see Table 7.1, p. 41**).
      2. Administer nebulizer treatments, *expectorants, mucolytics, bronchodilators*.
      3. Provide exercises that promote *position changes* and keep sputum moving up and out.
      4. Encourage *high fluid* intake to keep secretions liquefied.
      5. Suction, administer oxygen prn.
   B. Goal: *maintain adequate nutrition.*
      1. *Diet*: well-balanced, *high* calorie, *high* protein to prevent malnutrition.
      2. Administer *pancreatic enzyme* (*Pancrease, Cotazym, Ultrase*) immediately before *every* meal and *every* snack to enhance the absorption of vital nutrients, especially fats.
         a. If child is unable to swallow tablets, mix pancreatic enzyme powder with cold applesauce.
      3. Administer water-miscible preparations of fat-soluble vitamins (*A, D, E, K*), multivitamins, and *iron*.
      4. Encourage *extra salt* intake to compensate for excessive sodium losses in sweat.
      5. Encourage *extra fluid* intake (e.g., Gatorade) to prevent dehydration/electrolyte imbalance.
      6. Daily I&O and weights to monitor nutritional and hydration status.
      7. Encourage child to assume gradually increasing responsibility for choosing own foods within dietary restrictions.
   C. Goal: *prevent infection.*
      1. Standard precautions to prevent infection.
      2. Evaluate carefully, check continually for potential infection (especially respiratory); report to MD promptly
      3. Limit contact with staff or visitors with infection.
      4. Administer *antibiotics* as ordered, to treat respiratory infections and prevent overwhelming sepsis.
         a. May be placed on prophylactic antibiotic therapy between episodes of infection.
      5. Teach importance of prevention of infection at home: adequate nutrition, frequent medical check-ups, stay away from known sources of infection.
   D. Goal: **health teaching.** *Teach child and family about cystic fibrosis.*
      1. Discuss *diagnostic procedures*: sweat test, stool specimens.
      2. Review multiple medications: use, effects, side/toxic effects.

TABLE 7.1 ☞ GUIDELINES FOR THE USE OF POSTURAL DRAINAGE AND CHEST PHYSIOTHERAPY IN CHILDREN

1. Postural drainage is done to help a child clear the air passages of excess mucus caused by a variety of disease conditions, e.g., cystic fibrosis.
2. A variety of positions can be used to facilitate drainage of mucus from the lungs; however, not all positions should be used for every session. Most children tolerate 4–6 different positions per session. The nurse should monitor the child's tolerance for a session by checking: quality and rate of respirations, color, and *pulse oximetry*.
3. Postural drainage should be done 3–4 times daily. The length of treatment is usually 20–30 min, depending on the child's condition and tolerance level.
4. Postural drainage should be done *before* meals (or 60–90 min pc) and repeated at *bedtime*. It should *not* be done immediately pc because of the risk of vomiting and aspiration.
5. The nurse should provide the child with tissues and a waste receptacle for the mucus expectorated during the treatment.
6. Following the treatment, the nurse should provide oral hygiene for the child to remove the taste of foul secretions from the mouth. The child should then be left undisturbed for a period of rest.
7. If possible, bronchodilator and/or nebulizer treatments should be done shortly *before* postural drainage is performed to open up air passages and allow mucus to be expectorated more easily.
8. Chest physiotherapy can be done in conjunction with postural drainage to facilitate expectoration of mucus; it is used primarily for clients with increased mucus production. Chest physiotherapy can include any combination or all of the following:
   a. *Percussion*: the practitioner gently but firmly strikes the chest wall with a cupped hand.
   b. *Vibration*: handheld vibrators of various sizes can be applied to the chest wall.
   c. *Squeezing*: the child first takes a deep breath, then exhales rapidly and completely while the practitioner applies brief, firm pressure and uses hands to compress the client's chest.
   d. *Deep breathing*: may also use an *incentive spirometer* or incorporate with play for younger child, i.e., blowing bubbles, pinwheel.
   e. *Cough*: 1–2 hard coughs after a deep breath are most effective; chest may need to be splinted if painful.
9. *Contraindications* for postural drainage/chest physiotherapy:
   a. Pulmonary hemorrhage.
   b. Pulmonary embolism.
   c. End-stage renal disease.
   d. Increased intracranial pressure.
   e. Osteogenesis imperfecta ("brittle bones").
   f. Minimal cardiac reserves.

Source: Adapted from Wong DL. *Wong's Nursing Care of Infants and Children* (7th ed). St. Louis: Mosby.

---

3. Stress need to care for pulmonary systems (major cause of mortality/morbidity).
☞ 4. Teach various treatments: postural drainage, nebulizers, oxygen therapy, breathing exercise.
5. Encourage child to assume as much responsibility for own care as possible: medications, treatments, diet.
6. Promote development of healthy attitude toward disease/prognosis (no known cure).
7. Refer to appropriate community agencies for assistance with home care.
8. Assist with genetic counseling.
9. Discuss sexual concerns with adolescent.
⊂▭10. Keep influenza immunization current.
11. Prepare for possible lung transplant in adolescent years.

E. Goal: *promote compliance with treatment regiment*.
   1. Encourage child to verbalize anger or frustration at being "different"/body image alterations.
   2. Suggest alternatives to postural drainage, e.g., yoga, standing on head.
   3. Offer "rewards" for compliance: going swimming with friends or other types of peer activities.

▶ V. **Evaluation/outcome criteria:**
   A. Child can clear own airway, expectorate sputum.
   B. Adequate nutrition is maintained.
   C. Child is maintained in infection-free state.
   D. Child and family verbalize understanding of the disease.
   E. Child complies with rigors of treatment.

TABLE 7.2 PEDIATRIC RESPIRATORY INFECTIONS

Name	Definition	Age Group	Etiology	Definitive Clinical Signs and Symptoms	Specifics of Treatment	Prognosis
Bronchiolitis (RSV)	Acute viral infection of lower respiratory tract (small, low bronchioles), with resultant trapping of air.	Infants 2–12 mo (peak; 2–5 mo).	Respiratory syncytial virus (80% of cases).	Hyperinflation of alveoli. Scattered areas of atelectasis. Acute, severe respiratory distress for first 48–72 hours. Followed by rapid recovery.	Supportive care during acute phase: ■ Hospitalization for children with complicating conditions (e.g. heart or lung disease). ■ Humidity. ■ Clear liquids. *Ribavirin x 3 days.* *Respi Gam (prophylactically) in high-risk infants.*	Excellent (less than 1% mortality).
Croup (acute spasmodic laryngitis)	Paroxysmal attacks (spasms of larynx).	3 mo–3 yr.	Viral (with allergic component).	Most common onset at *night.* Inspiratory stridor. "Croupy" barking cough. Dyspnea. Anxiety.	Humidity. Common to treat at home.	Excellent (but likely to recur). Symptoms disappear during the day.
Epiglottitis	Extremely acute, severe, and rapid, progressive swelling (from infection) of epiglottis and surrounding tissue.	1–8 yr.	Bacterial (*H. influenzae* type b).	Abrupt onset—rapid progression. Dyspnea, dysphagia. Sit up/chin thrust/mouth open. Thick muffled voice. Cherry red, swollen epiglottis. Children look worse than they sound (e.g. toxic appearance).	☞ ***Do not*** visualize epiglottis unless airway support is immediately available. Will need endotracheal tube or tracheostomy for 24–48 h to maintain patent airway. IV *ampicillin* for 10–14 d to treat bacterial infection. IV *corticosteroids* (e.g., Solucortef) to reduce inflammation.	Very good, if detected and treated early. Preventable via *Hib* vaccine.
Laryngotracheo-bronchitis (LTB)	Acute infection of lower respiratory tract: larynx, trachea and bronchi.	3 mo–8 yr.	Viral (possible secondary bacterial infection).	Inspiratory stridor. *High* fever. Signs and symptoms of severe respiratory distress. Hoarseness, progressing to aphonia and respiratory arrest without treatment. Children sound worse than they look (e.g. nontoxic appearance).	Hospitalization: ■ Tracheostomy set at bedside. ■ Racemic epinephrine/*steroids.* *Antibiotics* if cultures are positive. ■ Humidity.	Good.

Adapted from: *Wong's Nursing Care of Infants and Children* (7th ed.) St. Louis, Mosby.

TABLE 7.3 ADVANTAGES AND DISADVANTAGES OF VARIOUS OXYGEN DELIVERY SYSTEMS

System	Advantages	Disadvantages
Cannula	Provides *low*-moderate oxygen concentration (22–40%) Child can eat/talk without altering F_1O_2 Possibility of more complete observation of child because nose and mouth remain unobstructed Relatively comfortable and inexpensive	Difficulty in controlling O_2 concentration if child breathes through mouth Must have patent nasal passages Possibility of causing abdominal distension/discomfort/vomiting Can cause drying/bleeding of nasal mucosa
Hood	Achievement of *high* O_2 concentration (F_1O_2 up to 1.00) Quick recovery time of F_1O_2 Free access to infant's chest for assessment	Moist environment may lead to skin irritation and prevent quick assessment of color or respiratory effort Need to remove infant for feeding and weighing
Mask	Various sizes available Delivers higher, more precise F_1O_2 concentration than cannula Comfortable for older children who are quiet and do not struggle	Accumulation of moisture on face leading to skin irritation Possibility of aspiration of vomitus Eating disrupts O_2 delivery Not well tolerated by most children due to fear of suffocation
Tent	Achievement of lower O_2 concentrations (F_1O_2 of 0.3–0.5) Child receives *increased* inspired O_2 concentrations even while eating Child can move around in bed and play while receiving O_2 and humidity	Necessity for tight fit around bed to prevent leakage of O_2 and maintain specific O_2 concentrations Child is difficult to see/assess Cool/wet tent environment will *decrease* body temperature, thus increasing O_2 requirements Inspired O_2 levels will fall whenever tent is entered for caregiving purposes

Pediatric Respiratory Infections

I. **Assessment:** general assessment of infant/child with respiratory distress. *Note:* Additional information about specific respiratory infections may be found in **Table 7.2, p. 42.**

   A. Restlessness—*earliest* sign of hypoxia.
   B. Difficulty sucking/eating—parents may state the infant or child has "poor appetite."
   C. Expiratory grunt, flaring of nasal alae, retractions.
   D. Changes in *vital signs*: fever, tachycardia, tachypnea.
   E. Cough: productive/nonproductive.
   F. Wheeze: expiratory/inspiratory.
   G. Hoarseness or aphonic crying.
   H. Dyspnea or prostration.
   I. Dehydration—related to increase in sensible fluid loss and poor PO intake.
   J. Color change (pallor, cyanosis)—*later* sign of respiratory distress.

II. **Analysis/nursing diagnosis:**

   A. *Ineffective airway clearance* related to infection and/or obstruction.
   B. *Fluid volume deficit* related to excessive losses through normal routes, discomfort and inability to swallow.
   C. *Anxiety* related to hypoxia.
   D. *Risk for injury* related to spread of infection.
   E. *Knowledge deficit* related to disease process, infection control, home care, follow-up.

III. **Nursing care plan/implementation:**

   A. Goal: *relieve respiratory distress by reducing swelling and edema and liquefying secretions.*
      1. Environment: cool, *high*-humidity.
      2. Administer oxygen as ordered. **Table 7.3**
      3. *Position:* semi-Fowler's position or in infant seat to provide maximum expansion of the lungs; small blanket or diaper roll under neck to keep airway patent; *change* position at least *q2h* to prevent pooling of secretions.
      4. Suction/postural drainage prn.
      5. Pin diapers loosely and use only loose-fitting clothing to *avoid* pressure on abdominal organs, which could impinge on diaphragm and impede respirations.
      6. Administer medications: *antibiotics, bronchodilators, steroids.*
      7. Monitor temperature q4h/prn; reduce fever via acetaminophen, cool sponges, hypothermia blanket.
   B. Goal: *maintain normal fluid balance.*
      1. May be NPO initially to prevent aspiration.
      2. IVs until severe distress subsides and child is able to suck and swallow.

3. Monitor hydration status: I&O, urine specific gravity, weight.

4. When resuming PO fluids—start with sips of *clear liquids*, advance slowly as tolerated: "Pedialyte," clear broth, Jello, popsicles, fruit juices, ginger ale, cola.

5. **Avoid** milk/milk products, which may cause increased mucus production.

C. Goal: *provide calm, secure environment.*

1. During acute distress: remain with child/family (do *not* leave unattended).

2. Keep crying to a minimum to prevent severe hypoxia and to reduce the body's demand for oxygen.

3. *Avoid* painful/intrusive procedures if possible.

4. Organize nursing care to provide planned periods of uninterrupted rest.

5. Allow parents to room-in; encourage their participation in care of their child to keep the child relatively calm and reduce anxiety.

6. Allow child to keep favorite toy or security object.

D. Goal: *observe for potential respiratory failure related to exhaustion or complete airway obstruction.*

1. Place in room near nurses' station for maximal observation.

2. Monitor *vital signs*: q1h during acute phase, then q4h.

3. Place emergency equipment near bedside prn: endotracheal tube, tracheostomy set.

4. Monitor closely for signs of impending *respiratory failure:* ↑ rapid, shallow respirations, progressive hoarseness/aphonia, deepening cyanosis.

5. Report adverse changes in condition stat to physician.

E. Goal: **health teaching**.

1. *Short term*: discuss equipment, treatments, procedures; offer frequent progress reports, answer parents' questions.

2. *Long term*: how to handle recurrences, how to check temperature at home, medications for fever, when to call physician about respiratory problem.

IV. **Evaluation/outcome criteria:**

A. No further evidence of respiratory distress.

B. Resumption of normal respiratory pattern.

C. Calm, secure environment is maintained and anxiety is reduced.

D. Injury is prevented.

E. Family verbalizes knowledge of disease process.

Asthma

I. *Introduction*: Asthma is generally considered a chronic, lower airway disorder characterized by heightened airway reactivity with bronchospasm and obstruction. The exact cause of asthma is unknown; however, it is believed to include an *allergic* reaction to one or more allergens and have psychogenic factors and perhaps other factors. The child usually exhibits other symptoms of allergy, such as infantile eczema or hayfever; in addition, 75% of children with asthma have a positive *family* history for asthma. The onset is usually before age 5 yr and remains with the child throughout life, although some children experience dramatic improvement in their asthma with the onset of puberty.

II. **Assessment:**

A. Expiratory wheeze.

B. General signs and symptoms of *respiratory distress*: anxiety, cough, shortness of breath, crackles, cyanosis from obstruction within the respiratory tract, use of accessory muscles of respirations.

C. Cough: hacking, paroxysmal, nonproductive; occurs especially at night.

D. *Position* of comfort for breathing: sitting straight up and leaning forward (orthopneic), which is the position for optimal lung expansion.

E. Peak expiratory flow rate (PEFR) is in the yellow zone (50-80% of personal best) or in the red zone (below 50% of personal best).

Peak expiratory flow rate (PEFR) is the greatest flow velocity that can be obtained by a forced expiration; it is measured by use of a peak flow meter.

Uses: Identify asthma attack.
Monitor asthma.
Make decisions about participation in sports.

"Personal Best" value is determined by measuring PEFR 2 times a day for 2-3 wk.

Zones:
Green = 80-100% of personal best; no signs, routine treatment.
Yellow = 50-80% of personal best; "caution", notify MD.
Red = less than 50% of personal best; **medical emergency**!

III. **Analysis/nursing diagnosis:**

A. *Ineffective airway clearance* related to bronchospasm.

B. *Anxiety* related to breathlessness.

C. *Knowledge deficit,* actual or potential, related to disease process, treatment, and prevention of future asthmatic attacks.

D. *Activity intolerance* related to dyspnea and bronchospasm.

IV. Nursing care plan/implementation:

A. Goal: *provide patent airway and effective breathing patterns*.

☞ 1. Initiate oxygen therapy, as ordered, to relieve hypoxia, with *high* humidity (to liquify secretions).

🔵 2. Medications to treat asthma are categorized in two general classes:

  a. *Long-term* control medications (AKA *preventor* medications) to achieve and maintain control of inflammation. Examples: corticosteroids, cromolyn sodium, nedocromil, long-acting B_2–agonists, methylxanthines, leukotriene modifiers.

  b. *Quick-relief* medications (AKA *rescue* medications) to treat acute symptoms and exacerbations. Examples: short-acting B_2–agonists, anticholinergics, systemic corticosteroids.

  Note: B_2–agonists can be used as both quick-relief and long-term medications.

🔵 3. Many medications used to treat asthma are given via *inhalation* with a nebulizer, *metered-dose inhaler* (MDI), turbuhaler.

🔵 4. *Concurrent use of corticosteroids* assists in reducing inflammation and decreasing symptoms.

B. Goal: *relieve anxiety*.

1. Provide relief from hypoxia (refer to Goal A), which is the chief source of anxiety.
2. Remain with child, offer support.
3. Encourage parents to remain with child.

🏠 C. Goal: **health teaching.** *Principles of prophylaxis*:

1. Review home medications, including cromolyn sodium.
2. Review breathing exercises.
3. Discuss precipitating factors and offer suggestions as to how to avoid. Keep annual influenza immunization current.
4. Introduce need for child to assume control over own care.
5. Discuss need for increased activity tolerance.

  a. Discuss benefits of exercise program (especially swimming) with child.

  b. Discuss asthma camp experience with child and family.

V. Evaluation/outcome criteria:

A. Adequate oxygenation provided, as evidenced by pink color of nailbeds and mucous membranes and ease in respiratory effort.

B. Anxiety is relieved.

C. Child verbalizes confidence in, and demonstrates mastery of, skills needed to care for own asthma.

D. Activity tolerance is increased.

Disorders of Unknown Etiology

I. Apnea of Infancy

A. *Introduction*: Apnea of infancy is the unexplained cessation of breathing for *20 sec or longer* in an apparently healthy, full-term infant (of more than 37 wk) gestation. Apnea is usually diagnosed by the *second* month of life and is generally thought to resolve during the *first 12-15 mo*. The exact cause is unknown. The association between apnea of infancy and sudden infant death syndrome (SIDS) is still controversial. However, infants experiencing significant apnea without a known cause are thought to be at *increased risk for SIDS* and must be treated accordingly.

B. **Assessment:**

1. Unexplained cessation of breathing (apnea) for 20 sec or longer.
2. Bradycardia.
3. Color change: cyanosis or pallor.
4. Limp, hypotonic.
5. *Diagnostic tests* include: cardiopneumogram, pneumocardiogram, and polysomnography.

C. **Analysis/nursing diagnosis:**

1. *Ineffective breathing patterns* related to apnea.
2. *Anxiety, fear* related to apnea and threat of infant's death.
3. *Knowledge deficit* regarding home care of infant on an apnea monitor and infant cardiopulmonary resuscitation (CPR).

D. **Nursing care plan/intervention:**

1. Goal: *maintain effective breathing pattern*.

  a. Apnea monitor on infant at all times, including at home.

  b. Possible use of *methyxanthines* (respiratory stimulant drugs such as theophylline or caffeine).

  c. Place in room near nurses' station for maximal observation with a nurse or parent present at all times.

  d. Suction, oxygen, and resuscitation equipment readily available if needed.

  e. Observe for apnea and/or bradycardia; note duration and associated symptoms—color change, change in muscle tone.

  f. If apnea occurs use gentle stimulation to start infant breathing again. If ineffective, begin CPR (**Table 7.4, p. 47** and **Figure 7.1, p. 48**)

  g. If suctioning is needed, do it gently and for the *shortest* time and *least* number of times possible to maintain patent airway. Note: repeated, vigorous suctioning is associated with periods of apnea.

  h. *Position*: supine, **NEVER** prone, to prevent SIDS.

🍎 i. Feedings: smaller and more frequent; *avoid* overfeeding, which can lead to reflux and apnea.

2. Goal: *reduce anxiety and fear.*
   a. Allow parents to "ventilate" feelings/concerns.
   b. Offer reassurance.

🏠 3. Goal: **health teaching.** *Care for their infant at home* (**Table 7.5, p. 49**).
   a. Thoroughly explain discharge plans to parents; encourage questions and discussion.
   b. Begin teaching use of apnea monitor and infant CPR techniques several days before discharge; allow parents to handle the monitor and become thoroughly familiar with its use.
   c. Provide parents with emergency response numbers and community health care nurse referral.
   d. Stress need for at least *1 yr of ongoing care* with constant use of monitor.
   e. Discuss need for support and refer to local self-help/support group.
   f. Encourage parents to take time for themselves if a reliable caregiver is available who is trained in use of monitor and infant CPR.

◀ E. **Evaluation/outcome criteria:**
   1. Effective breathing pattern is established.
   2. Anxiety and fear is controlled.
   3. Parents verbalize their concerns and express confidence in their ability to care for their infant at home.

II. **Sudden Infant Death Syndrome**
   A. *Introduction*: SIDS is the *sudden, unexpected* death of an apparently healthy infant under 1 yr which remains *unexplained* after a complete postmortem exam. Various theories have been suggested, none proven; research is ongoing. SIDS is the second leading cause of death in infants 1 mo–1 yr, and affects 2500 infants annually.

◀ B. **Assessment:**
   1. Sudden, unexplained death in otherwise "normal" infant; occurs *exclusively* during sleep.
   2. Note overall appearance of infant (differentiate from child abuse).

3. Obtain history from parents—note affect or how parents are dealing with grief.

◀ C. **Analysis/nursing diagnosis:**
   1. *Dysfunctional grieving* related to loss of infant.
   2. *Knowledge deficit* related to SIDS.
   3. *Interrupted family process* related to loss of infant.

◀ D. **Nursing care plan/implementation:**
   1. **Immediate goal**: *support grieving parents.*
      a. Stress that nothing could have been done to prevent the death.
      b. Allow parents to express grief emotions; provide privacy.
      c. Offer parents opportunity to see, hold infant.
      d. Explain purpose of autopsy (physician to obtain consent).
      e. Contact spiritual advisor: priest, rabbi, minister.
      f. Assist parents to plan what to tell siblings.
   2. Goal (**ongoing**): *provide factual information regarding SIDS.*
      a. Offer information that is known about SIDS in simple, direct terms (**Table 7.6, p. 49**).
      b. Answer questions honestly.
      c. Give parents printed literature on SIDS.
      d. Refer to local/national SIDS foundation group.
   3. Goal (**long-term**): *assist family to resolve grief.*
      a. Track progress of other siblings.
      b. Refer to local perinatal bereavement group.
      c. Consider subsequent pregnancy to be at risk for:
         (1) Attachment/bonding.
         (2) SIDS recurrence.

◀ E. **Evaluation/outcome criteria:**
   1. Parents are able to express their grief and receive adequate support.
   2. Parents raise questions about SIDS and can understand answers.
   3. Family's grief is resolved; in time, normal family dynamics resume.

TABLE 7.4 CPR: COMPARISON OF HCP VERSUS LR BLS ABCD MANEUVERS: (ADULTS, CHILDREN, AND INFANTS)[1]

Age:	Adults[2] HCP: Adolescent and older LR: > 8 yr	Children HCP: 1 yr to adolescent LR: 1–8 yr	Infants HCP: < 1 yr LR: < 1 yr
Maneuver: Check for response; activate EMS; position victim, begin **ABCD**			
AIRWAY	HCP: Head tilt/chin lift; suspected trauma: use jaw thrust LR: Head tilt/chin lift	HCP: Head tilt/chin lift; suspected trauma: use jaw thrust LR: Head tilt/chin lift	HCP: Head tilt/chin lift; suspected trauma: use jaw thrust LR: Head tilt/chin lift
BREATHING Initial	HCP: 2 b @1 s/b LR: As above	HCP: 2 effective b @1 s/b LR: As above	HCP: 2 effective b @1 s/b LR: As above
Rescue Breathing: without chest compressions	HCP: 10–12 b/m LR: N/A	HCP: 10–20 b/m LR: N/A	HCP: 10–20 b/m LR: N/A
Rescue Breaths for CPR: with advanced airway	HCP: 8–10 b/m LR: N/A	HCP: 8–10 b/m LR: N/A	HCP: 8–10 b/m LR: N/A
CIRCULATION Pulse check (< 10 s)	HCP: Carotid LR: N/A	HCP: Carotid LR: N/A	HCP: Brachial/femoral LR: N/A
Compression Landmarks	HCP: Lower half of sternum; between nipples LR: As above	HCP: Lower half of sternum; between nipples LR: As above	HCP: Lower half of sternum; just below nipple line LR: As above
Compression Method: • Push hard & fast • Allow complete recoil	HCP: Heel of one hand, other hand on top LR: As above	HCP: Heel of one hand or as for adults LR: As above	HCP: 2–3 fingers (**one HCP**); 2-thumb-encircling technique (**2 HCPs**) LR: 2–3 fingers
Compression Depth	HCP: 1½–2 in LR: As above	HCP: ¹/₃–¹/₂ the depth of the chest LR: As above	HCP: ¹/₃–¹/₂ the depth of the chest LR: As above
Compression Rate	HCP: 100/m LR: As above	HCP: 100/m LR: As above	HCP: 100/m LR: As above

Compression-Ventilation Ratio	HCP: 30:2 (**one HCP**)
	  30:2 (**2HCPs**)
	LR: 30:2
		HCP: 30:2 (**one HCP**)
		  15:2 (**2HCPs**)
		LR: 30:2
			HCP: 30:2 (**one HCP**)
			  15:2 (**2HCPs**)
			LR: 30:2

DEFIBRILLATION[3] AED	Use adult pads; DO NOT use pediatric pads	Use pediatric pads	No recommendation for infants < 1 yr

Key to Abbreviations:

ABCD: Airway, Breathing, Circulation, Defibrillation

Adolescent: Defined by the presence of secondary sexual characteristics

AED: Automated external defibrillator

b @ s/b: _breaths at_second/breath

b/m: breaths/minute

BLS: Basic life support

EMS: Emergency medical services

HCP: Health care provider

in: inch

LR: Lay rescuer

m: minute

N/A: not applicable or appropriate

[1]*For additional information regarding newborns, see ATI NurseNotes—Maternal–Newborn.*

[2]*For additional information regarding adults, see ATI NurseNotes—Medical–Surgical.*

[3]Cardiac arrest is not a single problem and the steps of cardiopulmonary resuscitation (CPR) may need to vary depending on the type or etiology of the cardiac arrest. *While the basic steps in CPR for both one and two rescuer (lay and health care provider) remain unchanged, significant changes have been made in the maneuvers. For sudden collapse (in or out of the hospital), the use of AED as soon as available/possible is recommended.*

Adapted from *Circulation*, Volume 112, Issue 21 Supplement: December 13, 2005.

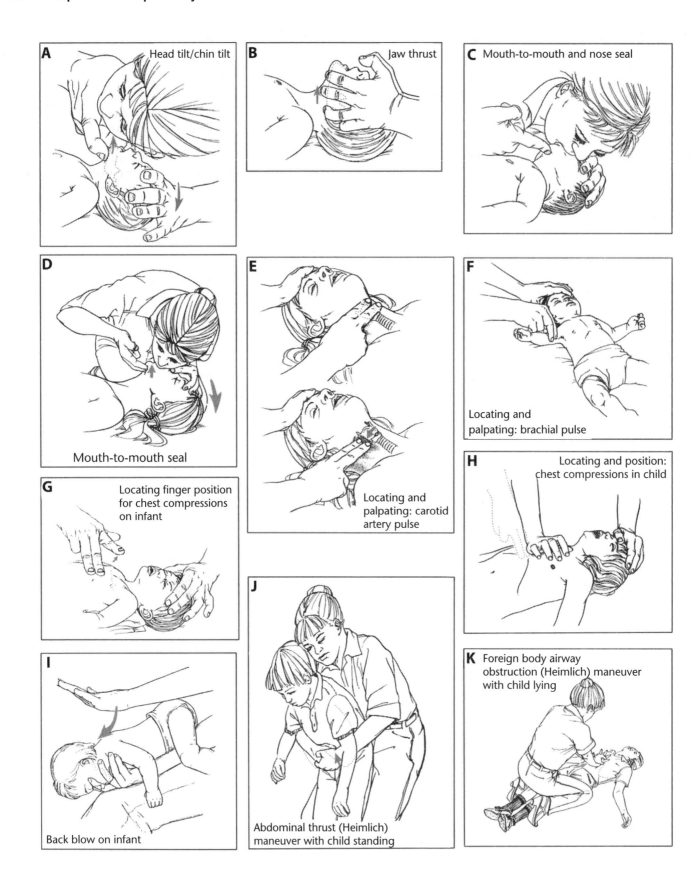

FIGURE 7.1 PROCEDURES FOR CARDIOPULMONARY RESUSCITATION (A TO H) AND FOREIGN BODY AIRWAY OBSTRUCTION (I TO K)

Source: *Wong's Nursing Care of Infants and Children* (7th edition), St. Louis: Mosby.

TABLE 7.5 📖 GUIDELINES FOR HOME CARE OF INFANT ON APNEA MONITOR

1. Demonstrate to parents how to connect monitor leads.
2. Remind parents to remove leads *unless* leads are connected to infant.
3. Stress that infant needs to be on monitor whenever respirations are not being directly observed and that a trained person needs to be present in the home at all times in case the alarm sounds. Caregiver must be able to reach an activated monitor within 30 seconds.
4. To eliminate false alarms, teach parents *not* to adjust monitor.
5. Explain that infant needs direct observation whenever loud noises could obscure the monitor alarm, e.g., dishwasher, vacuum cleaner.
6. Teach parents what to look for when the alarm sounds, i.e., loose monitor leads vs. apnea. Schedule regular maintenance of monitor. Keep power cord unplugged from electrical outlet when cord is not plugged into monitor. Use safety covers on electrical outlets to prevent children from inserting objects into the socket.
7. Teach parents how to assess the infant for an episode of apnea, i.e., lack of respirations, duration, color, muscle tone.
8. Teach parents to first use gentle physical stimulation if the infant experiences an apnea spell, e.g., touching the face or stroking the soles of the feet.
9. Demonstrate infant CPR to be used if tactile stimulation is not effective in re-establishing respirations.
10. Encourage parents to keep emergency numbers posted near their phone.
11. Explain that the monitor does not interfere with normal growth and development. Encourage parents to promote normal growth and development as much as possible.

Adapted from: Wong's Nursing Care of Infants and Children (7ᵗʰ ed.) St. Louis, Mosby.

TABLE 7.6 SIDS: WHAT TO TELL FAMILIES

Concern	*Facts*
Cause	Unknown (possibly related to delayed maturation of cardiorespiratory system).
Incidence	O.7:1000 live births (2500/year).
Occurence	During *sleep* (nap, night).
Age	Peak at 2–4 mo; 95% of cases occur by age *6 mo.*
Sex	More common in *boys.*
Race	More common in *African-Americans, Native Americans and Hispanics.*
Season	More common in *winter;* peak in January.
Siblings	May have greater incidence.
Perinatal factors	More common in *preterm* infants, in *multiple* births, and in infants with *low Apgar scores* or *low birth weight.* Maternal cigarette smoking (especially during pregnancy) and substance abuse may contribute to SIDS.
Socioeconomic level	More common in lower classes.
Feeding habits	Lower incidence in *breastfed* infants.

Adapted from: Wong's Nursing Care of Infants and Children (7ᵗʰ ed.) St. Louis, Mosby.

🔵 COMMONLY PRESCRIBED MEDICATIONS

Medication	Administration	Use/Action	⊨ Nursing Considerations

Antibiotics
Aminoglycosides
  Gentamicin
Cephalosporins/*Ancef;*
  Cefotan; Rocephin;
  Maxipime;
Penicillins/*Penicillin*
  V-K; Tegopen; Unasyn;
  Zosyn
	• Oral or parenteral
	• Calculate to child's weight
	  in kilograms
	• Administer in provided
	  dropper or calibrated
	  syringe
	• **NEVER** use household
	  measuring spoon
		Used for *bacterial infections* of respiratory system after cultures to determine sensitivity
		Kills bacteria
			• Assess for allergies prior to
			  administration
			• Obtain specimen for
			  〰 C & S prior to administration
			• Inform family of need to complete
			  entire course of therapy
			• Observe for superinfection (e.g. thrush
			  or monilial diaper dermatitis)

Anti-inflammatory
  Corticosteroids
Beclomethasone/*Vanceril*
Methylprednisolone
  Medrol
Prednisone/*Deltasone*
	• Oral, inhaled or parenteral
	• Calculate to child's weight
	  in kilograms
	• Administer in provided
	  dropper or calibrated
	  syringe
	• **NEVER** use household
	  measuring spoon
	• Shake metered-dose inhaler
	  (MDI) well before use
		Used in *asthma* to reduce inflammatory response *during* or to *prevent* an episode
		Reduces: inflammation and mucosal edema in airways
			• To prevent exercise-induced asthma
			  episode: give 15 minutes *before*
			  sustained activity
			• Use *lowest* possible dosage to prevent
			  side effects (e.g. growth and appetite
			  changes, etc.)
			• Take with milk or food to prevent
			  🍎 gastric upset
			• Rinse mouth *after* inhalation to
			  prevent oral candidiasis

Antivirals
Ribavirin/*Virazole*
	• Aerosolized
	• Calculate to child's weight
	  in kilograms
	• Administer via small-
	  particle aerosol generator
	  (SPAG) through hood,
	  tent, mask or ventilator
	  tubing
		Used for respiratory *syncytial virus* (RSV) and influenzae virus
		Inhibits replication of virus
			• Pregnant health care workers
			  should **not** care for child as drug is
			  teratogenic to fetus
			• Health care workers may experience:
			  headache, burning eyes,
			  crystallization of soft contact lenses;
			  (very expensive)

Bronchodilators
Albuterol/*Proventil*
Epinephrine/*Adrenalin*
Metaproterenol/*Alupent*
Terbutaline/*Brethaire*
	• Oral, inhaled or parenteral
	• Calculate to child's weight
	  in kilograms
	• Administer in provided
	  dropper or calibrated
	  syringe
	• **NEVER** use household
	  measuring spoon
		Used in *asthma* for *acute and daily* therapy
		Relaxes smooth muscles in airway
		Provides relief from bronchospasm
			• To prevent exercise-induced asthma
			  episode: give 15 minutes *before*
			  sustained activity
			• Assess for tachycardia and restlessness
			• Dosage may need to be decreased

Mucolytics
Acetylcysteine/Mucomyst
Dornase alfa/Pulmozyme
	• Inhaled
	• Calculate to child's weight
	  in kilograms
	• Administer via
	  recommended nebulizer
	  system
		Used in *cystic fibrosis* to loosen and thin pulmonary secretions
		Facilitates secretion removal by coughing
			• Prior to inhalation, have child cough
			  to clear airway
			• Does not replace other standard
			  therapies in treatment of cystic
			  fibrosis
			• Used in conjunction with other
			  therapies

(continued)

🔵 COMMONLY PRESCRIBED MEDICATIONS (continued)

Medication	Administration	Use/Action	🔀 Nursing Considerations
Nonsteroidal anti-inflammatories (NSAIDS) *Cromolyn/Intal* *Nedocromil /Tilade*	• Oral, nasal and inhaled (*Cromolyn*); inhaled (*Nedocromil*) • Calculate to child's weight in kilograms • Administer in provided dropper or calibrated syringe • **NEVER** use household measuring spoon • Shake metered-dose inhaler (MDI) well before use	Used in *asthma prophylactically* and for prevention of exercise-induced asthma episode Prevents activation and release of mediators of inflammation (e.g. histamine, leukotrienes, mast cells, eosinophils, monocytes)	• To prevent exercise-induced asthma episode: give 15 minutes *before* sustained activity • Stress need to take regularly for proper effect
Pancreatic enzymes *Pancrelipase/Pancrease; Cotazym; Ultrase*	• Oral; capsules that can be opened and the powder sprinkled on a small amount of food • Dosage is based on number and consistency of stools and adequate weight gain	Used in *cystic fibrosis* as a pancreatic enzyme replacement Aids in digestion and absorption of nutrients	• Enzymes must be consumed *before or with* every meal/snack • Do **not** sprinkle powder on hot food as enzyme activity will be compromised

💡 Study and Memory Aids

Cystic Fibrosis—Genetics

Cystic fibrosis = inherited trait from both parents

Cystic Fibrosis—Prognosis

Related to degree of pulmonary involvement

🔀 Cystic Fibrosis—Assessment

Newborn meconium ileus = cystic fibrosis or Hirschsprung's

Cystic Fibrosis—Diagnostic Test

 Sweat test (preparation: no powder or lotion; skin clean and dry)

Cystic Fibrosis—Nursing Care

🔵 Before postural drainage, give *bronchodilators*

Cystic Fibrosis—Medications

🔵 Pancreatic enzyme: **STAT** a.c.(powdered form mixed in cold applesauce)
Infancy, childhood—acute respiratory tract infection: most common illness

🍎 Respiratory Infections—Dietary Concerns

No dairy products with respiratory infection (due to ↑ mucus)

Asthma——Medication

🔵 *Cromolyn Na*—prevents asthma attacks; does not treat

SIDS—Risk Factors

Significant apnea → ↑ risk for SIDS

SIDS—Prevention

Position infant "back to sleep" supine, **never** prone

SIDS

A leading cause of death in infants aged 1-12 mo

Questions

1. A teenager with chronic asthma asks the nurse, "How come I make so much noise when I breathe?" The nurse's best reply is:
   1. "It is the sound of air passing through fluid in your alveoli."
   2. "It is the sound of air passing through fluid in your bronchus."
   3. "It is the sound of air being pushed through narrowed bronchi on expiration."
   4. "It is the sound of air being pushed past a narrowed larynx on inspiration."

2. The nurse should instruct the parents of a child with asthma that on first signs of an attack the parents should:
   1. Call the pediatrician.
   2. Use appropriate inhaler.
   3. Urge the child to drink clear fluids.
   4. Perform chest physiotherapy.

3. Chest physiotherapy is a standard adjunct to the treatment of chronic asthma. When should the nurse administer the child's bronchodilator in conjunction with postural drainage?
   1. One hour before postural drainage.
   2. During postural drainage.
   3. One hour after postural drainage.
   4. Between postural drainage treatments.

4. Which school-related activity might the school nurse prohibit for a child with asthma?
   1. The swim team.
   2. The band.
   3. Pet "show-and-tell" day.
   4. An art class.

5. At-home care instructions for a child with asthma include instructing the parents that use of a bronchodilator can result in:
   1. Decreased activity levels.
   2. Growth suppression.
   3. Weight gain.
   4. Insomnia.

6. An infant has laryngotracheobronchitis. On assessment, which symptom should the nurse anticipate?
   1. Barking cough and inspiratory stridor.
   2. Low-grade fever.
   3. Cherry-red epiglottis.
   4. Drooling.

7. A child presents in the hospital emergency department with acute epiglottis. The immediate goal of care is to:
   1. Suppress the child's infection.
   2. Rehydrate the child.
   3. Maintain a patent airway.
   4. Allay the family's anxiety.

8. Which nursing diagnosis is most developmentally focused for an adolescent who has cystic fibrosis?
   1. *High risk for altered nutrition, less than body requirements.*
   2. *High risk for body-image disturbance.*
   3. *High risk for infection.*
   4. *High risk for aspiration.*

9. In planning care for a child with cystic fibrosis, the nurse should know that the child must be protected from infections because:
   1. Each infection increases damage to the respiratory system.
   2. Pulmonary therapy is not effective during infection.

3. The child is already immunocompromised because of diminished pancreatic function.
   4. The child with cystic fibrosis is ineligible for usual childhood immunizations.

10. In evaluating the outcome of pulmonary therapy for a child with cystic fibrosis, the nurse should expect that:
    1. Secretions have been cleared from the airways.
    2. Pulmonary infections have been avoided.
    3. Appetite has improved.
    4. Medications can be more easily administered.

11. A toddler with cystic fibrosis is placed in a high-humidity cool-mist tent operated with compressed air. The nurse should know that the primary reason for this therapy is to:
    1. Provide oxygen.
    2. Lower the child's temperature.
    3. Moisten the airway and help mobilize secretions.
    4. Provide additional fluids to the child.

12. For a child in a mist tent (oxygen tent), which toy should the nurse remove?
    1. Blocks.
    2. A vinyl doll.
    3. A stuffed teddy bear.
    4. Plastic toy figures.

13. When performing postural drainage, how much time should the nurse generally plan to allow for this procedure?
    1. 10-15 minutes.
    2. 20-30 minutes.
    3. 30-45 minutes.
    4. One hour.

14. The nurse should be aware that postural drainage is useful in three of the following respiratory conditions. Which condition is not usually treated with postural drainage?
    1. Cystic fibrosis.
    2. Asthma.
    3. Pneumonia.
    4. Epiglottis.

15. When assessing a child who is suspected of having asthma, the nurse should specifically ask the parents about which symptom that they may have noted?
    1. Coughing at night in the absence of a respiratory infection.
    2. Coughing throughout the day.
    3. Expiratory wheezing.
    4. Shortness of breath.

16. The nurse notes that a child with a tracheostomy tube appears to be having significant respiratory distress. After several unsuccessful attempts to suction the child, even with the instillation of saline, the nurse should immediately:
    1. Change the tracheostomy tube.
    2. Page the MD.
    3. Bag the child with 100% oxygen.
    4. Remove the tracheostomy tube.

17. When suctioning a child with a tracheostomy tube, the nurse should select a catheter that is approximately one-half the diameter of the tube and suction for no longer than:
    1. 2 seconds.
    2. 5 seconds.
    3. 10 seconds.
    4. 15 seconds.

18. A preschooler with a diagnosis of epiglottitis is admitted to the hospital. Which MD order should the nurse question for this child?
    1. Place a pediatric-size tracheostomy tray in the child's room.
    2. Monitor pulse oxygen saturation every 15 minutes.
    3. IV of D5W at 42 mL/hour.
    4. Obtain **stat** CBC and throat culture.

Answers/Rationale

1. **(3)** Wheezing is produced when there is decreased expiratory airflow. Airways narrow because of bronchospasm, mucosal edema, and mucus plugs, with air becoming trapped behind occluded or narrowed airways. As air is pushed through the narrowed bronchi on expiration, wheezing is heard. Wheezing does *not* occur as air passes through fluid in the alveoli **(1)** or the bronchus **(2)**. Nor does wheezing occur when air is pushed past a narrowed larynx on inspiration **(4)**. Because the bronchi normally dilate and elongate during inspiration and contract and shorten on expiration, respiratory difficulty is more pronounced during the expiratory phase of respiration; wheezing is then heard. **IMP, COM, 6, PhI, Physiological adaptation**

2. **(2)** The appropriate inhaler as prescribed in the child's individual treatment plan will provide immediate bronchodilation and/or anti-inflammatory effects to open the airways. Calling the pediatrician **(1)** is acceptable but may *not* be necessary because many early asthma attacks can be successfully cared for at home. **(3)** Fluids provide adequate hydration and liquify secretions for easier removal, but would *not* be the first action. Chest physiotherapy **(4)** should *not* be used during an acute episode because it may aggravate the episode, but may be used as soon as signs of airway obstructions significantly subside. **IMP, ANL, 6, PhI, Reduction of risk potential**

3. **(1)** Bronchodilators are given before postural drainage so that they may fully dilate the bronchus and thus allow maximum removal of secretions during chest physiotherapy. Bronchodilators administered during **(2)**, after **(3)**, and between **(4)** chest physiotherapy treatments do *not* enhance loosening of secretions during the actual therapy. Other PO medications should be given after chest physiotherapy to minimize the danger of aspiration. **IMP, APP, 6, PhI, Pharmacological and parenteral therapies**

4. **(3)** Animal dander, especially from cats and dogs, can precipitate or aggravate an asthmatic episode. Swimming **(1)** involves exhaling underwater, which prolongs each expiration and increases the end-expiratory pressure within the respiratory tree. Activities such as participating in the band **(2)** or in an art class **(4)** do *not* require endurance exercise for participation and *are* therefore appropriate. Music and art are also known to reduce stress, which can be another factor in asthmatic episodes. **IMP, APP, 6, PhI, Reduction of risk potential**

5. **(4)** Insomnia is a noted side effect of bronchodilators; therefore, this medication should *not* be given *immediately before* the child's bedtime. *Increased* activity levels **(1)** are another side effect of bronchodilator therapy. Steroids are frequently administered in conjunction with bronchodilator therapy; side effects of *steroids* include growth suppression **(2)** and weight gain **(3)**. **IMP, APP, 1, PhI, Pharmacological and parenteral therapies**

6. **(1)** As laryngotracheobronchitis progresses, there is a gradually increasing barking cough (like a seal's bark) and inspiratory stridor. Stridor is a harsh sound caused by increased rate and turbulence of airflow in the larynx or trachea. Stridor is predominantly inspiratory. Fever in laryngotracheobronchitis is high, *not* low-grade **(2)**. A cherry-red epiglottis **(3)** and drooling **(4)** are associated with *acute epiglottis*, rather than laryngotracheobronchitis. **AS, APP, 6, PhI, Physiological adaptation**

7. **(3)** Complete airway obstruction caused by epiglottis may occur within 6-12 hours of onset. Throat swabbing, by using a tongue depressor or placing the child in a recumbent position (activities that can precipitate complete airway obstruction), should therefore *not* be attempted until an airway is established. Suppressing the infection **(1)**, rehydrating the child **(2)**, and allaying the family's anxiety **(4)** **are** appropriate but *secondary* goals. **PL, ANL, 6, PhI, Physiological adaptation**

Key to Codes

Nursing process: AS, assessment; **AN**, analysis; **PL**, planning; **IMP**, implementation; **EV**, evaluation. (See **Appendix L** for explanation of nursing process steps.)

Cognitive level: RE/KN, recall/knowledge; **COM**, comprehension; **APP**, application; **ANL**, analysis; **EVL**, evaluation; **SYN**, synthesis. (See **Appendix L** for explanation.)

Category of human function: 1, protective; **2**, sensory-perceptual; **3**, comfort, rest, activity, and mobility; **4**, nutrition; **5**, growth and development; **6**, fluid-gas transport; **7**, psychosocial-cultural; **8**, elimination. (See **Appendix N** for explanation.)

Client need: SECE, safe, effective care environment; **HPM**, health promotion and maintenance; **PsI**, psychosocial integrity; **PhI**, physiological integrity. (See **Appendix O** for explanation.)

Client subneed: See **Appendix O** for explanation.

8. (2) Adolescents are acutely aware of every change in their bodies; they scrutinize their bodies and compare their bodies with those of others. Adolescents with cystic fibrosis are thin and are probably short in stature. They may be embarrassed by odorous flatulence and stools and by uncontrolled bouts of coughing. Altered nutrition (1) and infection (3) are *physiologically* centered, rather than developmentally focused nursing diagnoses for adolescents with cystic fibrosis. Aspiration (4) is an *injury prevention/safety-centered* nursing diagnosis for adolescents with cystic fibrosis. Aspiration is prevented by **NEVER** performing the required chest physiotherapy immediately after a meal. **AN, ANL, 7, HPM, Health promotion and maintenance**

9. (1) Scar tissue can form in the lungs of a child with cystic fibrosis after each pulmonary infection. All infections should be prevented or cared for promptly in such a child. Pulmonary therapy (2) *is* effective when the child with cystic fibrosis has a respiratory infection. A decrease in pancreatic productivity (3) does *not* cause immunosuppression. Children with cystic fibrosis *should* receive all usual childhood immunizations (4) and have annual immunization for influenza. **PL, APP, 6, HPM, Health promotion and maintenance**

10. (1) The primary purpose of pulmonary therapy in cystic fibrosis is to clear secretions from the airways. Clearing the secretions assists in preventing pulmonary infections (2) caused by trapped secretions and may improve appetite (3) because most children with cystic fibrosis find the effort of eating easier when their lungs are clear. Inhalation medications (4), usually bronchodilators, are often given just *before* pulmonary therapy to help mobilize secretions. **EV, ANL, 6, PhI, Reduction of risk potential**

11. (3) The primary purpose of a high-humidity cool-mist tent for a toddler with cystic fibrosis is to moisten the airway and help mobilize secretions. Compressed air is the air *everyone* breathes in the environment; it does *not* contain extra oxygen (1). The mist tent provides a cooler environment, but it does *not* directly treat fever (2). *Inhaled* mist does *not* directly supply additional fluids (4); *Intravenous* therapy and encouraging additional oral intake of fluids will supply the needed fluids. **PL, APP, 6, PhI, Reduction of risk potential**

12. (3) Stuffed animals can absorb moisture and are difficult to dry; they can be a source of bacterial growth. Toys that are allowed in an oxygen tent are those that can be easily dried, such as blocks (1), vinyl dolls (2), and plastic toy figures (4). There is no need to remove these items. **IMP, APP, 6, SECE, Safety and infection control**

13. (2) Depending on the client's condition and tolerance level, postural drainage normally takes 20–30 minutes. Ten to fifteen minutes (1) is *too short* a period of time, and 30–45 minutes (3) or an hour (4) is *too long* and could overly exhaust the client. **PL, APP, 6, PhI, Reduction of risk potential**

14. (4) Epiglottitis is inflammation of the epiglottis, the flap of flesh that separates the trachea and the esophagus. Postural drainage is used to remove fluid or mucus from the bronchi or lower airway; it would be completely *ineffective* in treating epiglottitis. Postural drainage is used to remove fluid or secretions from the bronchi in cystic fibrosis (1), asthma (2), and pneumonia (3). **EV, ANL, 6, PhI, Reduction of risk potential**

15. (1) Nighttime coughing without any evidence of respiratory infection is one of the most common signs of asthma and is considered almost diagnostic. The nurse should be sure to ask about this symptom, even if the parents do not report it. Coughing all day (2) may indicate a respiratory infection or any number of possible problems and is *not* specifically related to asthma. The parents may or may not recognize the presence of an expiratory wheeze (3), which may be so mild as to be inaudible. Shortness of breath (4) is *not* necessarily evident unless the child is severely symptomatic; it is a *later* symptom of asthma. **AS, APP, 6, PhI, Physiological adaptation**

16. (1) The symptoms indicate a life-threatening occlusion, requiring the nurse to immediately change the tube. Removing the tube (4) without reinserting another tube would *not* secure the airway and could lead to further respiratory distress. Paging the MD (2) would *not* help the child in this life-threatening emergency. Bagging the child with oxygen (3) would be *ineffective* if the child's airway is not patent. **IMP, ANL, 6, PhI, Physiological adaptation**

17. (2) The American Heart Association recommends suctioning no longer than 5 seconds. Suctioning for only 2 seconds (1) is *too short*, and suctioning 10 (3) or 15 (4) seconds is *too long*. **IMP, COM, 6, PhI, Reduction of risk potential**

18. (4) If epiglottitis is suspected, the nurse should *not* attempt to visualize the epiglottitis because this could precipitate laryngospasm and respiratory arrest. It would be *appropriate* to place a pediatric-size tracheostomy tray in the child's room (1), to monitor the child's oxygen saturation (2), and start an IV (3) for fluids and hydration. **EV, APP, 6, SECE, Management of care**

Cardiovascular Disorders

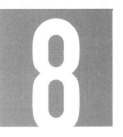

Chapter Outline

- Key Words
- Summary of Key Points
- Selected Cardiovascular Disorders
  - Congenital Heart Disease:
    Acyanotic: ASD, VSD, PDA, COA
    Cyanotic: Tetralogy of Fallot (TOF)
    Transposition of the Great Vessels
    (TGV)

- – Acquired Heart Disease:
    Rheumatic Fever
    Kawasaki's Disease
- Commonly Prescribed Medications
- Study and Memory Aids
- Questions
- Answers/Rationale

Key Words

cardiomegaly   enlargement of the heart.

clubbing   thickening of the fingers, and sometimes the toes, commonly found in diseases of the lungs and heart causing chronic hypoxia.

desquamation   peeling of skin or shedding of the epidermis in conditions such as Kawasaki's disease.

dyspnea   difficulty breathing.

ischemia   lack of adequate blood and oxygen supply to tissues or organs.

lymphadenopathy   swelling of the lymph glands, often related to disease.

orthopnea   difficulty breathing in any position except sitting straight up or standing.

panvasculitis   generalized inflammation of the vascular system (especially the coronary arteries in Kawasaki's disease).

petechiae   small, purplish, pinpoint hemorrhages caused by ruptured blood vessels; can occur anywhere on the body.

tachycardia   abnormally rapid heart rate.

tachypnea   abnormally rapid respiratory rate.

vasculitis   inflammation of the blood vessels.

🔑 Summary of Key Points

1. The most common cardiac problem in children is congenital heart disease.

2. The most common *acyanotic* defects are: atrial septal defect (ASD), ventricular septal defect (VSD), patent ductus arteriosus (PDA), and coarctation of the aorta (COA).

3. The most common *cyanotic* defects are tetralogy of Fallot (TOF) and transposition of the great vessels (TGF).

4. *Acyanotic* defects are characterized by the shunting of blood from *left to right* and the absence of cyanosis (unless congestive heart failure is present); treatment is generally accomplished by technically *simple* surgery that is completed in one stage.

5. The *cyanotic* defects are characterized by the shunting of blood from *right to left* and severe cyanosis; treatment is generally accomplished by technically *complex* surgery that requires two or more stages to complete.

6. The most frequent symptom that the nurse should observe in an infant with congenital heart disease is *tachycardia*; the most frequent complaint of parents of infants with congenital heart disease is *difficulty feeding*.

7. Acquired heart disease can be caused by *rheumatic fever* or *Kawasaki's disease*.

8. *Rheumatic fever* is an acute, systemic autoimmune disorder that is triggered by a strep infection (Group A B-hemolytic strep); the primary danger of rheumatic fever is that it can cause permanent damage to the valves of the heart, i.e., mitral stenosis.

9. The treatment of rheumatic fever includes: antibiotics to eradicate any lingering strep infection, aspirin, *digoxin*, and *furosemide* if CHF is present.

10. *Kawasaki's disease* is an acute, febrile, multisystem disorder of unknown etiology; it is characterized by high, unremitting fevers, desquamation of the palms of the hands and soles of the feet, and panvasculitis.

11. The treatment of *Kawasaki's disease* includes high-dose *gamma globulin* and aspirin along with *digoxin* and *furosemide* if CHF is present.

12. *Home care* for all children with cardiovascular disorders: **NEVER** allow tachycardia for more than 1 hour before seeking medical attention.

Selected Cardiovascular Disorders

Content has been synthesized for ease in review and recall; for the purpose of this review, only *six major* defects are given For additional study aids, refer to **Tables 8.1** and **Table 8.2, p. 57.** Also see **Figure 8.1, p. 58** for acyanotic heart defects and **Figure 8.2, p.59** for cyanotic heart defects.

Congenital Heart Disease

I. *Introduction*: There are more than 35 documented types of congenital heart defects, which occur in 5-8/1000 live births.

II. **Assessment:**
  A. *Risk factors/causes*: exact cause unknown, but related factors include:
    1. Familial history of congenital heart disease, especially in siblings, parents.
    2. Presence of other genetic defects in infant, e.g., Down syndrome, trisomy 13 or 18.
    3. History of maternal prenatal infection with rubella, cytomegalovirus, etc.
    4. High-risk maternal factors:
      a. Age: under 18, over 40 yr.
      b. Weight: under 100 pounds, over 200 pounds.
      c. Insulin-dependent diabetes.
    5. Maternal history of drinking during pregnancy, with resultant fetal alcohol syndrome.
    6. Extracardiac defects, including: tracheoesophageal fistula, renal agenesis, and diaphragmatic hernia.
  B. Most frequent parental complaint: *difficulty feeding*.
    1. Infant must be awakened to feed.
    2. Has weak suck.
    3. May turn blue when eating, especially with cyanotic defects.
    4. Infant takes overly long time to feed (↑ 20 minutes).
    5. Falls asleep during feeding, without finishing.
  C. *Nursing observations*
    1. *Most frequent symptom—tachycardia*, as body attempts to compensate for lack of oxygen (hypoxia); i.e., heart rate over 160 bpm.
    2. Tachypnea, corresponding to heart rate, i.e., respirations over 60/min.
    3. Cyanosis due to hypoxia:
      a. *Not* with acyanotic defects (unless CHF is present).
      b. *Always* with cyanotic defects ("blue babies").
    4. Failure to grow at a normal rate, i.e., slow weight gain, height and weight below the norm due to difficulty feeding and hypoxia.
    5. Developmental delays related to weakened physical condition.
    6. Frequent respiratory infections associated with increased pulmonary blood flow and/or aspiration.
    7. Dyspnea on exertion due to hypoxia, shunting of blood.
    8. Murmurs may or may not be present, e.g., PDA—machinery murmur.
    9. Changes in blood pressure, e.g., coarctation: increased blood pressure in arms; decreased blood pressure in legs.
    10. Possible congestive heart failure. *Note*: infants may *not* demonstrate distended neck veins.
    11. **Cyanotic heart defects** (see **Figures 8.2 A and 8.2 B, p. 59**):
      a. *"Tet. spells"*—choking spells with paroxysmal dyspnea: severe hypoxia, deepening cyanosis; relieved by squatting, or placing infant in *knee-chest* position, which alters cardiopulmonary dynamics, thus increasing the flow of blood to the lungs. Trend toward early surgical repair decreases occurrence of "tet. spells."
      b. Clubbing of fingers and toes—due to chronic hypoxia.
      c. *Polycythemia* (↑ RBC) with possible thrombi/emboli formation.

TABLE 8.1 COMPARISON OF ACYANOTIC AND CYANOTIC HEART DISEASE

Feature	Acyanotic	Cyanotic
Shunting of blood	L→R	R→L
Cyanosis	Not usual (unless congestive heart failure)	Always: "blue babies"
Surgery	Usually done in one stage—technically simple	Usually done in several stages—technically complex
Prognosis	Very good/excellent	Guarded
Major types	1. ASD (atrial septal defect) 2. VSD (ventricular septal defect). 3. PDA (patent ductus arteriosus) 4. COA (coarctation of the aorta)	1. TOF (tetralogy of Fallot) 2. TGV (transposition of the great vessels)

TABLE 8.2 OVERVIEW OF THE MOST COMMON TYPES OF CONGENITAL HEART DISEASE

Type of Defect	Medical Treatment	Surgical Treatment	Prognosis
Acyanotic **ASD (atrial septal defect)**	May be closed, using devices during cardiac catheterization	Open chest/open heart surgery with closure via patch (recommended age: preschooler)	Excellent, with survival greater than 99%
VSD (ventricular septal defect)	Clinical trials using device closure during cardiac catheterization	*Palliative treatment*: pulmonary banding; *definitive repair*: same as for ASD	Excellent, with 96-99% survival rate
PDA (patent ductus arteriosus)	In newborns—attempt pharmacologic closure with *indomethacin* (prostaglandin inhibitor)	Open chest: surgical ligation or division (recommended age: 1–2 yr)	Excellent with survival greater than 99%
COA (coarctation of the aorta)	Infants or children with CHF: *digitalis and diuretics*	Open chest: resection of coarcted portion of aorta with end-to-end anastamosis within first 2 yr	Fair—less than 5% mortality
Cyanotic **TOF (tetralogy of Fallot)**	None—supportive prn.	Often done in *stages* with definitive repair accomplished within first yr.	Fair—less than 5% mortality
TGV (transposition of the great vessels)	None—supportive prn.	Often done in *stages, with definitive repair* within first yr.	Guarded—less than 5% mortality

III. Analysis/nursing diagnosis:

A. *Ineffective breathing pattern* related to tachypnea and respiratory infection.

B. *Activity intolerance* related to tachycardia and hypoxia.

C. *Altered nutrition, less than body requirements,* related to difficulty in feeding.

D. *Risk for infection* related to poor nutritional status.

E. *Knowledge deficit* related to diagnostic procedures, condition, surgical/medical treatments, prognosis.

IV. Nursing care plan/implementation:

A. Goal: *promote adequate oxygenation.*

  1. Administer oxygen per MD order/prn.

  2. Use loose-fitting clothing; pin diapers loosely to *avoid* pressure on abdominal organs, which could impinge on diaphragm and impede respiration.

  3. *Position*: neck slightly hyperextended to keep airway patent; place in *knee-chest* (squatting) position to relieve "Tet. spell."

  4. Suction prn, to clear the airway.

  5. Administer *digoxin*, per MD order, to slow and strengthen heart's pumping action (refer to **Chapter 1, Table 1.5, p. 7** for pediatric pulse rate norms).

B. Goal: *reduce workload of heart to conserve energy.*

  1. *Position*: infant seat, *semi-Fowler's* position to provide maximal expansion of the lungs.

  2. Provide pacifier to promote psychological rest.

  3. Organize nursing care to provide periods of uninterrupted rest.

  4. Adjust physical activity according to child's condition, capabilities to conserve energy. Limit p.o. feedings to 20 minutes to prevent exhaustion.

  5. Provide diversion, as tolerated, to meet developmental needs yet conserve energy.

  6. *Avoid* extremes of temperature to avoid the stress of hypothermia/hyperthermia, which increases the body's demand for oxygen.

  7. Administer *diuretics*: furosemide (*Lasix*), per MD order, to eliminate excess fluids, which increase the work load of the heart. May alternate with potassium-sparing diuretic (e.g. spironolactone/aldactone) to decrease need for potassium supplement.

C. Goal: *provide adequate nutrition.*

  1. Offer *high calorie* formulas to meet nutritional needs without increasing fluids; e.g. 3hr feeds usually effective ($\bar{q}$ 2 hr prevents sufficient rest between feedings while $\bar{q}$ 4 hr requires an increased volume of feeding which may not be well tolerated).

  2. Discourage foods with *high* or added *sodium* to minimize fluid retention.

  3. I&O, daily/weekly weights, and monitor for rate of growth.

  4. Supplement PO feeding with gavage feeding (prn with MD order) to meet fluid and caloric needs.

  5. Encourage foods *high in potassium* (prevent hypokalemia) and *high in iron* (prevent anemia).

D. Goal: *prevent infection.*

  1. Standard precautions to prevent infection.

  2. Use good handwashing technique.

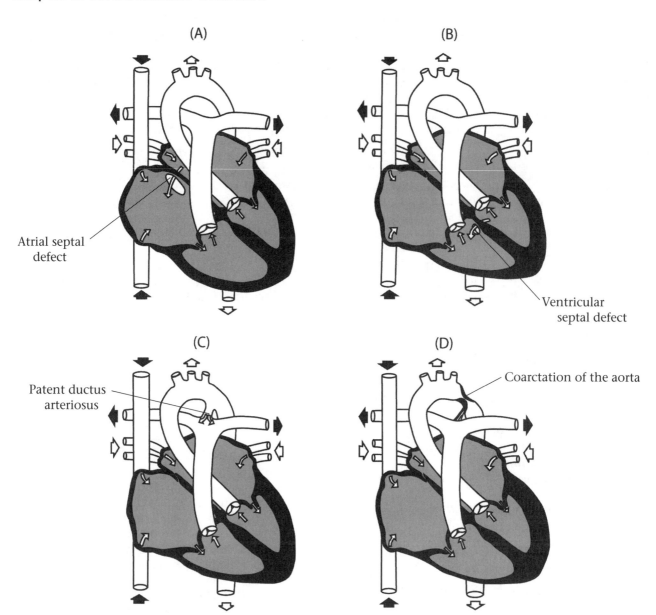

FIGURE 8.1 ACYANOTIC HEART DEFECTS.

(A) Atrial septal defect. **(B)** Ventricular septal defect. **(C)** Patent ductus arteriosus. **(D)** Coarctation of the aorta.

(From *Clinical Education Aid No. 7*. Columbus, Oh: Ross laboratories. Reproduced with permission.)

3. Limit contact with staff/visitors with infections.
4. Monitor for early symptoms and signs of infection; report stat.

📖 E. Goal: **health teaching**.

〰️ 1. Explain *diagnostic procedures*: blood tests, x-rays, urine, ECG, echocardiogram, cardiac catheterization.
2. Explain condition/treatment/prognosis (refer to **Table 8.2, p. 57**).
3. Review dietary restrictions, medications.
4. Discuss how to realistically adjust to life with heart disease, activity restrictions, etc.

▶️ V. **Evaluation/outcome criteria:**

A. Child's level of oxygenation is maintained, as evidenced by pink color in nailbeds and mucous membranes (for both light- and dark-skinned children) and ease in respiratory effort.
B. Energy is conserved, thus reducing the workload of the heart, as evidenced by vital signs within normal limits.
C. The child's fluid and caloric requirements are met, allowing physical growth to occur at normal or near-normal rate.
D. The child remains in an infection-free state.
E. The family (and child, when old enough) verbalize their understanding of the type of CHD, its treatment and prognosis.

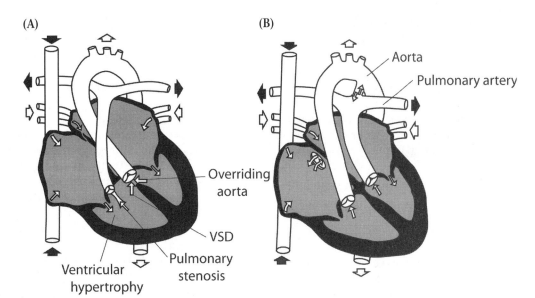

FIGURE 8.2 CYANOTIC HEART DEFECTS.

(A) Tetralogy of Fallot.   **(B)** Transposition of the great vessels.

(From Clinical Education Aid No. 7. Columbus, OH: Ross Laboratories. Reproduced with permission.)

Acquired Heart Disease

I. **Rheumatic Fever**

   A. *Introduction*: Rheumatic fever is an acute, *systemic, inflammatory* disease affecting *multiple* organs and systems: heart, joints, CNS, collagenous tissue, etc. Thought to be autoimmune in nature, it most commonly *follows* a strep infection (see **Chapter 10, Figure 10.1, p. 88**) and occurs primarily in *school-aged* children. In addition, it tends to *recur*, and the risk of permanent heart damage increases with each subsequent attack of rheumatic fever.

   B. **Assessment:**

   1. **Major manifestations** (modified *Jones criteria*)

      a. *Carditis*: tachycardia, cardiomegaly, murmur, congestive heart failure (CHF).

      b. *Migratory polyarthritis*: swollen, hot, red, and excruciatingly painful large joints; migratory and reversible.

      c. *Sydenham chorea* (*St. Vitus Dance*): sudden, aimless, irregular movements of the extremities; involuntary facial grimaces, speech disturbances; emotional lability; muscle weakness; completely reversible.

      d. *Erythema marginatum*: reddish pink rash most commonly found on the trunk; nonpruritic, macular, clear center, wavy but clearly marked border; transient.

      e. *Subcutaneous nodules*: small, round, freely movable, painless swellings usually found over the extensor surfaces of the hands/feet or bony prominences; resolves without permanent damage.

   2. **Minor manifestations**

      a. Clinical.

         (1) Previous history of rheumatic fever.

         (2) Arthralgia.

         (3) Fever—*normal* in morning, *rises* in mid-afternoon, *normal* at night.

      b. Laboratory:

         (1) *Increased* erythrocyte sedimentation rate (ESR).

         (2) *Positive* C-reactive protein.

         (3) Leukocytosis.

         (4) Anemia.

         (5) *Prolonged* P-R/Q-T intervals on ECG.

   3. Supportive evidence

      a. Recent history of streptococcus infection:

         (1) Strep throat/tonsillitis.

         (2) Otitis media.

         (3) Impetigo.

         (4) Scarlet fever.

      b. Positive throat culture for strep.

      c. *Increased* ASO titer: indicates presence of streptococcus antibodies; begins to rise in 7 d, reaches maximal level in 4-6 wk. ↑ 333 Todd units confirms recent streptococcal infection (normal value is 0-120 Todd units).

   C. **Analysis/nursing diagnosis:**

   1. *Decreased cardiac output* related to carditis.

   2. *Pain* related to migratory polyarthritis.

   3. *Risk for injury* related to chorea.

   4. *Diversional activity deficit* related to lengthy hospitalization and recuperation.

   5. *Knowledge deficit* related to preventing cardiac damage, relieving discomfort, and preventing injury.

   6. *Ineffective management of therapeutic regimen* with long-term antibiotic therapy and follow-up care.

D. Nursing care/plan implementation:

1. Goal: *prevent cardiac damage.*

   a. Hospitalization, with *strict bedrest* during acute phase.

   b. Monitor apical pulse for changes in rate, rhythm, murmurs.

   c. Evaluate tolerance of increased activity via apical rate: if heart rate increases by more than 20 bpm over resting rate, child should return to bed.

   d. Offer *low sodium* diet to prevent fluid retention.

   e. Administer *oxygen, digoxin/furosemide* per MD order (if CHF develops).

2. Goal: *relieve discomfort.*

   a. Use bed cradle to keep linens from resting on painful joints.

   b. Administer *aspirin* as ordered to relieve pain.

   c. Move child carefully, minimally—support joints.

   d. *Do not* massage; *do not* perform ROM exercises; *do not* apply splints; *do not* apply heat/cold. All these treatments cause increased pain and are *not needed* since no permanent deformities result from this type of arthritis.

3. Goal: *promote safety and prevent injury related to chorea.*

   a. Use side rails: elevated, padded.

   b. Restrain in bed if necessary.

   c. *No* oral temperatures—child may bite thermometer.

   d. Spoonfeed—*no* forks or knives, to prevent injury to oral cavity.

   e. Assist with all aspects of activities of daily living (ADL) until child can care for own needs.

4. Goal: *provide diversion as tolerated.*

   a. Encourage quiet diversional activities: hobbies, reading, puzzles.

   b. Get homework, books; provide tutor as condition permits.

   c. Encourage contact with peers: telephone calls, letters, cards.

5. Goal: *encourage child and family to comply with long-term antibiotic therapy.*

   a. Begin antibiotics immediately to eradicate any lingering streptococcus infection.

   b. Prepare child/family for minimum of 5 yr of intramuscular injections of *penicillin* on a monthly basis or daily p.o. antibiotic.

   c. Stress need for exact schedule: every 4 wk. The duration of long-term prophylaxis varies, depending on cardiac involvement; can extend into adulthood or be lifelong.

   d. Enlist child's cooperation with therapy, e.g., "hero" badge.

6. Goal: **health teaching.**

   a. To encourage compliance with prolonged bedrest, stress that ultimate prognosis depends on amount of cardiac damage.

   b. Teach necessity for long-term prophylactic therapy for 5 yr initially (with lifetime follow-up), e.g., during dental work, childbirth, surgery (to prevent subacute bacterial endocarditis).

   c. Teach rationale: permanent cardiac damage is more likely to occur with subsequent attacks of rheumatic fever.

E. Evaluation/outcome criteria:

1. No permanent cardiac damage occurs.

2. Child is free from discomfort or is able to tolerate discomfort.

3. Injuries are avoided.

4. Child's need for diversional activity is met.

5. Child/family comply with long-term antibiotic therapy/prophylactic therapy.

II. Kawasaki's Disease

A. *Introduction*: Kawasaki's disease (*mucocutaneous lymph node syndrome*) is an acute, febrile, *multisystem* disorder believed to be *autoimmune* in nature. Affecting primarily the skin and mucous membranes of the *respiratory* tract, *lymph nodes*, and *heart*, Kawasaki's disease has a low fatality rate (< 2%), although vasculitis and cardiac involvement (coronary artery changes) may result in major complications in as many as 20-25% of the children with this disease. The disease is not believed to be communicable, and the exact cause remains unknown; geographic (living near *fresh water*) and *seasonal* (late winter, early spring) outbreaks do occur. Kawasaki's disease occurs in both boys and girls 1-14 yr; 80% of cases occur in children *under* the *age of 5 yr, preceded by upper respiratory illness* (URI) or *exposure to a freshly cleaned carpet*. A complete and apparently spontaneous recovery occurs within 3-4 wk in the majority of cases. Treatment, which is primarily symptomatic, does not appear to either enhance recovery or prevent complications, although recent research indicates that life-threatening complications and long-term disability may be avoided or minimized with early treatment (i.e., *gamma globulin*) to reduce cardiovascular damage.

B. **Assessment:**

1. Abrupt onset with high fever (102°-106°F) lasting more than 5 days and does *not* remit with the administration of antibiotics.

2. Conjunctivitis—bilateral, nonpurulent.

3. Oropharyngeal manifestations:

   a. Dry, red, cracked lips.

   b. Oropharyngeal reddening and "strawberry" tongue.

4. Peeling (*desquamation*) of palms of hands and soles of feet; begins at fingertips and tips of the toes; as peeling progresses, hands and feet become very red, sore, and swollen.
5. Cervical lymphadenopathy.
6. Generalized erythematous rash on trunk and extremities, without vesicles or crusts.
7. Irritability, anorexia.
8. Arthralgia and arthritis.
9. Panvasculitis of coronary arteries: formation of aneurysms and thrombi; **CHF**, myocarditis, pericardial effusion, arrhythmias, mitral insufficiency, myocardial infarction (**MI**).
10. Laboratory tests:
    a. *Elevated*: ESR.
    b. *Elevated*: WBC count.
    c. *Elevated*: platelet count.
C. **Analysis/nursing diagnosis:**
   1. *Hyperthermia* related to high, unremitting fever.
   2. *Altered oral mucous membrane and impaired swallowing* related to oropharyngeal manifestations.
   3. *Impaired skin integrity* related to desquamation.
   4. *Fluid volume deficit* related to high fever and poor oral intake.
   5. *Altered tissue perfusion* (cardiovascular, potential/actual) related to vasculitis and/or thrombi.
   6. *Knowledge deficit* related to disease course, treatment, prognosis.
D. **Nursing care plan/implementation:**
   1. Goal: *reduce fever.*
      a. Monitor rectal temperature every 2 h or prn.
      b. Administer *aspirin* (*not* acetaminophen) per MD order. (*Note*: aspirin is the drug of choice to reduce fever; also has anti-inflammatory effect and anti-platelet effect. Dosage is 100 mg/kg/d in divided doses q6h. Monitor for signs of salicylate toxicity.)
      c. Tepid sponge baths or hypothermia blanket per MD order.
      d. Offer frequent *cool fluids.*
      e. Apply cool, loose-fitting clothes; use cotton bed linens only (*no* heavy blankets).
      f. Seizure precautions.
   2. Goal: *provide comfort measures to oral cavity to ease the discomfort of swallowing.*
      a. Good oral hygiene with soft sponge toothbrush.
      b. Apply petroleum jelly to lips.
      c. *Bland* foods in small amounts at frequent intervals.

d. *Avoid* hot, spicy foods.
e. Offer favorite foods from home or preferred foods from hospital selection.
   3. Goal: *prevent infections and promote healing of skin.*
      a. Monitor skin for desquamation, edema, rash.
      b. Keep skin clean, dry, well lubricated.
      c. *Avoid* soap to prevent drying.
      d. Gentle handling of skin to minimize discomfort.
      e. Provide sheepskin to lie on.
      f. Prevent scratching and itching—apply cotton mittens if necessary.
      g. Bedrest; *elevate* edematous extremities.
   4. Goal: *prevent dehydration and restore normal fluid balance.*
      a. Strict I&O.
      b. Monitor urine specific gravity q8h for *increase* (dehydration) or *decrease* (hydration).
      c. Monitor *vital signs* for: fevers, tachycardia, arrhythmia.
      d. Monitor for dehydration: skin turgor, mucous membranes, anterior fontanel.
      e. *Force* fluids.
      f. IV fluids per MD order.
   5. Goal: *prevent cardiovascular complications.*
      a. ECG monitor—report arrhythmias or tachycardia.
      b. Administer *aspirin* (see Goal 1) and high-dose IV *gamma globulin.*
      c. Monitor for signs and symptoms of CHF: tachycardia, tachypnea, dyspnea, crackles, orthopnea, distended neck veins, dependent edema.
      d. Monitor circulatory status of extremities—check for possible development of thrombi.
   6. Goal: **health teaching.**
      a. Stress need for long-term follow-up, including ECGs and echocardiograms.
E. **Evaluation/outcome criteria:**
   1. Fever returns to normal.
   2. Oral cavity heals and child is able to swallow.
   3. Skin heals and no infection occurs.
   4. Normal fluid balance is restored.
   5. Normal cardiovascular functioning is reestablished and no complications occur.
   6. Parents/child verbalize their understanding of Kawasaki's disease.

⬭ COMMONLY PRESCRIBED MEDICATIONS

Medication	Administration	Use/Action	🏴 Nursing Considerations
ACE Inhibitors Captopril/*Capoten* Enalapril/*Vasotec* Lisinopril/*Zestil*	• Oral • Calculate to child's weight in kilograms • Administer in provided dropper or calibrated syringe • **NEVER** in household measuring spoon	Used in treatment of *hypertension* and as an adjunctive therapy for congestive heart failure Suppresses renin-angiotensin-aldosterone system Produces reduction in peripheral arterial resistance, increases cardiac output with little/no change in heart rate	• Monitor blood pressure; if hypotension occurs, hold next dose • Assess potassium level • *Avoid high sodium* and *potassium* foods • *Avoid* sudden changes in position
Antibiotics Penicillin/Penicillin G Penicillin V	• Oral and parenteral • Calculate to child's weight in kilograms • Administer in provided dropper or calibrated syringe • **NEVER** in household measuring spoon	Used in treatment of *rheumatic* fever (primary prevention of streptococcal infections as well as prevention of recurrent attacks) Kills bacteria	• Assess for allergies prior to administration • Substitute macrolides or cephalosporins in penicillin-sensitive children • Long-term therapy involves monthly IM injections or two daily oral doses • Duration of long-term therapy depends on cardiac involvement
Cardiac Glycosides Digoxin/*Lanoxin*	• Oral or parenteral • Calculate to child's weight in kilograms • Administer in provided dropper or calibrated syringe • **NEVER** in household measuring spoon	Used in *congestive heart failure* Increases force of contraction; decreases heart rate Slows conduction of impulses through AV node Indirectly enhances diuresis by increased renal perfusion	• Check heart rate for one minute prior to administration and withhold if less than normal for age or prescribed parameters • Maintain serum drug level within therapeutic range (e.g. 0.8–2.0 ng/mL) • Monitor potassium level and correct to normal level before administering digoxin
Diuretics **Loop Diuretics** Furosemide/*Lasix*	• Oral and parenteral • Calculate to child's weight in kilograms • Administer in provided dropper or calibrated syringe • **NEVER** in household measuring spoon	Used in treatment of *severe congestive heart failure* Blocks reabsorption of sodium and water	• Administer in AM to *avoid* sleep interruption • Monitor I&O and weight to prevent dehydration caused by profound diuresis • Assess potassium level • Encourage *high* potassium foods
Potassium-sparing Diuretics Spironolactone/*Aldactone*	• Oral • Calculate to child's weight in kilograms • Administer in provided dropper or calibrated syringe • **NEVER** in household measuring spoon	Used in conjunction with Furosemide/*Lasix* therapy in treatment of *severe congestive heart failure* Blocks action of aldosterone; allows retention of potassium	• Monitor I&O and weight to prevent dehydration caused by profound diuresis • Assess potassium level • Encourage *low potassium* foods

(continued)

COMMONLY PRESCRIBED MEDICATIONS *(continued)*

Medication	Administration	Use/Action	Nursing Considerations
Nonsteroidal Anti-inflammatories (NSAIDS) Acetylsalicylic acid/ *Aspirin*	• Oral or rectal • Calculate to child's weight in kilograms • Administer in provided dropper or calibrated syringe • **NEVER** in household measuring spoon	Used in Kawasaki's disease for anti-inflammatory and platelet aggregation inhibition effect Decreases synthesis of endoperoxides and thromboxanes-substances that mediate platelet aggregation	• Assess chickenpox status prior to beginning drug (e.g. Reye syndrome) • Administer *with* food/fluids • Assess for ringing in ears or difficulty hearing • If child develops coronary abnormalities, therapy may continue indefinitely

Study and Memory Aids

Acyanotic Defects—Types

1. ASD—atrial septal defect
2. VSD—ventricular septal defect
3. PDA—patent ductus arteriosus
4. COA—coarctation of the aorta

Cyanotic Defects—Types: T²

1. TOF—Tetralogy of Fallot
2. TGV—Transposition of the great vessels

Congenital Heart Disease—Assessment

Difficulty in *feeding*: most frequent *parental* complaint
Tachycardia: most frequent *nursing* observation

CHD—Treatment: Digoxin

Monitor: normal therapeutic serum digoxin levels: 0.8-2.0 ng/mL.
When giving digoxin to infant or child, *always* check dose and calculation with another nurse to avoid errors.
When an infant or child is taking both *digoxin* and *furosemide*, the nurse should be particularly alert for the possible complication of hypokalemia; symptoms include: muscle weakness, hyporeflexia, tachycardia and hypotension.
Normal serum potassium levels: 3.5-5.0 mEq/L.

CHD—Diagnostic Test

After cardiac catheterization, nurse must especially
monitor pulse rate to check for dysrhythmia or bradycardia.

Rheumatic Fever—Characteristics

Autoimmune disorder
Antecedent cause: strep
Major complication: mitral stenosis

Rheumatic Fever—Medications

Aspirin is given to children with rheumatic fever for both its analgesic effect as well as its anti-inflammatory effect. The risk of cardiac damage rises with each subsequent attack of rheumatic fever; long-term prophylactic *antibiotic* therapy is given to prevent recurrent attacks.

Kawasaki's Disease—Assessment. Main Symptoms:

Desquamation of hands and feet
Fever
Panvasculitis

Panvasculitis—Medication

Aspirin is given to children with Kawasaki's disease for its anti-inflammatory effect as well as its anticoagulant effect.

Questions

1. In assessing a child with Kawasaki's disease, the nurse should recognize that the childhood communicable disease that poses the greatest danger for this child is:
   1. Measles.
   2. Mumps.
   3. Rubella.
   4. Chickenpox.

2. A parent of a toddler with Kawasaki's disease tells the nurse, "I just don't know what to do with my child. He's never acted like this before." The nurse's best reply is:
   1. "Don't worry. This type of behavior is typical for a toddler."
   2. "Irritability is part of Kawasaki's disease. Please don't be embarrassed."
   3. "Perhaps your child would benefit from stricter limits."
   4. "You seem to be in need of a referral to our Child Guidance Clinic."

3. Which statement made by the parents of a child with Kawasaki's disease indicates that the parents have understood the nurse's teaching regarding signs of aspirin toxicity?
   1. "We'll call the pediatrician immediately if our child develops vomiting or a rash."
   2. "We'll call the pediatrician immediately if our child develops a fever or a rash."
   3. "We'll call the pediatrician immediately if our child tells us he hears ringing in his ears."
   4. "We'll call the pediatrician immediately if our child starts to breathe slowly."

4. When assessing a child for signs and symptoms of rheumatic fever, which symptoms should the nurse anticipate?
   1. Tachycardia and joint pain.
   2. Bradycardia and swollen joints.
   3. Loss of coordination and pruritic rash.
   4. Bradycardia and fever.

5. Which nursing intervention is most effective in preventing rheumatic fever in children?
   1. Refer children with sore throats for a throat culture.
   2. Include an ECG in the child's yearly physical examination.
   3. Assess the child for a change in the quality of the pulse.
   4. Assess the child's blood pressure.

6. A treatment modality for a child with rheumatic fever is a period of bedrest lasting several weeks. Which nursing diagnosis is the child at greatest risk for developing?
   1. *High risk for impaired skin integrity.*
   2. *High risk for altered nutrition, less than body requirements.*
   3. *High risk for social isolation.*
   4. *High risk for injury.*

7. Which at-home care instruction is essential for the nurse to teach the parents of a child with rheumatic fever?
   1. Monitor intake and output.
   2. Monitor apical pulse.
   3. Monitor blood pressure.
   4. Monitor oxygen therapy.

8. A common goal for children with cardiac disease is to reduce the workload of the heart to conserve energy. Attainment of this goal can best be evaluated by:
   1. Vital signs that are within normal limits.
   2. Intake that equals output.
   3. Weight stabilization.
   4. Pink nailbeds and warm extremities.

9. Which is most beneficial in achieving the goal of preventing infection in a child with cardiac disease?
   1. Give the child extra immunizations.
   2. Keep the child on prophylactic antibiotics.

3. Keep the child away from others who are ill.
4. Place the child in protective isolation.

10. Which statement should the nurse refrain from making to a preschooler who is about to undergo a cardiac catheterization?
    1. "You will be getting some dye which will sting a little while we look at your heart."
    2. "The light will be turned off for a little bit while we look at your heart on the TV screen. I will stay very close to you when it gets dark."
    3. "You must lie very still when we look at your heart. We'll pretend that you are Sleeping Beauty waiting for the prince to come."
    4. "The doctor will just look at your heart. He will not cut or hurt your heart."

11. A 3-year-old child undergoes a diagnostic cardiac catheterization. On conclusion of this procedure, the nurse's first action should be to assess:
    1. The IV site for patency.
    2. Peripheral pulses and observe the incision site.
    3. Body temperature.
    4. Pain status.

12. The nurse is instructing the parents of a 2-month-old infant with congenital heart disease how to administer digoxin to the infant at home. Which statement reflects a lack of knowledge on the nurse's part?
    1. "In case the baby spits up, give the digoxin 1 hour before or 2 hours after feeding to avoid a dose being lost."
    2. "Do not change the amount or timing of the dose without specific instructions from your pediatrician."
    3. "Always use the same measuring device each time so the dose given remains consistent."
    4. "Take the apical pulse before giving the drug and do not give it if the pulse is below 80 beats per minute."

13. A newborn with patent ductus arteriosus is scheduled to receive indomethacin. The nurse administers this medication to:
    1. Open the ductus arteriosus.
    2. Close the ductus arteriosus.
    3. Enlarge the ductus arteriosus.
    4. Maintain the present size of the ductus arteriosus.

14. Which congenital heart defect necessitates that the nurse take upper and lower extremity blood pressure readings?
    1. Coarctation of the aorta.
    2. Tetralogy of Fallot.
    3. Ventricular septal defect.
    4. Patent ductus arteriosus.

15. An infant with ventricular septal defect develops congestive heart failure and is placed on digoxin therapy twice a day. The infant vomits the morning dose of digoxin. The most appropriate nursing intervention is to:
    1. Notify the pediatrician as soon as possible.
    2. Take the infant's pulse for 1 minute and repeat the dose of digoxin.
    3. Skip the dose and give twice the amount at the next dose.
    4. Repeat the dose and chart that the infant vomited the first dose.

16. The parents of a newborn with ventricular septal defect ask why their baby is being sent home instead of undergoing immediate open heart surgery. The nurse's best response is:
    1. "Your baby's condition is too serious for immediate open heart surgery."
    2. "Ventricular septal defects are not repaired until the infant is older."
    3. "Your baby has a small defect, and we hope that it will close spontaneously."
    4. "Your baby must be fully immunized before surgery."

17. When reviewing the chart of an infant with tetralogy of Fallot, the nurse should anticipate which laboratory finding?
    1. Anemia.
    2. Polycythemia.
    3. Increased white blood cell count.
    4. Decreased hematocrit.

18. An infant with tetralogy of Fallot becomes hypoxic following a prolonged bout of crying. The nurse's first action should be to:
    1. Administer oxygen.
    2. Administer morphine.
    3. Place the infant in the knee-chest position.
    4. Comfort the infant.

19. The parents of an infant with tetralogy of Fallot ask the nurse why their infant's fingers and toes appear "clubbed." The nurse should inform the parents that clubbing is:
    1. Part of the anomaly.
    2. Because the infant's extremities are in a dependent position.
    3. The result of extra capillaries forming in the tips of the extremities.
    4. Caused by poor venous return.

20. To avoid making a medication error when administering digoxin to a child, the nurse should always:
    1. Ask the MD to check the dose before giving digoxin.
    2. Double check all calculations before giving digoxin.
    3. Verify the calculation with another nurse before giving digoxin.
    4. Give 1 mL or less of digoxin for any one dose.

21. While caring for a child who is receiving digoxin, the nurse should monitor the therapeutic serum digoxin level, which should range from:
    1. 10-20 mcg/mL.
    2. 0.8-2 mcg/mL.
    3. 0.8-2 mg/mL.
    4. 15-30 mg/dL.

22. In taking a history for a child with rheumatic fever, which finding should the nurse consider to be possibly related to the onset of this condition?
    1. Aspirin given for fever and sore throat.
    2. Impetigo 3 weeks earlier.
    3. Chickenpox 5 weeks earlier.
    4. Mother has a history of mitral stenosis.

23. After a child returns from the cardiac catheterization laboratory, the nurse should monitor for possible bleeding and monitor vital signs, with special emphasis on:
    1. Temperature.
    2. Pulse.
    3. Respiration.
    4. Blood pressure.

24. When caring for a child who is receiving both digoxin and furosemide (*Lasix*), the nurse should be particularly alert for signs or symptoms of:
    1. Hypokalemia.
    2. Hyponatremia.
    3. Hypoglycemia.
    4. Hypocalcemia.

Answers/Rationale

1. **(4)** Salicylate therapy is the current therapy for Kawasaki's disease. If the child is exposed to chickenpox, aspirin should be stopped and the pediatrician notified immediately because of the drug's possible association with Reye syndrome. Measles (**1**), mumps (**2**) and rubella (**3**) are *not* associated with use of aspirin to control fever and the potential danger of developing Reye syndrome. **AN, ANL, 1, PhI, Physiological adaptation**

2. **(2)** Irritability and inconsolability are classic behaviors associated with the acute phase of Kawasaki's disease. Parents need to be informed and supported in their efforts to comfort an often inconsolable child. Placing the child in a quiet environment that promotes rest is of value, as is offering respite care to the family. Toddlers are a difficult age group to deal with when ill, but, the irritability associated with Kawasaki's disease exceeds "normal" toddler irritability (**1**). Increasing limits (**3**) is inappropriate during time of illness. The source of the irritability is *physiologic, not developmental*, although a referral (**4**) may be appropriate if it is presented in a supportive, uncritical manner. **IMP, APP, 7, PsI, Psychosocial integrity**

3. (3) Ringing in the ears (tinnitus), headache, dizziness, hyperpnea, and confusion are signs of aspirin toxicity. Vomiting and rash (1), fever and rash (2), and slow breathing (4) are *not* associated with aspirin toxicity. **EV, APP, 1, PhI, Pharmacological and parenteral therapies**

4. (1) Tachycardia, fever, migratory polyarthritis, loss of coordination, subcutaneous nodules, and a nonpruritic rash are classic signs and symptoms of rheumatic fever. Bradycardia (2, 4) and a pruritic rash (3) are *not* associated with rheumatic fever. **AS, COM, 1, PhI, Physiological adaptation**

5. (1) Rheumatic fever occurs after an infection and is usually upper respiratory in nature because of Group A beta-hemolytic streptococcus. Therefore, the cause of all sore throats in children should be documented via culture to prevent untreated infections from occurring. Follow-up ECGs (2), assessing for changes in the quality of the pulse (3), and assessing blood pressure (4) are appropriate interventions *after* an episode of rheumatic fever because carditis and its associated potential for permanent cardiac damage requires careful follow-up and management. **IMP, ANL, 1, SECE, Management of care**

6. (3) Because prolonged bedrest takes the child out of the classroom and away from normal peer activities, the child is at risk for social isolation. This is especially important because the child with rheumatic fever is usually between ages 6 and 15 years, with a peak incidence at about age 8 years—the age range in which school and peers become most important. Skin integrity (1) can be maintained by basic nursing interventions such as hygiene and frequent repositioning. Deficits in nutrition (2) can be prevented by a high protein and high caloric diet served in small frequent meals. Risk of injury (4) to the heart is prevented by the ordered bedrest. **AN, ANL, 7, PsI, Psychosocial integrity**

7. (2) A child with rheumatic fever is often discharged home on digoxin, so the parents need to be taught to take an apical pulse. Digoxin slows conduction, and therefore the heart rate, and strengthens the contractions of the myocardium, thereby improving cardiac efficiency. If there are changes in pulse rate or quality, particularly if there is a decrease in rate, the digoxin should be withheld. Intake and output (1), blood pressure (3), and oxygen therapy (4) are monitored carefully during the *acute* phase of the disease, when the child is hospitalized. **IMP, ANL, 1, PhI, Reduction of risk potential**

8. (1) Vital signs, especially the pulse, that are within normal limits are the best indicators that the goal of reducing the workload of the heart to conserve energy has been achieved. Fluid balance (2) and weight stabilization (3) correlate with *nutritional* goals for a child with cardiac disease. Pink nailbeds and warm extremities (4) correlate best with *oxygenation* goals for children with cardiac disease. **EV, ANL, 6, PhI, Reduction of risk potential**

9. (3) Other children (as well as adults) can often be a source of infection for the child with cardiac disease. Although friends and family are important for the child with cardiac disease, they should have contact with the child only if they are well themselves. Extra immunizations (1) are unnecessary and do *not* provide extra protection. Prophylactic antibiotics (2) can compromise the child's immune system and actually increase vulnerability to future infections. Protective isolation (4) is costly and frightening for the child with cardiac disease, who does *not* require isolation precautions unless medically indicated. **PL, APP, 1, HPM, Health promotion and maintenance**

10. (1) The nurse should prepare the child for the stinging sensation caused by the injection of dye but *avoid* the word "dye," because it may frighten young children who may think that dying is what this procedure is about. The nurse should say "medicine" instead. Fear of the dark (2) and its associated monsters is common among preschoolers. Reassuring them that they will not be alone in the dark is essential. Preschoolers love pretend and fantasy, so turning the procedure into a "Sleeping Beauty" game (3) would appeal to the child. Even preschoolers recognize that the heart is vital to the body. Preschoolers have many body mutilation fears, so reassurance that their heart will not be cut or hurt is essential (4). **IMP, APP, 5, PsI, Psychosocial integrity**

11. (2) Assessing peripheral pulses and observing the incision site should be the nurse's first action, especially when an artery was used for catheterization. A loose dressing on an artery can cause a large blood loss from the incision site in a relatively short time. Peripheral pulses must be assessed to ensure that blood flow to the extremity is not obstructed. The child will have been NPO during the procedure with an IV to prevent dehydration, so the IV site should be assessed (1) when time permits, but this is *not* the *priority* action. The IV can usually be discontinued as soon as the child is taking adequate oral fluids. The child may have slight hypothermia (3) from being uncovered during the

---

Key to Codes

Nursing process: AS, assessment; **AN**, analysis; **PL**, planning; **IMP**, implementation; **EV**, evaluation. (See **Appendix L** for explanation of nursing process steps.)

Cognitive level: RE/KN, recall/knowledge; **COM**, comprehension; **APP**, application; **ANL**, analysis; **EVL**, evaluation; **SYN**, synthesis. (See **Appendix L** for explanation.)

Category of human function: 1, protective; **2**, sensory-perceptual; **3**, comfort, rest, activity, and mobility; **4**, nutrition; **5**, growth and development; **6**, fluid-gas transport; **7**, psychosocial-cultural; **8**, elimination. (See **Appendix N** for explanation.)

Client need: SECE, safe, effective care environment; **HPM**, health promotion and maintenance; **PsI**, psychosocial integrity; **PhI**, physiological integrity. (See **Appendix O** for explanation.)

Client subneed: See **Appendix O** for explanation.

procedure, but a blanket usually corrects this *minor* problem. Incisional pain (**4**) is usually *minimal* and can be controlled with acetaminophen. **IMP, ANL, 6, PhI, Reduction of risk potential**

12. (**4**) Digoxin should be withheld if the infant's pulse is less than 100 beats per minute; 80 beats per minute is a safe range for an older child. Timing (**1, 2**) and amount of dosage (**2, 3**) must be consistent if the child is to receive the zaximum therapeutic benefit of the digoxin therapy. This information *should* be included in the nurse's discharge instructions. **EV, APP, 6, PhI, Pharmacological and parenteral therapies**

13. (**2**) Normally, the ductus arteriosus closes spontaneously immediately following birth because of a rise in arterial oxygen saturation with respiration, and the fall in circulating prostaglandins with the removal of the placenta. For an infant with a patent, or open, ductus arteriosus, one conservative means of effecting closure is to administer the drug indomethacin, a prostaglandin inhibitor. By inhibiting prostaglandin, indomethacin allows the ductus arteriosus to close. Keeping the ductus open (**1**), enlarging the ductus (**3**), or maintaining the present size of the ductus (**4**) are undesirable because they can lead to irreversible pulmonary vascular disease. **PL, APP, 6, PhI, Pharmacological and parenteral therapies**

14. (**1**) Because it is difficult for blood to pass through the narrowed lumen of the aorta, pressure is *high* proximal to the coarctation and *low* distal to it. This results in increased blood pressure in the upper portions of the body, because of increased pressure in the subclavian artery, and decreased blood pressure in the lower extremities. High blood pressure of the upper body produces headache and vertigo; diminished blood supply to the lower extremities may cause leg pain on exertion. Tetralogy of Fallot (**2**), ventricular septal defect (**3**), and patent ductus arteriosus (**4**) require monitoring *only* of *upper* body blood pressure. Blood pressure readings should be part of *all* pediatric health screenings, especially if a congenital heart defect is suspected. **AN, APP, 6, PhI, Reduction of risk potential**

15. (**1**) If the infant vomits, the nurse should *not* repeat the dose until a pediatrician confirms that it is safe to do so. Vomiting can be an early sign of digoxin toxicity. Repeating the dose (**2, 4**) or doubling the next dose (**3**) both present a danger to the infant because some of the medication may have been absorbed before emesis. The nurse should also take care not to allow the infant to become dehydrated through loss of fluid via vomiting because the effects of digoxin on the infant's body may be altered. **IMP, APP, 6, PhI, Pharmacological and parenteral therapies**

16. (**3**) 75-80% of all small ventricular septal defects close spontaneously, usually during the first 2 years of life. As long as the infant does not experience failure-to-thrive or congestive heart failure, the repair of the ventricular septal defect can be safely delayed. If the infant were in critical condition (**1**), the infant would *not* be discharged. Many small ventricular septal defect repairs can be successfully done when the infant is older (**2**), but this can not be generalized to all infants with ventricular septal defect. Because these infants are prone to infection, immunizations (**4**) are critical, but an urgent need for surgery outweighs the need for immunizations; moreover, it is likely that surgery will be unnecessary. **IMP, APP, 7, PhI, Physiological adaptation**

17. (**2**) Polycythemia, an increase in the number of red blood cells, occurs as the body attempts to provide enough red blood cells to supply oxygen to all body parts. This is a potential danger because the increased concentration causes the blood to become too thick, and clots in the blood vessels may occur, with consequent complications of thrombophlebitis, embolism, or brain attack. Anemia (**1**), elevated white cell count (**3**), and decreased hematocrit (**4**) are *not* associated with an otherwise healthy infant with tetralogy of Fallot. **AN, ANL, 6, PhI, Reduction of risk potential.**

18. (**3**) Hypoxic or "tet" spells are caused by decreased blood supply to the brain and are usually brought about by prolonged crying, exertion, or defecation. The infant should immediately be placed in the knee-chest position, which enhances systemic venous return and, in turn, helps to dilate the right ventricle, which decreases obstruction. The other interventions listed should take place *after* positioning of the infant. Oxygen (**1**) helps relieve the hypoxia. Administering morphine (**2**) helps to decrease infundibular spasms and to calm the infant; propranolol (Inderal, a beta blocker) may also be used to reduce heart spasm. Comforting the infant (**4**) is usually of little help during the actual episode. **IMP, ANL, 6, PhI, Physiological adaptation**

19. (**3**) Clubbing of the fingers and toes (distended and flat tips) occurs because of an increase in the number of capillaries formed in the tips of extremities as the body attempts to send blood to all body parts. Informing the parents that clubbing is part of the anomaly (**1**) is accurate but does *not* explain why this is happening to their infant. Clubbing of the extremities should *not* be confused with edema of the extremities, which can be caused by dependent positions (**2**) and poor venous return (**4**). **IMP, APP, 6, PhI, Physiological adaptation**

20. (3) To ensure safety, the nurse should always verify the calculation with another staff member before administering the drug. It would be inappropriate to ask the MD to check the calculation (1). Although the nurse should *always* check *all* calculations of medications (2), the nurse giving digoxin should check the calculation with *another* nurse because of the potency of the drug. Infants *rarely* receive more than 1 mL digoxin (4), but this question says "always"; on occasion, the nurse might give more than 1 mL of this medication, but the dose should be carefully calculated and checked with another nurse before it is administered. **IMP, APP, 1, PhI, Pharmacological and Parenteral therapies**

21. (2) The normal therapeutic serum digoxin level ranges from 0.8 to 2 mcg/mL. A range of 0.8 to 2 mg/mL (3) is much higher than normal. A serum level of 10–20 mcg/mL (1) is appropriate for theophylline, *not* digoxin. A serum level of 15–30 mg/dL (4) is appropriate for salicylates, *not* digoxin. **EV, APP, 6, PhI, Pharmacological and Parenteral therapies.**

22. (2) Rheumatic fever is preceded by a recent strep infection 2–6 weeks before onset. The strep infection can take the form of a strep throat, impetigo, or scarlet fever. The nurse should make a notation of this finding in the nurse's notes and also inform the MD. Taking aspirin for a sore throat and fever (1) and a history of chickenpox (3) are *not* associated with the onset of rheumatic fever. The maternal history of mitral stenosis (4) is *unrelated* to the onset of rheumatic fever in the child. **AN, ANL, 6, PhI, Reduction of risk potential**

23. (2) Following a cardiac catheterization, the nurse must carefully monitor all the child's vital signs, but especially the pulse. In addition to placing the child on a cardiac monitor, the nurse should count the apical pulse for 1 minute for any evidence of dysrhythmia or bradycardia. Although all vital signs should be monitored after a cardiac catheterization, there is less concern regarding the temperature (1), respiration (3), or blood pressure (4). **AS, ANL, 6, PhI, Reduction of risk potential**

24. (1) Furosemide (*Lasix*) is a non-potassium-sparing loop diuretic that causes loss of potassium. A fall in the serum potassium level enhances the effects of digoxin and increases the risk of digoxin toxicity; therefore, the nurse must be particularly alert to the development of hypokalemia when caring for a child receiving both medications. There is *no* particular concern regarding sodium (2), blood sugar (3), or calcium (4) when caring for a child receiving both furosemide and digoxin. **AN, APP, 6, PhI, Pharmacological and Parenteral therapies**

Gastrointestinal Disorders

Chapter Outline

- Key Words
- Summary of Key Points
- Selected Gastrointestinal Disorders
  - Hypertrophic Pyloric Stenosis
  - Acute Gastroenteritis
  - Hirschsprung's Disease
  - Intussusception
  - Celiac Disease (Gluten-Sensitive Enteropathy)
  - Appendicitis
  - Diabetes
- Commonly Prescribed Medications
- Study and Memory Aids
- Questions
- Answers/Rationale

Key Words

abdominal girth   measurement of the circumference of the abdomen.

obstinate constipation   history of inability to have a bowel movement without stool softeners, laxatives, or enemas.

peristalsis   progressive wavelike movements that occur along the GI tract to move nutrients along from the stomach to the rectum.

projectile vomiting   forceful expulsion of stomach contents.

sphincter   a circular muscle around an opening; e.g., the pyloric sphincter is the circular muscle between the stomach and the small intestine.

Summary of Key Points

1. *Hypertrophic pyloric stenosis* is characterized by: projectile vomiting of non-bile-stained stomach contents, an olive-shaped mass in the right upper quadrant of the abdomen and metabolic alkalosis.

2. *Acute gastroenteritis* is a common acute illness in infants and young children and can quickly produce dehydration. Treatment consists of rehydration with IV fluids and/or oral rehydration therapy.

3. *Hirschsprung's disease* is characterized by obstinate constipation that persists in spite of all medical attempts at treatment; the surgical treatment is a temporary colostomy.

4. *Intussusception* is characterized by colicky abdominal pain and "currant-jelly" stools; it is most often reduced with a barium enema.

5. *Celiac disease* is characterized by a permanent intolerance for *gluten*; it is treated by a gluten-free diet.

6. *Appendicitis* is the most common *surgical emergency* in children.

7. *Appendicitis* is characterized by severe and constant pain at the McBurney point; the pain is aggravated by movement.

8. Signs and symptoms of *peritonitis* include: a rigid, board-like abdomen, guarding, fever, and shock.

9. Signs and symptoms of *obstruction of the GI tract* include: nausea and vomiting, abdominal distention, constipation, and abdominal pain.

10. Signs and symptoms of *dehydration* include: poor skin turgor, dry mucous membranes, depressed anterior fontanel, sunken eyeballs, and *decreased* urine output with *increased* specific gravity.

11. *Home care* for all children with gastrointestinal disorders: **NEVER** allow vomiting and/or diarrhea to persist for more than 12–24 hours before seeking medication attention.

Selected Gastrointestinal Disorders

See **Chapter 16** for gastrointestinal malformations (tracheoesophageal fistula) and cleft lip and palate.

Hypertrophic Pyloric Stenosis

I. *Introduction*: Pyloric stenosis is an *acquired* disorder of the *upper* GI tract, but the infant frequently does not present with symptoms until 2–4 wk. Basically the condition involves thickening, or hypertrophy, of the pyloric sphincter located at the distal end of the stomach (**Figure 9.1, p. 70**); this causes a mechanical intestinal obstruction that becomes increasingly evident as the infant begins to consume larger amounts of formula during the early weeks of life. Pyloric stenosis is 4–6 times more common in *boys* than in girls and is most often found in full-term Caucasian infants; the exact etiology remains unknown.

II. Assessment:

A. Classic symptom is *vomiting*:
1. Begins as nonprojectile at 2–4 wk.
2. Advances to projectile at 4–6 wk.
3. Vomitus is non-bile-stained (stomach contents only).
4. Most often occurs shortly *after* a feeding.
5. Major problem is the mechanical obstruction of the flow of stomach contents to the small intestine due to the anatomical defect of stenosis of the pyloric sphincter.
6. *No* apparent nausea or pain, as evidenced by the fact that infant eagerly accepts a second feeding after episode of vomiting.
7. Metabolic alkalosis develops as a result of loss of hydrochloric acid.

B. *Inspection of abdomen reveals:*
1. Palpable olive-shaped mass in right upper quadrant (RUQ).
2. Visible peristaltic waves, moving from left to right across upper abdomen.

C. *Weight*: fails to gain or loses.

D. *Stools*: constipated, diminished in number and size—due to loss of fluids with vomiting.

E. Signs of *dehydration* may become evident (**Table 9.1, p. 71**).

F. Upper GI series reveals:
1. Delayed gastric emptying.
2. Elongated and narrowed pyloric canal.

III. Analysis/nursing diagnosis:

A. *Fluid volume deficit* related to vomiting.

B. *Altered nutrition, less than body requirements*, related to vomiting.

C. *Impaired skin integrity* related to dehydration and altered nutritional state.

D. *Knowledge deficit* related to cause of disease, treatment and surgery, prognosis and follow-up care.

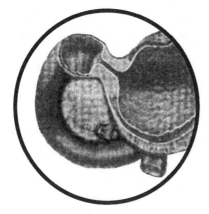

FIGURE 9.1 HYPERTROPHIC PYLORIC STENOSIS

(From *Clinical Education Aid* No. 4. Columbus, OH: Ross Laboratories. Reproduced with permission.)

IV. Nursing care plan/implementation:

A. Goal (**preoperative**): *restore fluid and electrolyte balance.*
1. Generally NPO, with IVs preop: IVs to provide fluids and electrolytes.
2. Observe and record I&O, including vomiting and stool.
3. Weight: check every 8 h or daily.
4. Monitor laboratory data especially for ↓ in *chloride* level with ↑ in *pH* and *bicarbonate* levels indicating *metabolic alkalosis.*

B. Goal: *provide adequate nutrition.*
1. Maintain NPO with IVs for 4-6 h postop, as ordered (*can* offer pacifier).
2. Follow specific *feeding regimen* ordered by MD—generally start with *clear fluids* in small amounts hourly, increasingly slowly as tolerated. Full feeding schedule reinstated within 48 h. Offer pacifier between feedings.
3. *Fed only by nurse* for 24–48 h, as vomiting tends to continue in immediate postop period.
4. *Burp* well—before, during, and after feeding.
5. *Position* after feeding: *high*-Fowler's position, turned to right side; *minimal* handling to prevent vomiting.

C. Goal (**pre- and postoperative**): *institute preventive measures to avoid infection or skin breakdown.*
1. Use good handwashing technique.
2. Administer good *skin care*, especially in diaper area (urine is highly concentrated); special care to any reddened areas.
3. Give mouth care when NPO or after vomiting.
4. Tuck diaper down *below* suture line to prevent contamination with urine (postoperatively).
5. Note condition of suture line—report any redness or discharge immediately.
6. Screen staff and visitors for any sign of infection.

D. Goal: **health teaching**. *Prepare parents to care for infant at home.*
1. Teach parent that defect is anatomic and unrelated to their parenting behavior/skill.
2. Demonstrate *feeding techniques*, and remind parent that vomiting may still occur.
3. Stress that repair is complete; condition will *never* recur.
4. Instruct parents in *care of the suture line*: no baths for 10 d, tuck diaper down, report any signs of infection promptly.
5. Offer follow-up referrals as indicated.

TABLE 9.1 SEVERITY OF CLINICAL DEHYDRATION

▶ *Clinical Assessment*	Mild	*Moderate*	*Severe*
Percent of body weight lost	Up to 5% (40–50 mL/kg)	6%–9% (60–90 mL/kg)	10% or more (100 + mL/kg)
Level of consciousness	Alert, restless, thirsty	Irritable or lethargic (*infants and very young children*); alert, thirsty, restless, (*older children and adolescents*)	Lethargic to comatose (*infants and young children*); often conscious, apprehensive (*older children and adolescents*)
Blood pressure	Normal	Normal or *low*; postural hypotension (*older children and adolescents*)	*Low* to undetectable
Pulse	Normal	*Rapid*	*Rapid, weak* to not palpable
Skin turgor	Normal	Poor	Very poor
Mucous membranes	Moist	Dry	Parched
Urine	May appear normal	*Decreased output* (< 1 mL/kg/hr) dark color, *increased* specific gravity	*Very decreased* or *absent* output
Thirst	Slightly increased	Moderately increased	Greatly increased unless lethargic
Fontanel	Normal	Sunken	Sunken
Extremities	Warm; normal capillary refill	Delayed capillary refill (> 2 sec)	Cool, discolored; delayed capillary refill (> 3–4 sec)
Respirations	Normal	Normal or rapid	Changing rate and pattern

Source: Ball J, Dinder R, *Pediatric Nursing: Caring for Children*, 3rd. ed. Prentice Hall, New Jersey.

▶ **V. Evaluation/outcome criteria:**
  A. Hydration is established and maintained pre and post operatively.
  B. Adequate nutrition is maintained, and infant begins to grow and gain weight.
  C. Skin integrity is restored.
  D. Parents verbalize confidence in their ability to care for their infant on discharge.

Acute Gastroenteritis

  I. *Introduction*: In infants and young children, acute gastroenteritis (AGE) is a very common acute illness that can rapidly progress to: dehydration, hypovolemic shock, and severe electrolyte disturbances.

▶ **II. Assessment:**
  A. *Diarrhea*: often watery, green, explosive, contains mucus and blood.
  B. Abdominal cramping and pain, often accompanied by bouts of diarrhea.
  C. *Dehydration*: see **Table 9.1**.
  D. Irritability, restlessness, alterations in level of consciousness.
  E. Electrolyte disturbances.

▶ **III. Analysis/nursing diagnosis:**
  A. *Infection* related to gastrointestinal pathogens.
  B. *Fluid volume deficit* related to vomiting and diarrhea.
  C. *Impaired skin integrity* related to diarrhea.

  D. *Knowledge deficit* regarding diagnosis, dietary restrictions, treatment.

▶ **IV. Nursing care plan/implementation:**
  A. Goal: *prevent spread of infection.*
    1. Standard precautions to prevent infection.
    2. Enforce strict handwashing.
    3. Institute and maintain *enteric precautions*—follow policies regarding linens, excretions, specimens ("double bag, special tag").
    4. Pin diapers snugly; keep patient's hands out of mouth.
    5. Obtain stool culture to identify causative organism; then administer *antibiotics* as ordered.
    6. Identify family members and others at high risk; obtain cultures.
  B. Goal: *restore fluid and electrolyte balance.*
    1. Administer IV fluids and electrolytes as ordered.
    2. Monitor for appropriate response to therapy: decreased specific gravity, good skin turgor, normal vital signs.
    3. Monitor weight, I&O, specific gravity.
    4. Oral feedings—*oral rehydration therapy* (ORT) with *Pedialyte* or comparable solution; resume normal diet as quickly as possible.
    5. Ongoing assessment of stools: note **a**mount, **c**olor, **c**onsistency, **t**iming (ACCT).
  C. Goal: *maintain or restore skin integrity.*
    1. Frequent diaper changes.

2. Keep perineal area clean and dry.

3. Apply protective ointments, e.g., petroleum jelly, A&D ointment.

4. If feasible, expose reddened buttocks to air (but *not* with explosive diarrhea).

D. Goal: **health teaching.** *Provide discharge teaching to parents:*

1. Careful review of diet to be followed at home.

2. Review principles of food preparation and storage to prevent infection.

3. Instruct in disposal of stools at home.

4. Emphasize importance of good hygiene.

V. **Evaluation/outcome criteria:**

A. No spread of infection noted.

B. Fluid and electrolyte balance normal.

C. No skin breakdown noted.

D. Parents verbalize understanding of home care.

Hirschsprung's Disease

I. *Introduction*: Hirschsprung's disease (*congenital aganglionic megacolon*) is a congenital anomaly of the *lower* GI tract, but the diagnosis is often not established until the infant is age 6–12 mo. The major problem is a *functional obstruction* of the colon caused by the congenital anatomical defect of lack of nerve cells in the walls of the colon, resulting in the absence of peristalsis (see **Figure 9.2**). Hirschsprung's disease is *four times* more common in *boys* than in girls and is frequently noted in children with *Down syndrome*.

II. **Assessment:**

A. In the newborn, failure to pass meconium in addition to other signs and symptoms of intestinal obstruction (see also discussion of cystic fibrosis, **Chapter 7**).

B. *Obstinate constipation*—history of inability to pass stool without stool softeners, laxatives, and/or enemas; persists in spite of all attempts to treat medically.

C. Stools, while infrequent, tend to be thin and ribbonlike.

D. Vomiting: bile-stained, flecked with bits of stool (breath has fecal odor), caused by GI obstruction and eventual backing-up of stools.

E. Abdominal distention can be severe enough to impinge on respirations, caused by GI obstruction and retention of stools.

F. Anorexia, nausea, irritability from severe constipation.

G. Malabsorption results in *anemia, hypoproteinemia,* and loss of subcutaneous fat.

H. Visible peristalsis and palpable fecal masses may also be detected.

III. **Analysis/nursing diagnosis:**

A. *Constipation* related to impaired bowel functioning.

B. *Altered nutrition, less than body requirements,* related to poor absorption of nutrients.

C. *Knowledge deficit* regarding care of the child with a colostomy and follow-up care pre- and postoperatively.

IV. **Nursing care plan/implementation:**

A. Goal (**preoperative**): *relieve constipation.*

1. Bowel is cleansed via a series of isotonic saline (0.9%) enemas. Amount of solution varies according to child's age.

B. Goal (**preoperative**): *promote optimal nutritional status, fluid and electrolyte balance.*

1. Monitor for signs and symptoms of progressive intestinal obstruction: measure abdominal girth daily.

2. Administer IV fluids, as ordered—may include *hyperalimentation and/or intralipids.*

3. Daily weights, I&O, urine specific gravity.

4. Monitor for possible dehydration.

5. *Diet: low* residue, *high* calorie, *high* protein.

C. Goal (**preoperative**): *assist in preparing bowel for surgery.*

1. Teach parents what will be done and why—enlist their cooperation as much as possible.

2. Insert *NG tube*, connect to low suction to achieve and maintain gastric decompression.

3. *Position*: semi-Fowler's.

4. Administer oral antibiotics, colonic irrigations to decrease bacteria.

5. Take axillary temperatures *only.*

6. If child can understand, prepare for probable colostomy using pictures, dolls (usual age at surgery is 10–16 mo).

D. (General) **Postoperative goals**: *same as for adult having major abdominal surgery or a colostomy.*

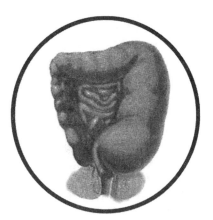

FIGURE 9.2 HIRSCHSPRUNG'S DISEASE

(From *Clinical Education Aid No. 4.* Colombus, OH: Ross Laboratories. Reproduced with permission.)

E. Goal (**postoperative**): **health teaching**. *Do discharge teaching to prepare parents to care at home for infant with a colostomy.*
  1. Home care for *colostomy* of infant is essentially same as for adult.
  2. Teach parents to keep written records of stools: number, frequency, consistency.
  3. Teach parents to tape diaper below colostomy to prevent irritation.
  4. Since colostomy is usually temporary, discuss:
      a. Second-stage repair (closure and pull-through) done when the child weighs about 20 pounds.
      b. Prepare parents for possible difficulties in toilet training.
  5. Stress need for long-term follow-up care.
  6. Make referral to home health nurse if indicated.

V. **Evaluation/outcome criteria:**
  A. Constipation is relieved preoperatively.
  B. Nutritional status is restored.
  C. Infant is prepared for surgery and tolerates procedure well.
  D. Postoperative recovery is uneventful.
  E. Parents verbalize confidence in ability to care at home for infant with a colostomy and verbalize their understanding that second surgery is needed to close the colostomy.

Intussusception

I. *Introduction*: Intussusception is the apparently *spontaneous telescoping* of one portion of the intestine into another, resulting in a mechanical obstruction of the lower GI tract (**Figure 9.3**). There is no known cause, and intussusception is *three times* more common in *boys* than in girls; the child with intussusception is usually 3–36 mo. The peak occurrence is between 5–9 months.

II. **Assessment:**
  A. Typically presents with *sudden* onset in healthy, thriving child.
  B. *Pain*: paroxysmal, colicky, abdominal, with intervals when the child appears normal and comfortable.
  C. *Stools*: "currant-jelly," (in 15-20% of children) bloody, mixed with mucus.
  D. *Vomiting* caused by intestinal obstruction.
  E. *Abdomen*: distended, tender, with palpable, sausage-shaped mass in RUQ.
  F. *Late signs*: fever, shock, signs of peritonitis as the compressed bowel wall becomes necrotic and perforates.

III. **Analysis/nursing diagnosis:**
  A. *Fluid volume deficit* related to diarrhea and vomiting.
  B. *Pain* related to bowel-wall ischemia necrosis, and death.

C. *Risk for injury/infection* related to bowel-wall perforation and peritonitis.
D. *Knowledge deficit* regarding the disease, medical and/or surgical treatment, and prognosis.

IV. **Nursing care plan/implementation:**
  A. Goal: *restore hydration status.*
    1. Obtain child's weight.
    2. Calculate % of dehydration and begin IV therapy with bolus fluids followed by maintenance fluids.
  B. Goal: *relief of pain.*
    1. Administer *analgesic* prn.
    2. Provide diversional activities.
  C. Goal: *risk of injury/infection* is minimized by early intervention.
    1. Explain to parents that a *barium enema* will be given to the child in an attempt to reduce the telescoping via hydrostatic pressure (successful in 75% of cases).
    2. Stress that, if this treatment is not successful, or if perforation of the bowel wall has already occurred, surgery is necessary.
    3. If medical treatment is apparently successful, monitor child for 24–36 h for recurrence before discharge.
    4. Stress that recurrence is rare (10%) and most often occurs within the first 24–36 h after reduction.
  D. Goal: *do pre and post operative and discharge teaching.*
    1. Same as for an adult with major abdominal surgery.

V. **Evaluation/outcome criteria:**
  A. Hydration status is restored.
  B. Child is pain-free upon discharge.
  C. Child tolerates medical-surgical treatment and recovers without incident (e.g. injury/infection).
  D. Parents verbalize confidence in ability to care for child after discharge.

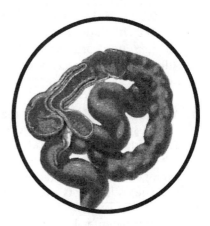

FIGURE 9.3 INTUSSUSCEPTION

(From *Clinical Education Aid No. 4.* Colombus, OH: Ross Laboratories. Reproduced with permission.)

Celiac Disease (Gluten–Sensitive Enteropathy)

I. *Introduction*: Celiac disease is a *malabsorption syndrome* characterized by abnormal mucosa in the small intestine and results in a *permanent* intolerance to gluten. Gluten is found in the grain of wheat, barley, rye, and oats. The exact incidence of celiac disease is unknown because statistics vary greatly from 1:3000-1:4000 population. Celiac disease is seen less frequently in the United States than in Europe, and is *rare* in African-Americans and Asians. A chronic disease whose severity varies greatly among children, celiac disease seems to cause the most severe symptoms in early childhood (*1–5 yr*) and again in the *adult* years.

II. **Assessment:**

A. *Stool*: steatorrhea, foul-smelling stools; chronic diarrhea.

B. *GI*: anorexia, nausea, vomiting, abdominal pain.

C. *Nutritional status*: slow or no weight gain, failure to grow, malnourishment, abdominal distention, muscle wasting, anemia, and secondary vitamin deficiencies.

D. *Behavioral changes*: irritable, cranky, uncooperative, becoming apathetic and lethargic.

E. *Diagnostic procedures:* stool collection, jejunal biopsy, gluten challenge.

III. **Analysis/nursing diagnosis:**

A. *Risk for injury* related to intestinal mucosa irritation.

B. *Altered nutrition*, less than body requirements, related to malabsorption syndrome.

C. *Altered family processes* related to care of the child with a chronic illness.

IV. **Nursing care plan/implementation:**

A. Goal: *decrease intestinal mucosa irritation.*

1. *Diet*: gluten-free
   a. *Avoid*: wheat, rye, barley, oats (**Table 9.2, p. 75** lists hidden sources of gluten in a child's diet).
   b. *Substitute*: corn, rice, millet.

2. Administer *steroids* (i.e., prednisone) per MD order.

B. Goal: *provide adequate nutrition.*

1. Administer supplements as ordered to correct specific nutritional deficiencies such as: *iron* deficiency, *folic acid* deficiency, *fat-soluble* vitamin deficiencies.

2. Arrange dietary consultation to select foods that the child prefers and that are allowed on gluten-free diet.

3. Monitor parenteral nutrition if ordered by MD.

C. Goal: **health teaching**. *Teach child/family self-management in preparation for discharge and home care.*

1. Discuss why gluten must be eliminated, or minimized, in the diet; discuss pathophysiology.

2. Provide written information concerning diet, including foods to be avoided as well as acceptable substitutes. Encourage new recipes with acceptable substitutes.

3. Stress the importance of carefully reading food labels to discover hidden sources of gluten.

4. Give referrals as needed, including dietician and home care.

V. **Evaluation/outcome criteria:**

A. Intestinal mucosa is irritation–free.

B. No evidence of malabsorption is noted and nutritional status improves.

C. Child and family comply with dietary restrictions and family processes are restored.

Appendicitis

I. *Introduction*: Appendicitis is defined as inflammation of the appendix, a small sac at the end of the cecum. It is the most common surgical emergency in children, and occurs most often in *children 10–12 yr of age*. Although early diagnosis is essential to prevent perforation and peritonitis, diagnosis is frequently delayed because children may be unable to verbalize symptoms accurately. The exact cause of appendicitis is unknown, but it is usually related to a fecalith (hardened feces) within the lumen of the appendix. After a simple appendectomy, complications are rare and recovery is generally rapid and complete. After *perforation*, mortality is rare (1%), but morbidity from *peritonitis* and wound abscesses is high.

II. **Assessment:**

A. *GI*: abdominal pain, tenderness, guarding; the pain becomes localized to the *McBurney* point (midway between the right anterior superior iliac crest and the umbilicus, in the right lower quadrant [RLQ]); the pain is described as severe and constant, aggravated by movement; after the pain starts, the child may complain of nausea, vomiting, and anorexia as well as diarrhea (or constipation).

B. *Systemic*: lethargy, irritability, pallor, complaints of difficulty walking, low-grade fever.

C. *Perforation*: fever higher than 102°F, sudden relief from pain later followed by: increase in diffuse pain, rigid abdomen, distention, chills, rapid shallow breathing, irritability and restlessness, absence of bowel sounds.

D. Lab: white blood cell count generally *elevated* to 15,000-20,000 mm³ with a *shift to the left* as indicated by increased bands; abdominal x-rays.

III. Analysis/nursing diagnosis:
  A. *Pain* related to inflammation of the appendix.
  B. *High risk for fluid volume deficit* related to decreased intake (anorexia and nausea) and increased output (vomiting).
  C. *High risk for injury* related to possible perforation.
  D. **With perforation:** *Infection* related to infectious organisms present within abdominal cavity.

IV. Nursing care plan/implementation:
  A. Goal: *relieve pain.*
    1. Allow child to assume a comfortable position.
    2. Administer *analgesics* as ordered and monitor effects.
    3. Prepare child for surgery as soon as possible.
  B. Goal: *restore fluid and electrolyte balance.*
    1. Generally NPO preoperatively with IVs to provide fluids and electrolytes; maintain integrity of IV site and maintain desired drip rate.
    2. Observe and record I&O, *urine specific gravity*, vomiting, and stool.
    3. Weight: monitor every 8 h or daily.
    4. Monitor laboratory data.
  C. Goal: *prevent perforation.*
    1. Assist with diagnostic procedures to ensure rapid diagnosis.
    2. Prepare for surgery as quickly as possible to ensure rapid treatment.
    3. *Avoid* palpating the abdomen.
  D. Goal (**with perforation**): *treat infection and prevent spread of infection.*

TABLE 9.2 🍎 HIDDEN SOURCES OF GLUTEN IN A CHILD'S DIET

Bread
Breakfast cereals
Cake, cookies, crackers
Catsup
Chocolate candy (certain types)
Doughnuts, pies
Gravy
Hamburgers, (commercially prepared)
Hot dogs, luncheon meats
Hydrolyzed vegetable protein
Ice cream, processed
Malted milk
Malt flavoring
Mayonnaise
Modified food starch
Soups, (commercially prepared, instant)
Spaghetti, pizza
Vinegar (*except* apple cider vinegar)

---

    1. *Position*: *low*-Fowler's position to localize infection and prevent upward spread.
    2. IV antibiotics, including *gentamicin, ampicillin*, and *metronidazole* or *clindamycin*.
    3. If infection is present, provide care of the drain and surrounding skin; *care of wound*, and proper disposal of infected, soiled dressings; maintenance of NG tube for gastric decompression.

V. Evaluation/outcome criteria:
  A. Discomfort is relieved.
  B. Fluid and electrolyte balance is restored.
  C. Perforation is prevented.
  D. **With perforation**: infection remains localized to the RLQ of the abdomen.

Diabetes

I. *Introduction*: Diabetes refers to a *heterogeneous* group of diseases involving the disruption of the metabolism of *carbohydrates, fats and protein.* If uncontrolled, serious vascular and neurologic changes occur. Both types of diabetes occur in children/adolescents. (See **Table 9.3, p. 76**)

II. **Types:**
  A. *Type 1*: *Previously* known as: insulin-dependent diabetes mellitus (**IDDM**) and as juvenile-onset or Type I. Characterized by destruction of pancreatic beta cells leading to absolute insulin deficiency. Believed to be *autoimmune* in nature; usually found in children/adolescents under the age of 20 yr.
  B. *Type 2*: *Previously* known as: non-insulin-dependent diabetes mellitus (**NIDDM**); adult-onset, maturity-onset diabetes of the young (**MODY**) or **Type II.** Characterized by insulin resistance and/or insulin secretory defect in the pancreas leading to relative insulin deficiency. Believed to be an *inherited* defect; usually found in children/adolescents under age of 25 yr. in ethnic minority populations (e.g. African-American, Hispanic-American, Asian-American or Native American).

III. **Pathophysiology:**
  A. *Type 1: absolute* deficiency of insulin as a result of destruction of pancreatic beta cells caused by the interaction of genetic, environmental and autoimmune factors.
  B. *Type 2*: relative deficiency of insulin as a result of insulin *resistance* and/or insulin *secretory defect* caused by *heredity* and *lifestyle* factors.

IV. **Risk factors/causes:**
  A. *Type 1*: genetic predisposition (e.g., child/adolescent inherits a susceptibility to the disease rather than the disease itself); exposure to a precipitating event (e.g., *viral infection*).
  B. *Type 2:* first-degree relative with type 2 disease; obesity; sedentary/low exercise lifestyle; ethnicity.

TABLE 9.3 COMPARISON OF TYPE 1 AND TYPE 2 DIABETES MELLITUS IN CHILDREN/ADOLESCENTS

	Type 1	Type 2
Age	↓ 20 yr. of age; *girls*: 10–12 yr. *boys*: 12–14 yr. ⟩ peak	↓ 25 yr. of age; Peaks in adolescence
Onset	Sudden	Gradual
Contributing factors	Occasional family history. Ethnic distribution: primarily Caucasian population	Frequent family history. Ethnic distribution: primarily minority populations
Weight	Underweight with recent weight loss	Overweight especially with central adiposity
Insulin values	Pancreatic content: none. Serum insulin: *low – absent*. Primary resistance: minimum	Pancreatic content: 50% normal. Serum insulin: *high–low*. Primary resistance: marked
Treatment	Insulin: required for remainder of life. Oral agents: *not* effective. Diet only: *not* effective	Insulin: required by 20–30% of clients or during acute illnesses/surgery/etc. Oral agents: often effective. Diet only: often effective
Complications	Nephropathy, neuropathy, retinopathy (the earlier the onset of Type 1 DM, the earlier the onset of complications)	Variable
Ketoacidosis	Frequent	Infrequent

Source: Adapted from *Wong's Nursing Care of Infants and Children*, 7th ed. St. Louis, Mosby.

V. Assessment:
   A. *Type 1*: polyuria, polydipsia and polyphagia (**3 P's**) with significant weight loss. Unexplained fatigue/lethargy, headaches, stomach aches, occasional enuresis in a child who was previously toilet-trained. *Candida vaginitis* in adolescent girls.
   B. *Type 2*: polyuria, polydipsia and polyphagia (**3 P's**) may be mild to absent with little or no weight loss or obesity. *Acanthosis nigricans* (e.g., hyperpigmentation and thickening of skin with velvety irregularities in skin folds of neck, axillae, elbows, knees, groin, abdomen); lipid disorders, hypertension; androgen-mediated disorders (e.g., acne, hirsutism, menstrual disturbances, polycystic ovary disease).
   C. *Laboratory values for* diagnosis of all types of diabetes mellitus in children/adolescents:
      1. Symptoms of diabetes (**3 P's**) plus plasma glucose concentration >200mg/dL taken at any time of the day regardless of time of last meal.
      2. Fasting plasma glucose >126mg/dL with no caloric intake for at least 8 hours.
      3. Two-hour plasma glucose >200mg/dL during an oral glucose tolerance test.
      Note: diagnosis of *type 1* includes unexplained weight loss; diagnosis of *type 2* includes *acanthosis nigricans* and obesity.

VI. Analysis/nursing diagnosis:
   A. *Knowledge deficit* (child/adolescent and parents), related to lack of exposure to diabetic management in the newly diagnosed child/adolescent.
   B. *Risk for injury* related to periods of hypoglycemia and ketoacidosis.
   C. *Risk for altered nutrition,* less than body requirements, related to glycosuria.
   D. *Altered family processes* related to management of a chronic disease.
   E. *Ineffective individual coping* related to inadequate level of confidence in ability to cope.
   F. *Health seeking behaviors* (child/adolescent), related to learning self-management of chronic disorder.

VII. Nursing care plan/implementation:
   A. Goal: *acquire appropriate knowledge skills for home management.*
      1. Assess developmental level and select an age-appropriate approach (see **Table 9.5, p. 77**).
      2. Teach how to monitor vital signs, blood glucose, insulin injection, food guidelines, when to call pediatrician.
      3. Use demonstration/return demonstration until goal is achieved.
   B. Goal: *promote safety and prevention of injury.*
      1. Teach signs and symptoms of hypoglycemia and ketoacidosis and appropriate care.
         a. *Hypoglycemia* (see **Table 9.4, p. 77**): "quick sugar" followed by complex carbohydrate and protein.
         b. *Ketoacidosis*: insulin, fluids, electrolyte replacement.

(continued on p.78)

TABLE 9.4 COMPARISON OF DIABETIC COMPLICATIONS IN CHILDREN/ADOLESCENTS

	Hypoglycemia	*Hyperglycemia*
Risk factors/causes	1. Insulin dose too high for food eaten. 2. Insulin injected into muscle. 3. Too much exercise for insulin dose. 4. Too few carbohydrates eaten. 5. Illness (especially vomiting/diarrhea). 6. Emotional stress.	1. Insulin dose too low for food eaten. 2. Insulin injected just under skin or into hypertrophied areas. 3. Too little/decreased *activity*. 4. Too many carbohydrates eaten. 5. Illness. 6. Emotional stress.
Assessment: signs and symptoms	*Rapid onset* 1. Irritability, nervousness, tremors, "shaky", difficulty concentrating/speaking, confusion, repetitive speech. 2. Shallow breathing. 3. Diaphoretic, pale skin. 4. Moist mucous membranes. 5. Hunger. 6. Headache, blurred vision. 7. Tachycardia. 8. Mouth: lips/tongue tingling. 9. Coma.	*Gradual onset* 1. Lethargy, sleepiness, slowed responses, confusion, shock. 2. Rapid breathing. 3. Flushed, dry skin. 4. Dry mucous membranes. 5. Hunger and thirst (dehydration). 6. Headache, blurred vision. 7. Weaker, slowed heart rate. 8. Mouth: fruity odor to breath. 9. Coma.
Management	1. If conscious, give 15g of carbohydrate (e.g., orange juice, raisins, glucose tablets). Wait 15 minutes and re-check blood glucose level. Give another 15g of carbohydrate if < 70mg/dL. Re-check blood glucose level in 15 minutes. 2. When blood glucose level returns to 80mg/dL, give cheese/milk and crackers snack (especially important if meal will be eaten more than 30 minutes later or activity/exercise is planned). 3. If unconscious, administer *glucagon* (IM or SQ).	1. Additional *insulin* given at usual injection time. 2. *Sliding* scale insulin for specific blood glucose levels when ill/injured. 3. *Extra* injections if hyperglycemia and moderate to large ketones. 4. Increase fluids.

Source: Adapted from Ball J, Bindler P, *Pediatric Nursing; Caring from Children*, New Jersey, Prentice Hall.

TABLE 9.5 APPROPRIATE AGES AND DEVELOPMENTAL STAGES TO INITIATE DIABETES MELLITUS TECHNICAL SKILL TRAINING

Skill	Age	Developmental Stage
Urine testing	4–6 yr	*Initiative*; is toilet-trained and has fine motor skills and attention span needed to perform this task.
Blood testing	4–8 yr	*Industry*; has overcome body mutilation fears associated with "sticking" self; likes to "make" things work (e.g., glucose meter); has fine motor skills and attention span needed to perform this task.
Insulin injections	8–10 yr	*Industry*; wants to care for own needs; requires supervision but has fine motor skills and attention span needed to perform this task.
Nutrition and management decision	10–14 yr 12–28 yr	*Identity*; has hypothetical and abstract thinking abilities; must assume control and responsibility for actions and choices.

Adapted from Potts N, Mandleco B, *Pediatrics Nursing: Caring for Children and their Families*, 1st ed., Delmar, New York.

2. Wear MedicAlert bracelet; investigate implanted insulin pump in adolescence or transplant.

C. Goal: *well-balanced diet and achievement of normal weight and height.*
1. Plot weight and height regularly.
2. Consult nutritionist for appropriate list of foods; eat meals and snacks on schedule; 50–60% carbohydrates, 10–20% protein, 20–30% fat is recommended balance; implement exchange or carbohydrate counting food systems; supervised weight loss if recommended by pediatrician.
3. Vitamin supplements if recommended by pediatrician.

D. Goal: *family will manage the required medical regime.*
1. Evaluate family's lifestyle and modify as necessary.
2. Include ways to handle *"special occasions"* (e.g., birthdays and holidays) and vacations.

E. Goal: *child/adolescent will demonstrate coping skills.*
1. Identify *"stressors"*.
2. Teach coping skills via role-playing and problem solving.
3. Encourage involvement in previous social activities and hobbies while encouraging involvement in "diabetic" social activities and hobbies (e.g., DM summer camp, support group, etc.)

F. Goal: **health teaching.** *Help child/adolescent to develop independent ability to manage diabetic care.*
1. Teach what food is "allowed" as well as what is "restricted".
2. Teach administration of *medications* as well as desired and side effects, action, site rotation, etc.
3. Teach signs and symptoms of *complications* (see **Table 9.4, p. 77**).
4. Teach importance of *preventative* health care (e.g., compliance, exercise, routine check-ups, vision care, prevention of infection [especially foot/nail care]).

VIII. **Evaluation/outcome criteria:**
A. Demonstrates proper techniques of DM care.
B. Describes accurately and treats appropriately adverse signs and symptoms and prevents injury.
C. Demonstrates appropriate dietary choices as well as maintenance of age and condition-appropriate weight.
D. Minimal lifestyle changes made by family.
E. Child/adolescent demonstrates appropriate coping skills and positive attitude toward self.
F. Child/adolescent demonstrates age-appropriate self-management.

COMMONLY PRESCRIBED MEDICATIONS

Medication	Administration	Use/Action	Nursing Considerations
Antidiabetics: **Insulins:** **Intermediate Acting/** *NPH; Lente* **Long Acting/** *Ultralente; Lantos/ insulin glargine* **Rapid Acting/***Lispro; Humalog* **Short Acting/Regular**	• SQ ONLY except for regular insulin which can be given IV/IM for ketoacidosis • Calculate child's weight in kilograms • Evaluate dosage according to: child's weight, blood glucose level (BGL), nutritional and activity status • Administer in specially calibrated syringe	Used in treatment of insulin-dependent type 1 diabetes mellitus; Non-insulin-dependent type 2 diabetes mellitus when diet/ weight control therapy has failed to maintain satisfactory blood glucose levels (BGL) Also used in: acute situations, such as ketoacidosis, severe infections; major surgery for those who are otherwise non-insulin-dependent; individuals receiving parenteral nutrition Binds to cell surface receptors	Check dosage with another nurse prior to administration Check blood glucose level (BGL) and administer approximately 30 minutes *prior* to meal Dosage is highly individualized in children Teach rotation of sites
Biguanides Metformin/*Glucophage*	• Oral • Calculate child's weight in kilograms • Maximum dose in children is 2,000mg/ day • Can be monotherapy or given together with insulin	Used in treatment of non-insulin-dependent type 2 diabetes mellitus when hyperglycemia cannot be managed by diet/ weight loss/exercise alone Decreases liver production of glucose Decreases absorption of glucose Improves insulin sensitivity	Assess for lactic acidosis (hyperventilation, muscle aches, tiredness) Do **not** skip or delay meals Be alert to conditions (e.g., fevers, increased activity, surgery) that alter glucose requirements

(continued)

COMMONLY PRESCRIBED MEDICATIONS   *(continued)*

Medication	Administration	Use/Action	Nursing Considerations
Antiemetics: Dimenhydrinate/ *Dramamine* Metoclopramide/ *Reglan* Ondansetron/*Zofran* Promethazine/ *Phenergan* Trimethobenzamide/ *Tigan*	• Oral, rectal and parenteral • Calculate to child's weight in kilograms • Administer in provided dropper or calibrated syringe • **NEVER** in household measuring spoon	Used in *vomiting* that can be caused by improper feeding techniques, GI obstruction, infection or emotional factors Blocks receptors in chemoreceptor trigger zone (*Zofran* and *Tigan*) Enhances gastroduodenal peristalsis (*Reglan*) Competes for hi-receptor sites (*Phenergan*) Depresses labyrinthine and vestibular function (*Dramamine*)	Assess hydration status Assess for peristalsis Do **not** give in the presence of persistent vomiting Relief is usually experienced in 30 minutes Can cause drowsiness, dry mouth and paradoxical reactions in children

Study and Memory Aids

Pyloric Stenosis—Postoperative Care

Position: high-Fowler's, right side
Minimal handling to prevent emesis

Hirschsprung's—Assessment

Newborn: Meconium ileus

Stool—Assessment: ACCT

Amount
Color
Consistency
Timing

Barium Enema—Purpose in Intussusception

1. Visualization
2. Mechanical reduction by hydrostatic pressure

Surgical Emergency in Children

The most common is *appendicitis*

Appendicitis—Assessment

Severe, constant pain at *McBurney* point

Appendicitis—Warning

Sudden relief from pain—perforation, peritonitis

Questions

1. When taking the health history from the parents of an infant with pyloric stenosis, which classic symptom would the nurse expect to hear the parents describe?
   1. Chronic diarrhea.
   2. Chronic constipation.
   3. Refusal to eat after vomiting.
   4. Vomiting after a feeding.

2. Which evidence provides the nurse with essential evaluation criteria needed to establish the diagnosis of pyloric stenosis?
   1. Hematest-positive stool.
   2. Hematest-positive urine.
   3. Non-bile-stained vomitus.
   4. Bile-stained vomitus.

3. The mother of an infant with pyloric stenosis tells the nurse, "I feel like such a failure. My baby vomits everything that I feed him." The nurse's best response is:
   1. "The vomiting will stop as soon as your baby has the necessary surgery."
   2. "Show me how you feed the baby."
   3. "Does he vomit when his father feeds him?"
   4. "You sound frustrated. Let's talk about your feelings."

4. The major preoperative nursing concern for an infant with pyloric stenosis is:
   1. *Fluid volume deficit* related to vomiting.
   2. *Pain* related to abdominal cramping.
   3. *Anxiety* related to medical condition.
   4. *Altered nutrition*, less than body requirements, related to vomiting.

5. When feedings are resumed postoperatively for an infant with pyloric stenosis, the nurse should:
   1. Begin with small amounts of clear fluids.
   2. Begin with small spoonfuls of thickened cereal.
   3. Begin with small amounts of half-strength formula.
   4. Resume per feeding the amount appropriate for the infant's chronologic age.

6. A 10-month-old infant is admitted to the pediatric unit to rule out Hirschsprung's disease. The nurse should expect the infant's stools to be:
   1. Watery, green in appearance.
   2. Currant-jellylike in appearance.
   3. Steatorrheac in appearance.
   4. Ribbonlike in appearance.

7. The ultimate goal of nursing care for a child with Hirschsprung's disease is to:
   1. Reduce the trauma induced by daily enemas.
   2. Teach the family how to plan an age-appropriate, low fiber diet.
   3. Prepare the child and family for surgical removal of the affected portion of bowel.
   4. Assist the child and family in accepting the permanent need for colostomy.

8. Following a rectal biopsy that confirms the diagnosis of Hirschsprung's disease, a child is to begin on daily enemas. Which selection, made by the child's parents, indicates that they have understood the nurse's teaching regarding the type of solution to be administered?
   1. Tap water.
   2. Normal saline.
   3. Soap suds.
   4. Pediatric Fleet preparation.

9. The nurse prepares to administer an isotonic enema to a 3-year-old child with Hirschsprung's disease. The nurse could safely administer:
   1. 480-720 mL.
   2. 360-480 mL.
   3. 240-360 mL.
   4. 120-240 mL.

10. Immediately after the creation of a temporary colostomy for Hirschsprung's disease, the nurse's priority assessment is for:
    1. Constipation.
    2. Infection control.
    3. Nutritional status.
    4. Patency of the nasogastric tube.

11. Which nursing intervention is most effective in preparing a 3-year-old child for the second-stage repair (closure and pull-through) of a colostomy done for Hirschsprung's disease?
    1. A verbal explanation.
    2. A diagram of a child with a colostomy.
    3. A video of the procedure.
    4. A teaching doll with a colostomy.

12. A 3-year-old child has just undergone a second-stage repair (closure and pull-through) of a colostomy originally done for Hirschsprung's disease. Which order for this child, written by the pediatrician, should the nurse question?
    1. Bilateral wrist restraints.
    2. Nasogastric tube connected to low, intermittent suction.
    3. Turn every 2 hours.
    4. Rectal temperature every 4 hours.

13. The nurse should suspect intussusception in an infant who experiences:
    1. Constipation.
    2. Bloody diarrhea.
    3. Projectile vomiting and an olive-shaped mass in the epigastric area.
    4. Sudden onset of vomiting and severe, crampy, abdominal pain.

14. A 6-month-old infant with suspected intussusception passes a "currant jelly" stool. The nurse's first action is to:
    1. Note this finding in the patient's chart.
    2. Notify the pediatrician.
    3. Hematest the stool.
    4. Ask the parents to sign a surgical consent form for an immediate abdominal exploration.

15. Which statement made by the parents of an infant with intussusception indicates that they have understood the nurse's teaching regarding the rationale for a barium enema as a treatment modality?
    1. "The pressure of the barium enema may return our baby's bowel back to its normal position."
    2. "The barium enema will relieve our baby's constipation."
    3. "The pressure of the barium enema will stop our baby's bowel from bleeding."
    4. "The barium enema will prevent our baby from needing abdominal surgery."

16. Which finding, when a diaper check is performed, should alert the nurse that an infant with intussusception is successfully passing the barium left in the infant's bowel following a barium enema?
    1. A green, watery stool.
    2. A bulky, greasy stool.
    3. A black, tarry stool.
    4. A grayish-white stool.

17. An infant is admitted to the pediatric unit for dehydration caused by acute gastroenteritis. The priority nursing intervention is to:
    1. Obtain the infant's blood pressure.
    2. Take the infant's pulse.
    3. Weigh the infant.
    4. Check the infant's skin turgor.

18. The priority goal of nursing care for an infant with acute gastroenteritis is to:
    1. Rehydrate the infant.
    2. Contain the causative agent via enteric precautions.
    3. Restore skin integrity of the buttocks.
    4. Teach the parents how to prevent future occurrences.

19. When discharging an infant with acute gastroenteritis from the hospital, the nurse should instruct the parents that if diarrhea recurs, which fluid should they refrain from giving their infant?
    1. Water.
    2. Similac.
    3. Pedialyte.
    4. Rehydrate.

20. An 8-year-old child with type 1 diabetes actively played during recess but presents to the school nurse with complaints of a headache and feeling "shaky." The nurse's first action should be to:
    1. Notify the child's parents.
    2. Have the child lie down for a few minutes and see whether the symptoms subside.
    3. Give the child a simple-carbohydrate snack.
    4. Give the child a complex-carbohydrate and protein snack.

21. A 10-year-old with newly diagnosed type 1 diabetes asks why he must take "shots" every day, when his aunt with diabetes "gets to take pills." The nurse's best response is:
    1. "When you get older, you can take the pills, too."
    2. "When your pancreas gets bigger, you will be able to stop taking the shots."
    3. "You have a different type of diabetes than your aunt does. Your type needs insulin shots every day."
    4. "You don't understand diabetes. Have you read the pamphlet I gave you?"

22. Which characteristic of an adolescent must the nurse first consider in order to assist the teenager to deal with the diagnosis of type 1 diabetes?
    1. Desire for independence.
    2. Goals for the future.
    3. Need to be like peers.
    4. Wish to please parents.

Answers/Rationale

1. **(4)** Vomiting after a feeding is the classic symptom of pyloric stenosis. The emesis is usually projectile in nature. Diarrhea (**1**) is *not* associated with pyloric stenosis because there is a mechanical obstruction of the flow of stomach contents to the small intestine. Constipation (**2**) is a *secondary* symptom of pyloric stenosis and is caused by loss of fluids with vomiting. The infant usually *eagerly accepts* a second feeding after an episode of vomiting (**3**). **AS, COM, 4, PhI, Physiological adaptation**

2. **(3)** The vomitus contains no bile because the constriction is proximal to the ampulla of Vater, the site at which the common bile duct enters the duodenum. Blood-tinged stool (**1**) and urine (**2**) are *not* usually consistent with pyloric stenosis (however, on rare occasion, there is blood-tinged vomitus from the force and pressure of the emesis or the concurrent gastritis that can accompany pyloric stenosis). Bile-stained emesis (**4**) is *not* consistent with pyloric stenosis. **EV, ANL, 4, PhI, Physiological adaptation**

3. **(4)** Acknowledging the mother's feelings and offering her the opportunity to talk about her frustrations when attempting to feed her infant is a therapeutic, open response. Informing the mother that the vomiting will cease after the surgery (**1**) is accurate but *does not acknowledge* the mother's feelings and frustrations, and is *not* therapeutic. Asking to see how the mother feeds the baby (**2**), or if the baby vomits when fed by others (**3**), demonstrates a *lack of knowledge* regarding pyloric stenosis on the nurse's part, and may cause the mother to believe that she is doing "something wrong." Infants with pyloric stenosis vomit *regardless* of who feeds them *until* they are repaired surgically. **IMP, ANL, 4, PsI, Psychosocial integrity**

4. **(1)** Preoperatively, the emphasis is placed on restoring hydration and electrolyte balance. The infant is NPO, and an IV of sodium chloride, glucose, and electrolytes is administered (potassium is usually added when there is adequate urinary output). Pain (**2**) is *not* a preoperative component in pyloric stenosis. Anxiety (**3**) is always present during hospitalization but is a *secondary* concern until fluid and electrolyte balance is restored. Altered nutrition (**4**) is a concern, but because oral feeding cannot be resumed until approximately 8–12 hours after surgery, vomiting is unlikely immediately after surgery. **AN, APP, 4, PhI, Physiological adaptation**

5. **(1)** The nurse should begin feeding the infant small amounts of clear fluids at intervals determined by the pediatrician. The infant should be fed in an upright position, burped before, during, and after feeding, and not handled excessively. A pacifier may be offered between feedings. Thickened cereal (**2**) or half-strength formula (**3**) may be added to the infant's feeding regime as incisional healing occurs but *not* for *initial* feedings. The infant must be slowly advanced in resuming feeding; determining the amount by the infant's chronologic age (**4**) increases the risk of vomiting. **IMP, ANL, 4, PhI, Basic care and comfort**

6. **(4)** Ribbonlike stools are associated with Hirschsprung's disease because the stool must pass through areas of chronically constipated/impacted feces and through the narrow aganglionic distal segment of the bowel. Watery, green stools (**1**) indicate gastrointestinal *infections*. Currant-jellylike

---

Key to Codes

Nursing process: AS, assessment; **AN**, analysis; **PL**, planning; **IMP**, implementation; **EV**, evaluation. (See **Appendix L** for explanation of nursing process steps.)

Cognitive level: RE/KN, recall/knowledge; **COM**, comprehension; **APP**, application; **ANL**, analysis; **EVL**, evaluation; **SYN**, synthesis. (See **Appendix L** for explanation.)

Category of human function: 1, protective; **2**, sensory-perceptual; **3**, comfort, rest, activity, and mobility; **4**, nutrition; **5**, growth and development; **6**, fluid-gas transport; **7**, psychosocial-cultural; **8**, elimination. (See **Appendix N** for explanation.)

Client need: SECE, safe, effective care environment; **HPM**, health promotion and maintenance; **PsI**, psychosocial integrity; **PhI**, physiological integrity. (See **Appendix O** for explanation.)

Client subneed: See **Appendix O** for explanation.

stools (**2**) are associated with *intussusception*. Streatorrheac stools (**3**) are associated with conditions in which there is an alteration in fat metabolism, such as *cystic fibrosis*. **AS, ANL, 8, PhI, Basic care and comfort**

7. (**3**) The ultimate goal of nursing care is to promote a normal elimination pattern via the rectum by removing the diseased portion of the bowel. Measures to reduce the trauma of daily enemas (**1**) and learn about the necessary low fiber diet (**2**) are appropriate *interim* goals for a child with Hirschsprung's disease. Colostomy (**4**) is usually *temporary*. **PL, ANL, 8, PhI, Basic care and comfort**

8. (**2**) Normal saline is the choice for a child with Hirschsprung's disease because the child retains some of the solution, which will be absorbed through the bowel wall; the isotonic nature of the solution does *not* alter the child's fluid balance or lead to water intoxication. Tap water (**1**), soap suds (**3**) and pediatric Fleet preparation (**4**) are nonisotonic solutions that could *alter* the child's fluid balance or *lead to water intoxication*. **EV, ANL, 8, PhI, Reduction of risk potential**

9. (**3**) 240–360 mL may safely be administered to a 2–4-year-old child. 480–720 mL (**1**) is the correct amount of solution for children *11 years* of age and older. 360–480 mL (**2**) is the correct amount for children 4–10 years of age. 120–240 mL (**4**) is the correct amount for *infants*. **IMP, APP, 8, PhI, Reduction of risk potential**

10. (**4**) Patency of the nasogastric tube is critical to achieve and maintain gastric decompression until bowel motility resumes. Constipation (**1**), infection control (**2**), and nutritional status (**3**) are appropriate postoperative concerns but are *not* the nurse's *primary* focus of assessment. **AS, ANL, 8, PhI, Reduction of risk potential**

11. (**4**) Preschoolers are especially receptive to therapeutic play and teaching by use of dolls that the children can manipulate and experiment with. This method heightens their sense of control and comprehension when faced with stressful situations such as surgery. Verbal explanations (**1**), diagrams (**2**), and videos (**3**) are interventions better suited to *school-aged* children and *adolescents* who have more highly developed cognitive abilities. **IMP, APP, 5, HPM, Health promotion and maintenance**

12. (**4**) Rectal temperatures and rectal examinations must *not* be done postoperatively because of the possibility of traumatizing the surgical site. Wrist restraints (**1**) *are* usually in place to prevent the child from dislodging various tubes. A nasogastric tube (**2**) *is* in place to decompress the stomach and prevent pressure from a distended abdomen on the suture line. The nasogastric tube also reduces feelings of nausea and prevents vomiting. Frequent changes of position (**3**) *do* prevent atelectasis or pneumonia from developing. **AN, APP, 8, SECE, Management of care**

13. (**4**) Intussusception has symptoms that are frightening and disturbing to parents because an otherwise healthy infant suddenly shows symptoms of severe abdominal pain that recur at frequent intervals and is usually accompanied by vomiting. Constipation (**1**) and bloody diarrhea (**2**) are *not* associated with intussusception, but can be discriminating symptoms of other gastrointestinal disturbances. Projectile vomiting and an olive-shaped mass in the epigastric area (**3**) are associated with *pyloric stenosis*. **AS, COM, 8, PhI, Physiological adaptation**

14. (**2**) A "currant jelly" stool (a mix of blood and mucus as a result of intestinal irritation) occurs in approximately 50% of all patients with intussusception and indicates that the infant's condition has worsened. The pediatrician should be notified as soon as possible. Noting this finding in the client's chart (**1**) and hematesting the stool (**3**) are appropriate *secondary* nursing interventions. Initiating getting parental consent for surgery (**4**) is *not* the nurse's role at this time; other conservative measures, such as a barium enema, may be tried before subjecting the infant to surgery. **AN, ANL, 8, PhI, Physiological adaptation**

15. (**1**) The hydrostatic pressure of the barium enema can result in extension of the bowel to its normal position. The success rate for this procedure is approximately *70%* if done within the first 24 hours of the onset of symptoms. Constipation (**2**) is *not* associated with intussusception. Beliefs that a barium enema stops intestinal bleeding (**3**) or prevents additional abdominal surgery (**4**) are *incorrect* and indicate the need for additional teaching. **EV, APP, 8, PhI, Physiological adaptation**

16. (**4**) Barium causes feces to become grayish-white. It is essential that all the barium be removed from the bowel or additional obstruction may occur. A green, watery stool (**1**) is consistent with a gastrointestinal *infection*. A bulky, greasy stool (**2**) is consistent with unabsorbed fat in the gastrointestinal tract, such as that found in *celiac disease*. A black, tarry stool (**3**) is consistent with gastrointestinal *bleeding* or *iron* therapy. **EV, APP, 8, PhI, Basic care and comfort**

17. (**3**) In assessing an infant for dehydration, weight loss is the most important variable to determine. *Mild* dehydration is less than 5% weight loss; *moderate* dehydration is 5–9% weight loss; *severe* dehydration is 10–15% weight loss. Obtaining the blood pressure (**1**), pulse (**2**), and checking for skin turgor status (**4**) are essential but *secondary* elements of a dehydration assessment. **IMP, ANL, 8, PhI, Physiological adaptation**

18. (**1**) The priority goal of nursing care is to rehydrate the infant by administering IV fluids and electrolytes as ordered. As the infant returns to health, an oral rehydration solution may be added to the infant's feeding regimen. Containing the causative agent (**2**), restoring skin integrity (**3**), and preventing

recurrences (**4**) are appropriate *secondary* goals. **PL, ANL, 8, PhI, Physiological adaptation**

19. (**2**) Similac is a lactose-based formula and should be *avoided* in the presence of diarrhea. Water (**1**) and *Pedialyte* (**3**) and *Rehydrate* (**4**) are oral rehydration solutions that *can be* used in treating most infants with isotonic, hypotonic, or hypertonic dehydration. **IMP, APP, 8, PhI, Basic care and comfort**

20. (**3**) The nurse should give the child a simple-carbohydrate snack, such as honey, because headache, shakiness, palpitations, and dizziness are symptoms of hypoglycemia. A simple carbohydrate elevates the blood glucose level and alleviates the symptoms. The simpler the carbohydrate, the more rapidly it is absorbed. Notifying the child's parents (**1**) should be done *after* immediate first aid is rendered. The parents and nurse should confer about possible causes for the hypoglycemic episode. Having the child rest a few minutes (**2**) does *not* help to elevate the blood glucose level. A complex-carbohydrate snack (**4**), such as bread or crackers with peanut butter or cheese, should *follow* the simple-carbohydrate snack to maintain the blood glucose level. **IMP, ANL, 4, PhI, Physiological adaptation**

21. (**3**) "You have a different type of diabetes than your aunt does" is the best response. Diabetes is a complex subject, and a newly diagnosed 10-year-old child needs repeated explanations with reinforcement before he is able to grasp the concept of types of diabetes. Neither maturation (**1**) nor growth of the pancreas (**2**) supplies the insulin that the child is unable to produce. Lack of understanding of the disease process (**4**) is to be expected in anyone who is newly diagnosed with a disease such as diabetes. Also this answer sounds like a "put down," and asks a question that closes communication because it calls for a "yes" or "no" response. **IMP, APP, 7, PsI, Psychosocial integrity**

22. (**3**) The need to be like peers is a driving force for the adolescent and greatly influences acceptance of and compliance with a prescribed diabetic regime. Desire for independence (**1**) and future orientation of goals (**2**) are also important elements to consider when caring for an adolescent, but they do *not* outweigh the adolescent's need for acceptance and sameness with his peer group. Adolescents may not feel the need to please parents (**4**) and may, in fact, be somewhat hostile toward parents and other authority figures. **AN, APP, 5, PsI, Psychosocial integrity**

Genitourinary Disorders

Chapter Outline

- Key Words
- Summary of Key Points
- Selected Genitourinary Disorders
  - Nephrosis
  - Acute Poststreptococcal Glomerulonephritis
  - Urinary Tract Infections
- Commonly Prescribed Medications
- Study and Memory Aids
- Questions
- Answers/Rationale

Key Words

anasarca   severe generalized edema of the total body.

ascites   accumulation of fluid in the peritoneal cavity; it is usually related to cardiac disease or a disturbance in the electrolyte balance, such as the hypoproteinemia of nephrosis.

diuresis   passage of an abnormally large amount of urine related to fluid retention in the body. Diuresis may occur naturally in the course of a disease, as in acute poststreptococcal glomerulonephritis, or be induced with the administration of certain medications (e.g. diuretics, such as furosemide [*Lasix*] or bumetamide [*Bumex*]).

dysuria   painful or difficult urination; often a symptom of urinary tract infection.

exacerbation   return of symptoms or worsening of the severity of symptoms of a disease.

idiopathic   of unknown cause; may be spontaneous or a result of factors as yet unrecognized.

periorbital edema   swelling around the eyes, primarily on the eyelids.

remission   absence of symptoms or a lessening of the severity of symptoms of a disease.

turgor   resistance of skin to being grasped or pinched. In a healthy child, when the skin on the abdomen or thigh is grasped between the nurse's fingers and then released, it settles into its normal appearance fairly quickly. In a child who is dehydrated, the skin remains raised, indicating "poor" skin turgor.

🔑 Summary of Key Points

1. *Nephrosis, acute glomerulonephritis,* and *urinary tract infections* are the most common inflammatory conditions of the genitourinary tract.

2. *Nephrosis* is a chronic renal disease with no known cause or cure.

3. The symptoms that bring a child with *nephrosis* to the attention of the health care practitioner are *weight gain* and *edema*.

4. The treatment of *nephrosis* is primarily supportive, consisting of *steroids* and symptom management.

5. *Acute glomerulonephritis* is a bilateral inflammation of the glomeruli of the kidneys. It is thought to be the result of an antigen-antibody reaction to a strep infection.

6. The main symptom that brings a child with *acute glomerulonephritis* to the attention of the health care practitioner is *hematuria*, evidenced by dark urine often described as "tea-colored" or "cola-colored."

7. The treatment of *acute glomerulonephritis* includes eradicating any lingering strep infection, maintaining fluid balance, and treating hypertension.

8. A *urinary tract infection* is the presence of bacteria in the urine, with or without signs or symptoms of inflammation.

9. The incidence of *urinary tract infection* is 10–30 times greater in *girls* than it is in boys.

10. The *treatment of urinary tract infection* includes culturing the urine, administering *antibiotics*, and teaching clients to prevent recurrence.

11. *Home care* for all children with genitourinary disorders: NEVER allow changes in urinary output or type for more than 24 hours before seeking medical attention.

Selected Genitourinary Disorders

See **Chapter 16** for genitourinary malformation (hypospadias).

Nephrosis (Nephrotic Syndrome)

I. *Introduction*: Nephrosis (idiopathic nephrotic syndrome/*minimal-change nephrotic syndrome* [MCNS]) is a *chronic* renal disease having no known cause, variable pathology, and no known cure. It is thought that several different pathophysiologic processes adversely affect the glomerular membranes of the kidneys, resulting in increased permeability to protein. "Leakage" of protein into the urine results in massive *proteinuria*, severe *hypoproteinemia*, and total body edema. A chronic disease, nephrosis often has its onset during the preschool years but is characterized by periods of exacerbation and remission throughout the childhood years. Further information about nephrosis is found in **Table 10.1, p. 87**.

II. **Assessment:**

   A. *Weight* gain greater than expected, slowly progressing over several weeks; parents may report that the child's shoes or clothing appear to be too tight.

   B. *Edema*

   1. Initially presents as periorbital edema on waking, but decreases throughout the day as swelling of the abdomen and lower extremities occurs.

   2. Eventually presents as total body edema (*anasarca*) with ascites and labial or scrotal swelling.

   3. Edematous tissue is prone to breakdown.

   C. *Laboratory tests reveal*:

   1. Massive proteinuria (50 mg/kg/day).
   2. Hypoalbuminemia (< 2.5 g/dL).
   3. Hyperlipidemia (450-1500 mg/dL).

   D. *General*:

   1. Urine output is decreased; urine is dark and foamy in appearance.
   2. Pallor, fatigue.
   3. Anorexia, diarrhea.
   4. Blood pressure is normal or slightly decreased.
   5. Increased susceptibility to infection: cellulitis, pneumonia, septicemia.

III. **Analysis/nursing diagnosis:**

   A. *Fluid volume excess* related to shift of fluid from the plasma to the interstitial spaces.

   B. *Altered nutrition* less than body requirements, related to anorexia.

   C. *High risk for impaired skin integrity* related to edema and immobility.

   D. *High risk for infection* related to diminished body defenses.

   E. *Activity intolerance* related to fatigue.

   F. *Knowledge deficit* related to disease process, treatment, and long-term follow-up care.

IV. **Nursing care plan/implementation:**

   A. Goal: *prevent fluid retention.*

   1. Administer medications as ordered, including steroids (e.g., *prednisone*) and diuretics (e.g., loop diuretics such as *furosemide*) in combination with metolazone. Possible use of salt-poor albumin in children who are severely edematous; or oral alkylating agent (cyclophosphamide) in conjunction with prednisone.

   2. Monitor daily weights and abdominal girth.

   3. Urine: strict I&O, specific gravity and dipstick for protein for every void.

   4. Note edema: extent, location, progression.

   5. Diet:

      a. *Salt restriction* during periods of massive edema (e.g. no salt at the table; foods with very high salt content are excluded); regular diet when remission is achieved.

      b. Fluid restrictions are seldom necessary except during edematous period.

   B. Goal: *provide adequate nutrition.*

   1. *Diet*: high protein (unless renal failure is present).

   2. Stimulate appetite: offer small portions prepared attractively; meals with family or other children; offer prepared foods, if possible; encourage parents to bring in special foods, e.g., culturally related preferences.

   C. Goal: *maintain skin integrity.*

   1. Provide good skin care; turn and position frequently. Monitor for signs of breakdown.

   2. Support edematous organs, e.g., support swollen scrotal sac on soft towel or rolled blanket.

   3. Cleanse edematous eyelids with normal saline.

   D. Goal: *prevent further infection.*

   1. Use good handwashing technique.

   2. Screen staff, visitors, other clients to limit contact with persons who are infectious.

   3. Administer *antibiotics* as ordered when the child has an infection.

   4. Keep warm and dry; stress good hygiene.

   5. Note possible sites of infection: skin, lungs, blood.

   E. Goal: *conserve client's energy.*

   1. Maintain bedrest during acute exacerbations.

   2. Provide periods of rest between ambulations.

   3. Provide age-appropriate diversion as tolerated.

TABLE 10.1 COMPARISON OF NEPHROSIS & ACUTE POSTSTREPTOCOCCAL GLOMERULONEPHRITIS

Factor	Nephrosis (Nephrotic Syndrome/MCNS)	Acute Poststreptococcal Glomerulonephritis (APSGN)
Illness type	Chronic	Acute
Illness course	Characterized by periods of exacerbations and remissions during many years	Predictable, self-limiting, typically lasting 4–10 d (acute edematous phase)
Cause	Unknown	Group A beta hemolytic strep
Age at onset	2–4 yr	Early school-aged children; peaks at 6–7 yr
Sex	More common among boys	More common among boys
Major signs and symptoms:		
General	Syndrome with variable pathology: massive proteinuria, hypoalbuminemia, severe edema, hyperlipidemia	Hematuria, hypertension
Blood pressure	Normal or decreased	*Elevated*
Edema	Generalized and severe	Periorbital
Proteinuria	Massive	Moderate
Serum protein level	*Decreased (6.1–7.9 g/dL)*	*Increased*
Serum lipid level	*Elevated*	Normal
Potassium level	Normal (3.5–5 mEq/L)	*Increased*
Treatment	Symptomatic—no known cure; prednisone, cyclophosphamide, furosemide	Penicillin (EES), hydralazine, furosemide
Diet	↓ sodium, ↑ protein (if without renal failure)	↓ sodium, ↓ potassium, ↑ protein (if without renal failure)
Fluid restrictions	Seldom necessary	Necessary if output is significantly reduced
Specific nursing care	Treat at home if possible; good skin care; prevent infection	Treat in hospital during acute phase; monitor *vital signs*, especially BP; on discharge, stress need to restrict activity until microscopic hematuria is gone
Prognosis	Fair; subject to long-term steroid treatment and social isolation related to frequent hospitalizations/confinement during relapses; 20% suffer chronic renal failure	Good; stress that recurrence is *rare* because specific immunity *is* conferred

F. Goal: **health teaching.** *Teach child and family about nephrosis/discharge planning.*

1. Teach child and family that the child is usually treated at home with supportive care; hospitalizations are for the newly diagnosed child, assessment and treatment of infection, or response to therapy.
2. Teach general measures, diet, medications.
3. Arrange for long-term follow-up care.
4. Address concern for social isolation related to hospitalizations and treatment.

V. **Evaluation/outcome criteria:**

A. Normal fluid balance maintained/restored.
B. Adequate nutrition is maintained.
C. Skin integrity is maintained.

D. No secondary infections occur.
E. Energy is conserved.
F. Child/family verbalize their understanding of the disease, its treatment, and its prognosis.

Acute Poststreptococcal Glomerulonephritis

I. *Introduction*: Acute poststreptococcal glomerulonephritis (APSGN) is a *bilateral* inflammation of the glomeruli of the kidneys and is the most common *noninfectious* renal disease of childhood. It occurs most frequently in early school-aged children, with a peak age of onset of 6–7 yr; it is *twice* as common in *boys* than girls. Like rheumatic fever, APSGN is thought to be the result of an *antigen-antibody reaction to a strep infection*

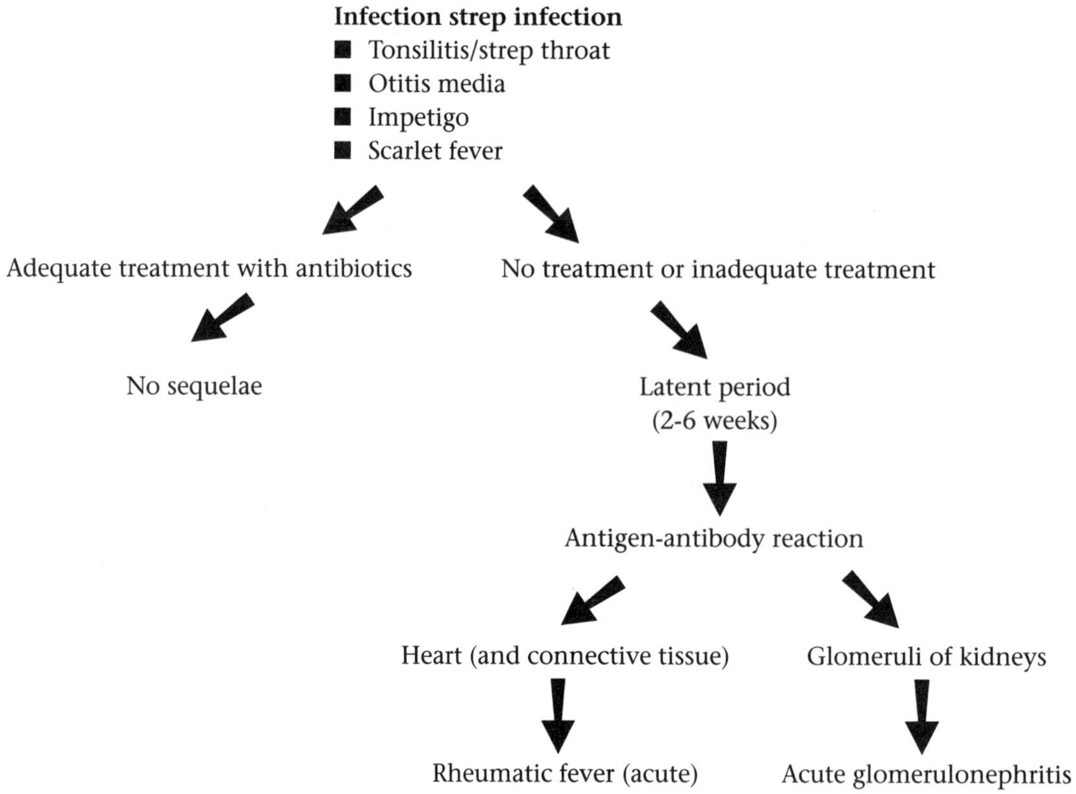

Infection strep infection
- Tonsilitis/strep throat
- Otitis media
- Impetigo
- Scarlet fever

Adequate treatment with antibiotics → No sequelae

No treatment or inadequate treatment → Latent period (2-6 weeks) → Antigen-antibody reaction

Heart (and connective tissue) → Rheumatic fever (acute)

Glomeruli of kidneys → Acute glomerulonephritis

FIGURE 10.1 SEQUELAE OF STREP INFECTIONS

(©Lagerquist, S., *Little, Brown's NCLEX-RN® Examination Review.* Boston: Little, Brown; out of print.)

(**Figure 10.1**); however, unlike rheumatic fever, it does *not* tend to recur because specific immunity is conferred after the first episode of APSGN. Further information about APSGN is found in **Table 10.1, p. 87.**

II. Assessment:

A. Typical concerns from family about urine: change in color/appearance of urine (thick, reddish brown; decreased amounts).

B. **Acute edematous phase**—usually lasts 4–10 d.

  1. Lab examination of urine:
    a. Severe **hematuria**.
    b. Mild proteinuria.
    c. *Increased* specific gravity.

  2. Blood tests reveal:
    a. *Increased* serum protein levels.
    b. *Increased* potassium levels.
    c. *Elevated* antistreptolysin O (ASO) titer: norm = 170-330 Todd U/mL.

  3. *Hypertension.*
    a. Headache.
    b. Potential hypertensive encephalopathy → seizures, increased intracranial pressure.

  4. Mild to moderate *edema*: chiefly periorbital; increased weight due to fluid retention.

  5. *General*:
    a. Abdominal pain.
    b. Malaise.
    c. Anorexia.
    d. Vomiting.
    e. Pallor.
    f. Irritability.
    g. Lethargy.
    h. Fever.

C. **Diuresis phase**:
  1. Copious diuresis.
  2. Decreased body weight.
  3. Marked clinical improvement.
  4. Decrease in gross hematuria, but microscopic hematuria may persist for weeks or months.

III. Analysis/nursing diagnosis:

A. *Fluid volume excess* related to decreased urine output.

B. *Altered nutrition, less than body requirements,* related to anorexia and vomiting.

C. *Pain* related to fluid retention.

D. *High risk for infection* related to diminished body defenses.

E. *Knowledge deficit* related to disease process, treatment, and follow-up care.

IV. Nursing care plan/implementation:

A. *Goal: monitor fluid balance, observing carefully for complications.*

  1. Check and record blood pressure (BP) at least every 4 h to monitor hypertension.

2. Monitor daily weights.

3. Urine: strict I&O; specific gravity and dipstick for blood every void.

4. Note edema: extent, location, progression.

5. Adhere to *fluid restrictions* if ordered.

6. *Bedrest*, chiefly due to hypertension: monitor for possible development of hypertensive encephalopathy (seizures, increased intracranial pressure); report any changes **STAT** to physician.

7. Administer medications as ordered:

   a. *Antibiotics*—eradicate any lingering strep infection.

   b. *Antihypertensives*, e.g., *hydralazine*.

   c. *Diuretics*, e.g., *furosemide*.

   d. If heart failure develops—may use digoxin.

B. Goal: *provide adequate nutrition*.

1. *Diet*: regular diet in uncomplicated cases but *no additional salt* (NAS) is added to foods. Possible *potassium restriction* if *oliguria*, and *protein restriction* if *azotemia*.

2. Stimulate appetite: offer small portions prepared attractively; meals with family or other children; offer preferred foods, if possible; encourage parents to bring in special foods, e.g., culturally related preferences.

C. Goal: *provide reasonable measure of comfort*.

1. Encourage parental visiting.

2. Provide for positional changes, give good skin care.

3. Provide appropriate diversion, as tolerated.

D. Goal: *prevent further infection*.

1. Use good handwashing technique.

2. Screen staff, other clients, visitors to limit contact with people who are infectious.

3. Administer *antibiotics* if ordered (usually only for children with positive cultures).

4. Keep warm and dry; stress good hygiene.

5. Note possible sites of infection: ↑ skin breakdown secondary to edema.

E. Goal: **health teaching**. *Teach child and family about APSGN discharge planning*.

1. Teach how to check urine at home: dipstick for protein and blood. (*Note*: Occult hematuria may persist for months.)

2. Teach activity restriction: *no* strenuous activity until hematuria is completely resolved.

3. Teach family how to prepare *low sodium, low potassium* diet.

4. Arrange for follow-up care: physician, community health nurse.

5. *Stress* that subsequent recurrences are *rare* because specific immunity is conferred.

V. **Evaluation/outcome criteria:**

A. Normal fluid balance is maintained/restored.

B. Adequate nutrition is maintained.

C. Comfort level is achieved/maintained.

D. No secondary infections occur.

E. Child/family verbalize their understanding of the disease, its treatment, and its prognosis.

Urinary Tract Infections

I. *Introduction*: A urinary tract infection (UTI) is the presence of bacteria in the urine, with or without signs or symptoms of inflammation. The peak age for UTIs is age 2–6 yr. *Girls* have an incidence 10–30 times greater than that of boys because a girl has a shorter urethra, which provides a ready pathway for invading bacteria. *E. coli* bacteria cause 80% of cases of UTI.

II. **Assessment:**

A. Nonspecific signs in infants or children under 2 yr:

1. *GI*: vomiting, diarrhea, poor feeding.

2. *GU*: frequent voiding, weak urine stream, dribbling of urine, straining with urination, foul-smelling urine, persistent diaper rash.

3. *Other*: irritability, lethargy, slow weight gain, jaundice.

B. Genitourinary:

1. *Lower* urinary tract infection: frequent and painful urination, dysuria, urgency, hematuria.

2. *Upper* urinary tract infection: chills, fever, flank pain.

3. Urine: cloudy, thickened with strands of pus and mucus, numerous white blood cells and possibly some red blood cells present, unpleasant odor.

III. **Analysis/nursing diagnosis:**

A. *High risk for injury* related to possible kidney damage from recurrent infection.

B. *Knowledge deficit* regarding drug administration, prevention of recurrent UTIs.

IV. **Nursing care plan/implementation:**

A. Goal: *eliminate infective organism(s)*.

1. Obtain urine culture before start of antibiotics.

2. Administer *antibiotics* as prescribed: *penicillin, sulfonamides, cephalosporins, nitrofurantoin*.

3. Assist with diagnostic tests as ordered; collect specimens as ordered.

B. Goal: **health teaching**. *Prevent recurrence of infection*.

1. *Home care/teach* preventive measures, including:

   a. Perineal hygiene: wipe from front to back.

   b. *Avoid* tight-fitting clothing or diapers; wear cotton panties or cotton-lined panties.

c. Encourage child to void frequently and to *avoid* "holding" urine for prolonged periods of time. Teach child to empty bladder completely with each void.

d. *Avoid* constipation, which can be related to UTIs.

e. Encourage *generous fluid intake*, especially fluids that cause the urine to be more acidic to decrease bacterial growth; *avoid* caffeinated/carbonated beverages which can cause bladder irritation.

f. Sexually active adolescent girls should void after sex to flush out bacteria.

g. *Avoid* bubble baths, which can be related to UTIs.

2. Answer questions the child or family may have; clarify any misconceptions.

3. Encourage follow-up care with MD.

V. **Evaluation/outcome criteria:**

A. No evidence of infection is present.

B. Family complies with treatment regimen; child does not have recurrent UTIs.

COMMONLY PRESCRIBED MEDICATIONS

Medication	Administration	Use/Action	Nursing Consideration
Alkylating Agents Cyclophosphamide/ *Cytoxan*	• Oral or parenteral • Calculate child's weight in kilograms • Administer in provided dropper or calibrated syringe • **Never** use household measuring spoon	Used in treatment of urinary tract infections caused by: a wide-range of gram-positive or gram-negative bacteria; natural or synthetic compounds that have the ability to kill or suppress the growth of microorganisms in a variety of ways	• Assess for allergy prior to administration • Obtain specimen for culture and sensitivity prior to administration • Maintain adequate fluid intake • Emphasize need to complete entire prescription
Antibiotics Aminoglycosides/ *Gentamicin* Cephalosporins/ *Keflex; Fortaz* Penicillins/ *Amoxicillin*	• Oral or parenteral • Calculate child's weight in kilograms • Administer in provided dropper or calibrated syringe • **NEVER** use household measuring spoon	Used in treatment of nephrotic syndrome (MCNS) Potent immuno-suppressant which prevents cell growth	• Obtain weekly white blood cell count (WBC) during therapy • Encourage *high fluid* intake and frequent voiding to prevent cystitis • Do **not** have immunizations without pediatrician's approval (as drug lowers body resistance) • Report signs of infection promptly • Teach that alopecia is reversible but new hair may have different color or texture

See also: **Chapter 8**: diuretics

Study and Memory Aids

Nephrosis (MCNS)—Assessment, Treatment

↑ weight, edema → seek medical attention.
↓ serum protein (normal = 6.1–7.9 g/dL).
Chronic, no cure.
Tx: supportive, symptomatic.

Acute Glomerulonephritis (APSGN)—Assessment

Hematuria → seek medical care.
Evidence of a recent strep infection can be found in the: antistreptolysin O (ASO) titer; a normal ASO titer is 170-330 Todd units.
Sudden ↓ wt = diuresis phase; ↑ improvement.
Microscopic hematuria continues.
Teach: dipstick test for hematuria; *no* sports until *no* hematuria.

UTI—Assessment, Pathophysiology, Tx

More common in *girls*.
Constipation → bladder, urethra pressure → urinary stasis, infection.
Cranberry juice → ↑ urine acid → ↓ bacterial growth.

Questions

1. When obtaining a health history from the parents of a child with acute glomerulonephritis, what should the nurse anticipate that the parents may report?
   1. The color of the child's urine.
   2. The child's weight loss.
   3. The child's increased energy level.
   4. The child's increased appetite.

2. A 4-year-old child with acute glomerulonephritis is placed on fluid restrictions. Which intervention would make fluid restriction less obvious to a child in this age group?
   1. Make a "tea party" game and serve the allowed liquids in small cups.
   2. Allow the child to have the full allotment of liquids in a large single container and instruct the child to drink just a little at a time.
   3. Fill regular cups and glasses half-full and say nothing if the child questions this presentation.
   4. Show the child how to record intake and output to keep the child distracted.

3. The parents of a child hospitalized with acute glomerulonephritis question the nurse about why their child is being disturbed during the night to have blood pressure taken. The nurse's best response is:
   1. "This is part of standard nursing care for a child who is hospitalized."
   2. "The pediatrician ordered blood pressures to be taken every 4 hours around the clock."
   3. "Elevations in blood pressure are a frequent complication of acute glomerulonephritis and can only be detected by checking the blood pressure at frequent intervals."
   4. "If you sign the necessary form releasing the hospital from responsibility for your child's well-being, we can discontinue taking blood pressures during the night."

4. Which is the best indicator to the nurse of a return to health in the child with acute glomerulonephritis?
   1. A weight gain of 3 pounds after 1 week of hospitalization.
   2. A weight loss of 5 pounds after 1 week of hospitalization.
   3. Unchanged gross hematuria.
   4. Slight increase in urinary output.

5. A child with nephrotic syndrome is on long-term steroid therapy. Which nursing diagnosis presents the greatest risk for this child?
   1. *High risk for altered nutrition, more than body requirements.*
   2. *High risk for infection.*
   3. *High risk for impaired skin integrity.*
   4. *High risk for body image disturbance.*

6. Which nursing intervention is most appropriate for a child hospitalized with nephrotic syndrome?
   1. Change the child's position frequently.
   2. Encourage age-appropriate activities.
   3. Weigh the child weekly.
   4. Invite the child's schoolmates to visit.

7. A child with nephrotic syndrome enters remission and is to be discharged home. The nurse should instruct the parents about the development of which symptom that would be a cause for concern?
   1. The child's shoes and clothes become tight.
   2. The child resists returning to school.

3. The child's behavior seems "younger" than it was before hospitalization.
4. The child craves junk food.

8. When caring for a child with nephrotic syndrome, which laboratory result should the nurse expect?
   1. Potassium = 3.6 mEq/L; serum protein = 5 g/dL.
   2. Potassium = 5.8 mEq/L; serum protein = 3.3 g/dL.
   3. Potassium = 2.9 mEq/L; serum protein = 9.0 g/dL.
   4. Potassium = 5.4 mEq/L; serum protein = 7.0 g/dL.

9. When assessing a 6-year-old child for the possibility of APSGN, the nurse should check the ASO titer for evidence of recent strep infection. Which finding should the nurse recognize as an abnormally high ASO titer, indicating recent strep infection?
   1. ASO = 200 Todd units.
   2. ASO = 250 Todd units.
   3. ASO = 300 Todd units.
   4. ASO = 400 Todd units.

10. A child is seen in the pediatric clinic for a variety of symptoms, including periorbital edema that is worse in the morning, loss of appetite, and dark-colored urine. Which diagnosis should the nurse anticipate?
    1. Nephrotic syndrome.
    2. Acute glomerulonephritis.
    3. Urinary tract infection.
    4. Wilms' tumor.

11. The MD orders a Fleet enema for a child with acute renal failure. The nurse should question the order because of the risk of:
    1. Fluid retention.
    2. Hyperkalemia.
    3. Hyperphosphatemia.
    4. Hypertension.

12. To detect a urinary tract infection in an infant, the nurse should check the baby's diaper every 30 min. Which findings would indicate this problem?
    1. Blood-streaked urine, highly concentrated urine, amber-colored urine.
    2. Sweet-smelling, "fruity" urine; large volume of highly dilute, clear urine.
    3. Minimal urine output or complete absence of urine output.
    4. Fretting before voiding begins, intermittent starting and stopping of the urine stream, frequent dripping of small amounts of urine.

13. The mother of a 5-year-old girl with a urinary tract infection (UTI) mentions to the clinic nurse that her daughter frequently seems to be constipated. She asks the nurse what can she do to relieve this annoying problem. The nurse's best response at this time is to:
    1. Ask the mother to explain what she means by "constipation."
    2. Discuss the relationship between constipation and UTIs in girls.

3. Encourage the mother to add more fiber and liquids to the child's diet.
4. Assure the mother this problem is common in preschoolers and should pass when the child enters school.

14. A child with a urinary tract infection is being treated with Bactrim. After instructing the parents, the nurse could confirm the teaching was effective if the parent(s) verbalized which information?
    1. "My child should drink extra fluids."
    2. "My child should stay out of the sun."
    3. "My child should take this medicine with meals or snacks."
    4. "My child may have reddish-colored urine."

15. When evaluating the urinalysis results of a child with UTI, the nurse can expect to find:
    1. White blood cells.
    2. Ketones.
    3. Protein.
    4. Glucose.

Answers/Rationale

1. **(1)** Signs and symptoms of acute glomerulonephritis are acute in onset. A puffy face (edema) and cola- or tea-colored urine (hematuria) are the two most common presenting complaints. The child's weight *increases* **(2)** because of fluid retention. The energy level **(3)** is markedly *depleted*, as evidenced by malaise and lethargy. The child usually becomes *anorexic* **(4)**. **AS, COM, 8, PhI, Physiological adaptation**

2. **(1)** Preschoolers enjoy "pretend" types of games and are less likely to notice or question restricted amounts of fluids if the serving size is in proportion to the container size. Expecting a preschooler to self-ration **(2)** is unrealistic. Ignoring questions **(3)** does not make the question go away. Preschoolers cannot yet tally numbers **(4)**, so this intervention is better suited to a school-aged child's sense of industry and knowledge of mathematics. **IMP, ANL, 5, PhI, Physiological adaptation**

3. **(3)** Hypertension is a frequent complication of acute glomerulonephritis and can be found only by checking the blood pressure frequently. Occasionally, hypertension can be severe enough to cause headaches, visual disturbances, seizures, and coma; thus, early detection is essential. Responses about standardized care **(1)** or physician's orders **(2)** shift the responsibility away from the nurse and do *not* correct the parent's knowledge deficit. It is *not* within the nurse's scope of practice to direct parents away from care and treatments needed by the child **(4)**. **IMP, APP, 6, PhI, Reduction of risk potential**

4. **(2)** Decreased weight is an indicator that the child is entering the diuresis phase of acute glomerulonephritis and thus is showing a return to health. An *increase* in weight **(1)** and unchanged gross hematuria **(3)** indicate that the child is *still* in the early edematous phase of acute glomerulonephritis. *Copious, not* slight, diuresis **(4)** must take place before a return to health is evidenced. **EV, ANL, 6, PhI, Physiological adaptation**

5. **(2)** Infection poses the greatest risk for this child because steroids are immunosuppressive in nature. Altered nutrition, excessive **(1)** because of increased appetite, impaired skin integrity **(3)**, and body image disturbance **(4)** caused by fluid retention are unfortunate side effects of the necessary steroids. The nurse should reassure the child and the family that these symptoms will disappear gradually after discontinuation of the drug. **AN, ANL, 1, HPM, Health promotion and maintenance**

6. **(1)** Changing the child's position frequently is essential to prevent skin breakdown secondary to massive edem**a**. The child's activity level **(2)** is usually limited to bedrest during the edema phase of the illness. Weight **(3)** is checked *daily* or more often to assess fluid retention. Inviting schoolmates to visit **(4)** is discouraged during the acute phase of the illness because the visitors may be a possible source of infection. Telephone calls and get-well cards from schoolmates are encouraged. **IMP, ANL, 3, PhI, Basic care and comfort**

7. **(1)** Tightness of shoes and clothes may indicate the onset of edema and a possible relapse. This could be documented by a weight gain over the expected, based on the child's previous pattern. Resisting returning to school **(2)** may indicate the social isolation that illness commonly produces in the child. Regressive or "younger" behavior **(3)** is *expected* in any child who has been acutely ill over a period of time. Junk food cravings **(4)** are *expected* as a side effect of steroid therapy and as a result of the restrictive nature of the child's diet during the acute phase of the illness. **IMP, ANL, 6, HPM, Health promotion and maintenance**

8. **(1)** In nephrotic syndrome, laboratory findings should reveal a normal potassium level, with a decreased serum protein level secondary to the massive proteinuria these children experience. Normal potassium level in a child is 3.5–5 mEq/L; a reading of 3.6 is within normal limits. Normal serum protein level in a child is 6.1–7.9 g/dL; a reading of 5 is well below the norm. The nurse should not expect the potassium level to vary, which eliminates the low **(3)** or high **(2 and 4)** levels. The nurse should not expect the serum protein levels to be normal **(4)** or above normal **(3)** because of the massive proteinuria these children experience. **EV, ANL, 6, PhI, Reduction of risk potential**

9. **(4)** In school-aged children, an ASO titer is normally 170–330 Todd units. A level of 400 Todd units is above the norm and indicates the presence of a recent (mild) strep infection. Levels of 200 **(1)**, 250 **(2)** and 300 **(3)** are all within *normal* limits and thus do *not* indicate the presence of a recent strep infection. **EV, ANL, 1, PhI, Reduction of risk potential**

10. **(2)** This choice most accurately describes the major signs and symptoms of acute glomerulonephritis; another major symptom the child also is likely to exhibit is hypertension. Nephrotic syndrome **(1)** is characterized by generalized severe edema and changes in the urine and blood. Urinary tract infections **(3)** are characterized by urgency, frequency, burning upon urination, foul-smelling urine, and vague systemic symptoms such as loss of appetite and fatigue. Wilms' tumor **(4)** is characterized by an abdominal mass, malaise, loss of weight, and anemia. **EV, APP, 8, PhI, Physiological adaptation**

11. **(3)** The use of a Fleet enema in a child with acute renal failure is contraindicated because of potentially fatal hyperphosphatemia. Use of a Fleet enema does *not* generally result in fluid retention **(1)**, hyperkalemia **(2)**, or hypertension **(4)**. **EV, APP, 8, SECE, Management of care**

12. **(4)** This choice most accurately describes signs and symptoms of a urinary tract infection (UTI) in an infant or toddler. Blood-streaked urine **(1)** is *not* usual in a UTI, although occult hematuria may be present. Concentrated, dark-colored urine **(1)** is associated with dehydration, *not* UTI. Sweet-smelling urine and dilute urine **(2)** are associated with diabetes, *not* UTI. Minimal or no output **(3)** is associated with renal failure, *not* UTI. **EV, APP, 8, PhI, Physiological adaptation**

13. **(1)** The best possible response is for the nurse to gather more data to clarify exactly what the mother means by "constipation." It is possible that the mother's description indicates normal stool pattern or it may be truly abnormal; however, without further data, taking any action would *not* be appropriate. Although there is a relationship between chronic constipation and urinary tract infections **(2)**, the nurse should *not* proceed with this explanation until the assessment is complete. At some point, dietary teaching **(3)** may be needed; however, since the child is being seen for UTIs, the nurse should *first* determine whether the child is truly constipated. The nurse should *not* offer the mother false reassurance **(4)** because, if the child continues to be constipated, UTIs are likely to continue. **AS, APP, 8, PhI, Basic care and comfort**

14. **(1)** Bactrim contains the sulfonamide, sulfamethizole, which can cause crystalluria and kidney damage. To prevent this, clients taking Bactrim should ensure adequate fluid intake by drinking at least 8 glasses of water daily. There are *no* precautions with Bactrim about staying out of the sun **(2)**, taking the medication with meals or snacks **(3)**, or about the medication turning the urine reddish **(4)**. If the parent(s) verbalize one of these statements, further teaching is needed. **EV, APP, 8, PhI, Pharmacological and parenteral therapies**

15. **(1)** The presence of white blood cells (WBC) is expected when a child has a urinary tract infection. The normal WBC count in urine is less than 1–2/mL; in UTI, 5–8 WBC/mL or more is considered diagnostic. In UTIs, the nurse should *not* expect to find ketones **(2)**, protein **(3)**, or glucose **(4)**. **EV, APP, 8, PhI, Reduction of risk potential**

Key to Codes

Nursing process: AS, assessment; **AN**, analysis; **PL**, planning; **IMP**, implementation; **EV**, evaluation. (See **Appendix L** for explanation of nursing process steps.)

Cognitive level: RE/KN, recall/knowledge; **COM**, comprehension; **APP**, application; **ANL**, analysis; **EVL**, evaluation; **SYN**, synthesis. (See **Appendix L** for explanation.)

Category of human function: 1, protective; **2**, sensory-perceptual; **3**, comfort, rest, activity, and mobility; **4**, nutrition; **5**, growth and development; **6**, fluid-gas transport; **7**, psychosocial-cultural; **8**, elimination. (See **Appendix N** for explanation.)

Client need: SECE, safe, effective care environment; **HPM**, health promotion and maintenance; **PsI**, psychosocial integrity; **PhI**, physiological integrity. (See **Appendix O** for explanation.)

Client subneed: See **Appendix O** for explanation.

Hematologic Disorders

11

Chapter Outline

Key Words

epistaxis nosebleed or hemorrhage from the nares.

glossitis inflammation of the tongue.

hemarthrosis bleeding into a joint.

jaundice a condition characterized by yellowing of the skin and whites of the eyes caused by the deposition of bile pigments resulting from excess bilirubin in the blood; usually related to *liver* disease.

koilonychia dystrophy of the fingernails in which they appear to be concave; may be described as "spoon" fingernails; condition is frequently seen in *iron deficiency* anemia.

pallor paleness or lack of color.

petechiae small, purplish, pinpoint hemorrhages caused by ruptured blood vessels; can occur anywhere on the body.

stomatitis inflammation of the mouth.

tachycardia abnormally rapid heart rate.

tachypnea abnormally rapid respiratory rate.

🔑 Summary of Key Points

1. *Iron deficiency anemia* is the most common nutritional disturbance in the United States; premature infants, children from lower-income families, and adolescents are at the *highest* risk for iron deficiency anemia.

2. *Iron supplements* should be administered *between* meals on an *empty* stomach, given with a fruit juice *high* in vitamin C, and given through a straw or dropper; iron should *never* be given with milk or milk products.

3. For the child with *sickle cell anemia*, conditions of *low* oxygen tension precipitate sickling of defective red blood cells, resulting in agglutination of red cells and obstruction of capillary flow, followed by tissue ischemia, necrosis, and death.

4. In sickle cell crisis, the *priority* nursing intervention is to *hydrate* the child; a primary concern is to *prevent* sickle cell crisis by maintaining adequate hydration and *preventing* dehydration.

5. *Hemophilia* is a *sex-linked recessive* disorder that is transmitted by symptom-free *female* carriers to their *male* offspring.

6. There is no known cure for *hemophilia*; symptomatic treatment for bleeding includes the administration of the clotting factor.

7. *Home care* for all children with hematologic disorders: **NEVER** allow pallor, listlessness, new-onset bruising (without explanation) for more than 1 week before seeking medical attention.

Selected Hematologic Disorders

Red Blood Cell Disorders

I. **Iron Deficiency Anemia**

   A. *Introduction*: Anemia is a blood disorder in which the number of red blood cells and/or the hemoglobin concentrate is below normal. Iron deficiency anemia is caused by: a decreased supply of iron, *or* an impaired absorption of iron, *or* an increased need for iron, *or* conditions that affect the synthesis of iron. Although there has been a decreased incidence of iron deficiency anemia during the past 30 yrs, it is still the most prevalent nutritional disturbance in the United States and around the world. Children who are at highest risk include: premature infants, toddlers, children from lower-income families, and adolescents.

   B. **Assessment**:

   1. *General signs and symptoms*: fatigue, exercise intolerance; pallor of skin and mucous membranes; menorrhagia (heavy menstrual bleeding) in adolescent girls.

2. *Central nervous system signs* and *symptoms*: headache, dizziness, irritability; impaired cognitive skills such as decreased attention span or sluggish thought processes.

3. Other: *koilonychia* (concave or "spoon-shaped" fingernails).

4. Lab: *decreased* hemoglobin, *decreased* red blood cell (RBC) count with microcytic and hypochromic cells, *decreased* mean corpuscular volume, *decreased* reticulocyte count; *decreased* serum iron concentration.

C. Analysis/nursing diagnosis:

1. *Activity intolerance* related to diminished oxygen-carrying capacity of RBCs.

2. *Altered nutrition*, less than body requirements, related to inadequate iron intake.

D. Nursing care plan/implementation:

1. Goal: *increase oxygen supply to body tissues and promote adequate rest.*

   a. *Position*: semi-Fowler's for maximum expansion of the lungs.

   ☞ b. Administer oxygen per MD order, monitor for therapeutic response.

   c. Observe for signs of overexertion: tachycardia, tachypnea, shortness of breath.

   d. Assist with activities of daily living (ADL).

   e. Provide diversionary activities within acceptable limits of tolerance.

   f. Select same-sex roommate of same developmental level and who is also on restricted activity.

   g. Organize nursing care to provide periods of uninterrupted rest.

TABLE 11.1 🍎 IRON-RICH FOODS

Bread and cereal, iron-enriched
Cereal and formula, iron-fortified
Egg yolks
Fruits, dried
Grains, whole
Kidney
Legumes, nuts, seeds
Liver: pork, calf, beef, chicken
Meats, red
Molasses
Potatoes
Poultry
Shellfish
Tofu
Vegetables, green leafy (except spinach)
Wheat germ

Adapted from Wong DL. *Nursing Care of Infants and Children* (7th ed). St. Louis, Mosby.

---

2. Goal: *increase intake of iron-rich foods to meet minimum daily requirements and increase iron stores in body.*

   a. Diet: high in iron (see **Table 11.1** for foods *high* in iron).

   b. Refer to dietician for teaching and counseling for iron-rich diet.

   c. Offer milk or formula *after* solid foods have been consumed; *limit* milk or formula in favor of *high* iron, solid foods.

   d. Administer *iron* supplements as ordered.

3. Goal: **health teaching.** *Teach the family how to administer iron correctly at home*:

> (1) Ideally, for maximal absorption, *iron* should be administered *between* meals to child who has an *empty* stomach; iron should be given in divided doses per MD order.
>
> (2) *Iron* should be administered with a fruit *juice high in vitamin C* to maximize absorption.
>
> (3) Iron should *not* be given with milk, milk products, or antacids, which decrease its absorption.
>
> (4) *Liquid iron* preparations should be given through a *straw* (or dropper) to *avoid* staining teeth.
>
> (5) Stools should be checked for color; if iron is being given in adequate amounts, stools should be a dark, tarry, blackish green.

E. Evaluation/outcome criteria:

1. Respiratory rate and depth are within normal limits and no signs of fatigue or overexertion are noted.

2. Minimum daily requirement of iron is consumed in the diet and iron supplements are taken, as evidenced by stool characteristics.

II. Sickle Cell Anemia

A. *Introduction*: Sickle cell anemia (SCA) is a *congenital* hemolytic anemia resulting from a defective hemoglobin molecule (*hemoglobin S*). It is most common in African-Americans (8% have sickle cell trait) and in people of Mediterranean descent. The diagnosis is usually made during the toddler or preschool years, during the first crisis episode following an infection. There is also the need to differentiate between *sickle cell trait* (Sickledex) and *sickle cell anemia* (hemoglobin electrophoresis). Sickle cell anemia has no known cure.

B. Assessment:

1. Increased susceptibility to infection (cause: unknown; most common cause of death in children under 5 yr with SCA).

2. Inherited as *autosomal recessive* disorder (**Figure 11.1, p. 97**).

3. Precipitated by conditions of *low* oxygen tension and/or dehydration.
4. *Signs of anemia*:
   a. Pallor (in dark-skinned children, do *not* rely on pallor alone—check Hgb and Hct).
   b. Jaundice, due to excessive hemolysis.
   c. Irritability, lethargy, anorexia, malaise.
5. *Vaso-occlusive crisis*: severe pain (variable sites), fever, swelling of hands and feet, joint pain and swelling, all related to hypoxia, ischemia and necrosis at the cellular level. Most common; *not* life-threatening.
6. *Splenic sequestration crisis*: blood is sequestered (pooled) in spleen; precipitous drop in BP, ↑ pulse, shock, and ultimately death from profound anemia and cardiovascular collapse.

C. **Analysis/nursing diagnosis**:
   1. *Altered tissue perfusion* related to anemia and occlusion of vessels.
   2. *High risk* for infection.
   3. *Pain* related to vaso-occlusion.
   4. *Knowledge deficit* related to disease process and treatment (e.g., prevention of sickling and/or infection; genetic counseling).

D. **Nursing care plan/implementation**:
   1. Goal: *prevent sickling*.
      a. *Avoid* conditions of *low* oxygen tension, which causes RBCs to assume a sickled shape.
      b. Provide continuous extra *fluids* to prevent dehydration, which causes sluggish circulation.
      c. *Avoid* activities that may result in overheating, to prevent dehydration; suggest appropriate clothes; limit time in sun.
      d. If dehydrated due to acute illness, supplement with IV fluids and additional oral fluids to reestablish fluid balance.
      e. MD may consider use of hydroxyurea to decrease sickling episodes.

FIGURE 11.1   GENETIC TRANSMISSION OF SICKLE CELL ANEMIA

(A) Normal parent and parent who carries trait

	A	A
A	AA	AA
S	AS	AS

1:2 (or 2:4) chance offspring will carry trait

(B) Two parents who carry trait

	A	S
A	AA	AS
S	AS	SS

1:4 chance offspring will be normal
1:4 chance offspring will have sickle cell anemia
1:2 (or 2:4) chance offspring will carry trait

(C) Normal parent and parent with sickle cell anemia

	A	A
S	AS	AS
S	AS	AS

4:4 (100%) chance offspring will carry trait

(D) Parent with sickle cell anemia and parent who carries trait

	A	S
S	AS	SS
S	AS	SS

1:2 (or 2:4) chance offspring will carry trait
1:2 (or 2:4) chance offspring will have sickle cell anemia

(E) Two parents with sickle cell anemia

	S	S
S	SS	SS
S	SS	SS

4:4 (100%) chance offspring will have sickle cell anemia

Key:
AA = normal hemoglobin
AS = sickle cell trait
SS = sickle cell disease (anemia)

Note: The odds cited here are for each pregnancy

(From ©Lagerquist S: Little, *Brown's NCLEX-RN® Examination Review. Boston*: Little, Brown—out of print.)

FIGURE 11.2 GENETIC TRANSMISSION OF HEMOPHILIA

(A) "Normal" male and female with trait		
	X	Y
X*	X*X	X*Y
X	XX	XY

1:4 chance will be female with trait
1:4 chance will be male with hemophilia
1:2 (or 2:4) chance will be "normal" female/male

(B) Male with hemophilia and "normal" female		
	X*	Y
X	X*X	XY
X	X*X	XY

1:2 (or 2:4) chance will be female with trait
1:2 (or 2:4) chance will be "normal" male

(C) Male with hemophilia and female with trait		
	X*	Y
X*	X*X*	X*Y
X	X*X	XY

1:2 (or 2:4) chance will be female with trait
1:4 chance will be "normal" male
1:4 chance will be male with hemophilia

Key:
XY = normal male
X*Y = male with hemophilia
XX = normal female
X*X = female carrying hemophilia trait
X*X* = female with possible relative lack of clotting factor—*not* a true hemophiliac (von Willebrand's disease).

Note: The odds cited here are for *each* pregnancy

(From ©Lagerquist S: *Little, Brown's NCLEX-RN® Examination Review.* Boston: Little, Brown—out of print.)

2. Goal: *maintain infection-free state*.
   a. Standard precautions to prevent infection.
   b. Use good handwashing technique.
   c. Evaluate carefully, check continually for potential infection sites, which may either lead to death due to sepsis or precipitate sickle cell crisis.
   d. *Teach* importance of *prevention*: adequate nutrition; frequent medical check-ups; keep away from known sources of infection; keep immunization up-to-date.
   e. Stress need to report early signs of infection promptly to physician.
   f. Need to balance prevention of infection with child's need for a "normal" life.
   g. Begin oral penicillin prophylaxis by 2 months of age.
3. Goal: *provide supportive therapy during crisis to minimize pain*.
   a. Provide *bedrest*/hospitalization during crisis to decrease the body's demand for oxygen.
   b. Relieve pain by administering *pain* medications as ordered; handle gently and use proper positioning techniques.
   c. Apply heat (**never cold**) to affected painful areas to increase blood flow (vasodilation) and oxygen supply.

   d. Administer oxygen, as ordered, to relieve hypoxia and prevent further sickling.
   e. Administer blood transfusions, as ordered, to correct severe anemia.
   f. Monitor fluid and electrolyte balance: I&O, weight, electrolytes.
   g. Perform ADL for child if unable to care for own needs; encourage self-care as soon as possible to promote independence.
4. Goal: **health teaching**. *Teach child and family about sickle cell anemia.*
   a. Provide factual information based on child's developmental level.
   b. When asked, offer information regarding prognosis (no known cure).
   c. Encourage child to live as normally as possible.
   d. Genetic screening and counseling (**Figure 11.1**). Investigate bone marrow transplant.
E. **Evaluation/outcome criteria:**
   1. Sickling is prevented or kept to a minimum.
   2. Child is maintained in infection-free state.
   3. Pain is prevented or kept to a minimum.
   4. Child/family verbalize their understanding about disease, its management and prognosis.

Defects in Hemostasis: Hemophilia

I. *Introduction*: Hemophilia is a bleeding disorder inherited as a *sex*-linked (X-linked) *recessive* trait; that is, it occurs *only* in men but is transmitted by symptom-free *women carriers* (refer to **Figure 11.2, p. 98**). Hemophilia results in a *deficiency of one or more clotting factors*; and it is necessary to determine which clotting factor is deficient and to what extent. In classic hemophilia (hemophilia A), a lack of *clotting factor* VIII accounts for 75% of all cases of hemophilia.

II. **Assessment:**

A. Major problem is bleeding.
1. In *newborn* boy: abnormal bleeding from umbilical cord, prolonged bleeding from circumcision site.
2. In *toddler* boy: excessive bruising, possible intracranial bleeding, prolonged bleeding from cuts or lacerations.
3. *General*: hemarthrosis, petechiae, epistaxis, frank hemorrhage anywhere in body, anemia.

B. Need to determine which clotting factor is deficient/missing and extent of deficiency:
1. *Mild*: child has 5–50% of normal amount of clotting factor.
2. *Moderate*: child has 1–5% of normal amount of clotting factor.
3. *Severe*: child has less than 1% of normal amount of clotting factor. 60–70% of children with hemophilia have this form.

III. **Analysis/nursing diagnosis:**

A. *Risk for injury* related to bleeding tendencies.
B. *Pain* related to hemarthrosis.
C. *Impaired physical mobility* related to bleeding and pain.
D. *Knowledge deficit* related to home care and follow-up.

IV. **Nursing care plan/implementation:**

A. Goal: *prevent injury and possible bleeding and control bleeding episodes when they occur*.
1. Provide an environment that is as safe as possible, e.g., toys with *no* sharp edges, child's safety scissors. Wear helmets and joint pads when playing actively.
2. Use soft toothbrush to prevent trauma to gums.
3. When child is old enough to shave, must use *only* electric razor (*no* straight-edge razors).
4. *Avoid* IMs/IVs—but when absolutely necessary, treat as arterial puncture; that is, apply direct pressure to the site for at least 5 min after withdrawing needle.
5. Do **not** use aspirin or medication containing aspirin (prolongs bleeding/clotting time).
6. *Local measures*: apply direct pressure, *elevate*, apply ice (vasoconstriction), keep immobilized during acute bleeding episodes

only. For epistaxis: child should *sit up and lean slightly forward.*
7. *Systemic measures*: administer clotting factor (antihemophilic factor, factor VIII) via IV infusion. *Note*: This is a blood product, so a transfusion reaction is possible.

B. Goal: *control pain appropriately*
1. *Non-steroidal anti-inflammatory* drugs (NSAIDS) are effective for relieving pain caused by synovitis. Use with *caution* as they inhibit platelet function.

C. Goal: *prevent long-term disability related to joint degeneration.*
1. Keep *immobilized* during period of acute bleeding and for 24–48 h afterward to allow blood to clot and to prevent dislodging the clot.
2. Begin passive range-of-motion exercises as soon as possible after acute phase.
3. Administer prescribed pain medications *before* physical therapy sessions.
4. Begin prescribed exercise program, starting with passive range of motion (ROM) and gradually advancing to active ROM, then full exercise program, as tolerated, to maintain maximum joint function.
5. **Avoid**: prolonged immobility, braces, and splints, which can lead to permanent deformities and loss of mobility.

D. Goal: **health teaching**. *Promote independence in management of own care.*
1. Encourage child to assume responsibility for choosing safe activities.
2. Encourage child to attend regular school as much as possible; provide support via school nurse.
3. Advise child to wear MedicAlert bracelet.
4. Caution parents to *avoid* overprotection of child.
5. Offer child chance to self-limit activities within appropriate limits (parents can offer guidance).
6. Assist child to cope with life-threatening disorder with no known cure.
7. From *9–12 yr*: child can be taught to self-administer clotting factor intravenously (prior to this, family can perform).
8. As child enters *adolescence*: begin to discuss issues such as realistic vocations, insurance coverage, genetic transmission (refer to **Figure 11.2, p. 98**).

V. **Evaluation/outcome criteria.**

A. Serious injuries are prevented; bleeding is kept to a minimum. Episodes of bleeding controlled by prompt, effective intervention.
B. Pain is prevented or kept to a minimum.
C. There are no long-term disabilities.
D. Child is able to manage own care independently, with minimal supervision.

COMMONLY PRESCRIBED MEDICATIONS

Medication	Administration	Use/Action	⋈ Nursing Consideration
Antihemophilic Agents Factor VIII/*ReFacto*	• IV ONLY • Calculate to child's weight in kilograms • Dosage is highly individualized depending on severity of bleeding and degree of deficiency	Used in treatment of hemophilia Accelerates conversion of prothrombin to thrombin Temporarily replaces the missing clotting factor	• Document baseline vital signs and monitor every 15 minutes during infusion • Assess urine for: quantity, color, occult blood • Pre-medicate with diphenhydramine (*Benadryl*)
Antineoplastic/ Antimetabolite Hydroxyurea/*Hydrea*	• Oral • Calculate to child's weight in kilograms • Administer for 6 weeks before efficacy is assessed	Used in treatment of sickle cell anemia Decreases formation of sickled cells Reduces frequency of crises	• Monitor complete blood count (CBC) every 2 weeks • Drink 8–10 glasses of fluid per day (excreted through urine) • Report signs of infection • Sexually active adolescents to practice contraception
Hematinics Ferrous sulfate/ *Fer-in-Sol*	• Oral • Calculate to child's weight in kilograms • Administer in provided dropper or calibrated syringe • NEVER use household measuring spoon	Used in treatment of iron deficiency anemia Essential component in formation of hemoglobin, myoglobin and enzymes	• Use dropper or straw to prevent staining of teeth • Allow solution to drop on back of tongue • Administer with citrus juice to maximize absorption • *Avoid* giving with milk which decreases absorption • Note color changes (darker) in stools

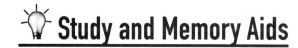

💡 Study and Memory Aids

Iron Deficiency Anemia (most common nutritional disturbance in the United States)—Children at High Risk:

1. Premature infants
2. Toddlers
3. Children of lower-income families
4. Adolescents

Iron Deficiency Anemia—Medications

Give iron supplements
- Through straw/dropper (prevents teeth stains)
- Between meals
- With vitamin C (e.g., fruit juice)

Sickle Cell Anemia—Genetics

To be born with sickle cell anemia, the child must have inherited the trait from *both* parents.

Progression of Sickle Cell Crisis—Pathophysiology

Low oxygen tension
↓
Sickling of defective red blood cells
↓
Agglutination of cells
↓
Obstruction of capillary flow
↓
Tissue ischemia, necrosis, death

Sickle Cell Crisis—Prevention

To prevent sickle cell crisis, prevent *dehydration*; if crisis occurs, hydration is the priority.

Hemophilia—Genetics

A father with hemophilia cannot pass the disease to his sons, but he passes *trait* to his *daughters*, who may in turn pass the disease to their sons.

Hemophilia—Treatment (Symptomatic)

1. Give antihemophilic factor VIII
2. *Avoid* injections
3. Do *not* give aspirin

Questions

1. An adolescent who has infrequent sickle cell crises is in pain but fears taking "too much" analgesia and becoming addicted. How should the nurse counsel this adolescent?
   1. Encourage the adolescent to use analgesics sparingly because children easily become addicted.
   2. Encourage the adolescent to use a sufficient amount of analgesia to remain sedated until the crisis resolves.
   3. Encourage the adolescent to use acetaminophen to control the pain.
   4. Encourage the adolescent to request analgesia before the pain becomes uncontrollable.

2. A nursing goal for a child with sickle cell anemia is to prevent sickling. Which action best indicates compliance by the family in achieving this goal?
   1. The family moves to a small town in the Rocky Mountains where there is less stress.
   2. The family takes up desert dirt-bike racing as a way of promoting family togetherness.
   3. The family goes to a weekly Sunday afternoon movie together.
   4. The family goes for a long midday walk three times a week.

3. Which is a critical nursing intervention when caring for a child with sickle cell anemia?
   1. Referring the child for genetic counseling.
   2. Teaching the child how to live a normal life.
   3. Teaching the child and the parents how to prevent sickling, which leads to crisis.
   4. Teaching the child how to correctly apply heat to painful areas.

4. A 10-year-old in sickle cell crisis is admitted to a hospital pediatric unit. Which of the child's activities during the past week indicates the need for further health teaching?
   1. Went to the movies with a friend.
   2. Studied in the school library.
   3. Visited a classmate who is sick.
   4. Went swimming in a heated pool.

5. A young child is in vaso-occlusive crisis secondary to sickle cell anemia. Which statement made by the child's parents indicates the need for further teaching by the nurse?
   1. "We will pay more attention to our child's fluid intake in the future."
   2. "Next time our child runs a temperature, we'll call the pediatrician right away."
   3. "We will apply ice to the painful areas on his hands and feet next time a crisis occurs."
   4. "We'll continue to avoid taking our child into high altitudes."

6. A parent of an infant newly diagnosed with hemophilia tells the nurse, "I won't let my baby have the treatment. I'm not going to lose him to AIDS!" The nurse's best response is:
   1. "The current blood supply is safe and you have nothing to worry about."
   2. "AIDS is not transmitted by the clotting factor."
   3. "Refusing the clotting factor puts your baby at risk for death from hemorrhage.
   4. "I understand your concerns. Let's talk about AIDS and hemophilia."

7. A goal in caring for a child with hemophilia is to prevent injury. How can this best be achieved?
   1. Pad the side of an active infant's crib.
   2. Restrict a preschooler from riding a Big Wheel tricycle.
   3. Restrict a school-aged child from all sports except karate.
   4. Encourage a teenager to grow a beard instead of shaving.

8. A child with hemophilia injures an ankle while playing soccer and comes to the hospital emergency department. The ankle is swollen and painful. The nurse's first action is to:
   1. Immediately elevate and immobilize the extremity.
   2. Apply slight pressure to the injury site.
   3. Apply a warm, moist compress to the ankle.
   4. Administer aspirin to control the pain.

9. Which intervention is contraindicated for a child with hemophilia during an episode of hemarthritis?
   1. Application of splints or other immobilizing devices.
   2. Administration of non-aspirin-based analgesics.
   3. Active range-of-motion exercises.
   4. Infusions of clotting factor.

10. An 11-year-old child with hemophilia tells the school nurse, "I'm not wearing this dumb Medic-Alert bracelet or that stupid helmet for sports." The best action by the nurse is to:
    1. Allow the child to ventilate his feelings.
    2. Inform the child that failing to cooperate will result in removal from the team.
    3. Contact the parent regarding the child's statement.
    4. Send the child to the principal's office.

11. A 10-year-old child should be involved in which aspect of the hemophilia regimen?
    1. Genetic transmission.
    2. Insurance coverage.
    3. Administration of the clotting factor.
    4. Appropriate career choices.

Answers/Rationale

1. **(4)** A goal in the treatment of sickle cell anemia is prevention of pain. Children with sickle cell anemia tend to be undermedicated, *not* overmedicated. The adolescent should request analgesia before the pain is out of control. Children rarely become addicted **(1)** despite high doses of analgesics. The adolescent should not be so sedated **(2)** that participation in activities that provide oxygenation and hydration necessary for recovery is precluded. Acetaminophen does *not* control the pain associated with sickle cell anemia **(3)**; the pain usually requires opioids. **IMP, ANL, 6, PhI, Physiological adaptation**

2. **(3)** Attending a movie together does *not* contribute to sickling in a child with sickle cell anemia and is therefore an appropriate activity. It does *not* expose the child to situations involving low oxygen tension or dehydration, which can precipitate sickling. Moving to a small town in the mountains **(1)** is *not* advised because conditions of *low* oxygen tension (found in *high* altitudes) can precipitate sickling. Activities performed in a hot environment, such as the desert **(2)**, can promote dehydration, which also precipitates sickling. Activities done in the direct sun **(4)** are also to be avoided because they can lead to dehydration. **EV, ANL, 6, HPM, Health promotion and maintenance**

3. **(3)** The most critical element in caring for the child with sickle cell anemia is teaching the child and the family how to prevent the sickling that leads to crisis. Teaching usually entails instruction on how to *avoid* infections and maintain hydration. Referring the child for genetic counseling **(1)** is usually *not* necessary until the child reaches the childbearing years. Teaching the child how to live a normal life **(2)** is *not* effective unless instructions about how to prevent sickling are given *first*. Repeated sickling episodes prevent a normal life from being achieved. Knowledge of the correct method to apply heat **(4)** is appropriate, but *not critical*. **IMP, ANL, 6, HPM, Health promotion and maintenance**

4. **(3)** Children with sickle cell anemia have increased susceptibility to infections, so visiting with a friend who is sick indicates the need for additional teaching. Sickle cell crisis is precipitated by conditions of low oxygen tension and dehydration. Going to the movies **(1)**, using the school library **(2)**, or swimming in a heated pool **(4)** would *not* precipitate a crisis. **EV, ANL, 6, HPM, Health promotion and maintenance**

5. **(3)** Heat, *not* cold, is applied to painful body areas such as the hands and feet during a vaso-occlusive crisis. The desired effect of heat is to increase blood flow (vasodilation) and oxygen supply to the affected area. Statements about providing fluids **(1)** to prevent dehydration; observing for elevations in temperature **(2)**, which can signal the start of an infection leading to sickling; and avoiding high altitudes **(4)** with low oxygen tension *all* signify an *appropriate* knowledge base and compliance by the parents. **EV, ANL, 6, HPM, Health promotion and maintenance**

6. **(4)** An empathetic response by the nurse and an offer to teach the parent about the relationship between AIDS and hemophilia should reassure and calm the parent. When the parent is less stressed and ready to learn, the nurse can then teach the other facts noted in options **1, 2,** and **3**. Individuals with hemophilia diagnosed and treated with blood products **(1)** or factor concentrates **(2)** since 1985 are at virtually no risk for developing HIV infection because of current purification techniques. Refusing treatment places the infant at risk for uncontrollable hemorrhage **(3)**. **IMP, ANL, 7, HPM, Health promotion and maintenance**

7. **(1)** Padding the crib rails of an active infant's crib helps prevent injury to the infant when the infant pulls up into the standing position using the rails. Padding also prevents facial injuries caused by teething on or falling into the crib rails. Pre-schoolers **(2)** need *not* be restricted from "Big Wheel" tricycles because this toy is low to the ground; falls and subsequent bleeding are usually prevented with this toy. School-aged children **(3)** may swim and hike, but activities, such as karate, that are strenuous on the child's joints should be avoided. Teenagers **(4)** need *not* refrain from shaving if an electric razor is used to prevent injury. **PL, ANL, 6, SECE, Safety and infection control**

8. **(1)** The nurse's first action is to immediately immobilize and elevate the extremity above the level of the heart to decrease blood flow because bleeding is occurring into the joint capsule. Direct pressure **(2)** must be applied to any noticeable *bleeding* for a period of at least 5-15 minutes. Ice, *not* heat **(3)**, is applied to the injury site because ice causes vasoconstriction. (To prevent skin damage, ice is used cautiously in young children.) Aspirin **(4)**, which prolongs bleeding time, is *not* used for analgesia in children and especially *not* in children with hemophilia. **IMP, ANL, 6, PhI, Physiological adaptation**

Key to Codes

Nursing process: AS, assessment; AN, analysis; PL, planning; IMP, implementation; EV, evaluation. (See **Appendix L** for explanation of nursing process steps.)

Cognitive level: RE/KN, recall/knowledge; COM, comprehension; APP, application; ANL, analysis; EVL, evaluation; SYN, synthesis. (See **Appendix L** for explanation.)

Category of human function: 1, protective; 2, sensory-perceptual; 3, comfort, rest, activity, and mobility; 4, nutrition; 5, growth and development; 6, fluid-gas transport; 7, psychosocial-cultural; 8, elimination. (See **Appendix N** for explanation.)

Client need: SECE, safe, effective care environment; HPM, health promotion and maintenance; PsI, psychosocial integrity; PhI, physiological integrity. (See **Appendix O** for explanation.)

Client subneed: See **Appendix O** for explanation.

9. **(3)** Active range-of-motion can aggravate the bleeding further by moving the affected area, particularly a painful joint. *After* bleeding has been controlled, *passive* range-of-motion exercises can be done to prevent stiffness and eventual contractures of the joint. Immobilization **(1)**, analgesia **(2)**, and clotting factor **(4)** are the basis of treatment for an active bleed into a joint. **IMP, ANL, 6, SECE, Safety and infection control**

10. **(1)** This child has had the burden of being "different" since birth, so outbursts are to be expected on occasion. The child must comply with certain things to ensure own safety; however, this can be discussed after the child has had a chance to "blow off steam." Developmentally, older school-aged children want to be like their peers; MedicAlert bracelets and helmets visibly demonstrate that they are not. Informing the child that the child must comply in order to continue participating on the team **(2)** is appropriate only *after* feelings have first been acknowledged. Parents should be informed **(3)** so that they, too, can be involved in assisting their child in coping with feelings, but this also should happen *later*. Punitive actions, such as involving the principal **(4)**, should be avoided. **IMP, ANL, 7, HPM, Health promotion and maintenance**

11. **(3)** Older school-aged children have both the fine and gross motor skills and the cognitive abilities to self-administer the needed clotting factor, with supervision. Future concerns, such as genetic transmission **(1)**, insurance coverage **(2)**, and career choices **(4)**, should be delayed until the child is well into adolescence. Choices that affect one's future begin to be made in adolescence. **IMP, APP, 5, HPM, Health promotion and maintenance**

Neoplastic Disorders

12

Key Words

anaphylaxis an allergic hypersensitivity reaction of the body to an offending allergen, which may be a foreign protein or drug. This is an acute, life-threatening emergency which requires prompt and aggressive intervention to avoid death.

hepatosplenomegaly enlargement of the liver and spleen, often related to disease.

leukoencephalopathy inflammation of the brain caused by the infiltration of white blood cells in conditions such as leukemia.

leukopenia abnormal decrease in white blood cells.

lymphadenopathy swelling of the lymph glands, often related to disease.

mesenchyme cells of mesodermal origin that are capable of developing into connective tissues, blood, and lymphatic and blood vessels.

metastasis spread of cancer from one part of the body to another.

nephrectomy surgical removal of a kidney.

neutropenia abnormally low number of neutrophils in the blood.

reticuloendothelial system (RES) the body's system of defense against invading organisms; it includes all cells scattered throughout the body that have the ability to phagocytose (ingest and destroy) foreign cells (bacteria).

stomatitis inflammation of the mouth.

thrombocytopenia abnormal decrease in the number of blood platelets.

Summary of Key Points

1. The most common type of childhood cancer is *leukemia*.

2. *Leukemia* is characterized by a malignant proliferation of immature and poorly functioning white blood cells, which invade other body systems such as the reticuloendothelial system, the central nervous system and bones.

3. *Bone tumors* are characterized by localized pain, which is relieved by a flexed position.

4. *Ewing's sarcoma* is treated with surgery, chemotherapy and radiation therapy; *osteosarcoma* is treated by amputation followed by chemotherapy.

5. *Brain tumors* are the second most common pediatric cancer. Prognosis is based on type and location of the tumor.

6. *Wilms' tumor* is characterized by a mass over the kidney area that is first felt by the parents and brings the child to the attention of the practitioner.

7. The treatment for *Wilms' tumor* is nephrectomy; preoperatively, the child should have a sign posted that says "Do Not Palpate Abdomen."

8. *Home care* for all children with neoplastic disorders: NEVER allow swollen lymph glands or fever for more than 24-48 hours before seeking medical attention.

Selected Neoplastic Disorders (Cancer)

Leukemia

I. *Introduction*: Known as "cancer of the blood," leukemia is the most common form of childhood cancer, with an incidence of 4/100,000. Acute leukemia is basically a malignant proliferation of white blood cell (WBC) precursors triggered by an unknown cause and affecting *all blood-forming organs and systems* throughout the body. The onset is typically insidious, and the disease is most common in preschoolers (ages 2–6 yr), occurring more frequently in *boys*.

II. **Assessment:**

A. Major problem: leukopenia: ↓ WBC/↑ blasts (over-production of immature, poorly functioning white blood cells).

B. Bone marrow dysfunction results in:
1. *Neutropenia*: multiple prolonged infections.
2. *Anemia*: pallor, weakness, irritability, shortness of breath.
3. *Thrombocytopenia*: bleeding tendencies (petechiae, epistaxis, bruising).

C. Infiltration of reticuloendothelial system (RES): hepatosplenomegaly → abdominal pain, lymphadenopathy.

D. Leukemic invasion of CNS: ↑ ICP/leukemic meningitis (leukoencephalopathy).

E. Leukemic invasion of bone: pain, pathologic fractures, hemarthrosis.

III. **Analysis/nursing diagnosis:**

A. *Risk for infection* related to neutropenia.

B. *Risk for injury* related to thrombocytopenia.

C. *Altered nutrition, less than body requirements*, related to loss of appetite, vomiting, mouth ulcers.

D. *Pain* related to disease process and treatments (e.g., hemarthrosis, bone pain, bone marrow aspiration).

E. *Activity intolerance* related to infection and anemia.

F. *Self-esteem disturbance* related to disease process and treatments (e.g., loss of hair with chemotherapy, moon face with prednisone).

G. *Anticipatory grieving* related to life-threatening illness.

H. *Knowledge deficit* related to diagnosis, treatment, prognosis.

IV. **Nursing care plan/implementation:**

A. Goal: *maintain infection-free state.*
1. Standard precautions to prevent infection.
2. Use good handwashing technique.
3. Ongoing evaluation of sites for potential infection, e.g., gums.
4. Provide meticulous oral hygiene.
5. Keep record of *vital signs*, especially temperature.
6. Provide good skin care.
7. Screen staff and visitors—restrict anyone with infection.
8. *Protective isolation/reverse isolation* to minimize exposure to potentially life-threatening infection.
9. Discharge planning: return to school, but isolate from chickenpox or known communicable diseases.

B. Goal: *prevent injury.*
1. *Avoid* IMs/IVs if possible, due to bruising and bleeding tendencies.
2. Do *not* give *aspirin* or medications containing aspirin, which interferes with platelet formation, thus increasing the risk of bleeding.
3. Use soft toothbrush to *avoid* trauma to gums, which may cause bleeding and infection.
4. *Avoid* "per rectum" suppositories, due to probable rectal ulcers.
5. Supervise play/activity carefully to promote safety and prevent excessive bruising or bleeding.

C. Goal: *promote adequate nutrition.*
1. *Diet*: high calorie, *high* protein, *high* iron. If neutropenic, *remove* fresh, raw fruits and vegetables from diet.
2. Encourage *extra fluids* to prevent constipation or dehydration.
3. I&O, daily weights, to monitor fluid and nutritional status.
4. Allow child to be involved with food selection/preparation; allow child almost any food he or she tolerates, to encourage better dietary intake.
5. Serve *frequent, small snacks* to increase fluid and caloric consumption.
6. Offer dietary supplements to increase caloric intake.
7. Encourage local anesthetics such as *dextromethorphan* lozenges before meals to allow child to eat without pain from oral mucous membrane ulcers.

D. Goal: *relieve pain.*
1. Offer supportive alternatives: extra company, back rub, etc.
2. Administer medications, regularly, before pain becomes excessive.
3. Administer medications that produce conscious sedation (*midazolam, fentanyl*) for painful procedures such as spinal taps or bone marrow aspiration.
4. Use bean bag chair for positional changes.
5. **Avoid** excessive stimulation (noise, light), which may heighten perception of pain.

E. Goal: *conserve energy.*
   1. Cluster care to prevent exhaustion.
   2. Provide rest periods between care.
F. Goal: *promote self-esteem.*
   1. Stress what child can still do to keep the child as independent as possible.
   2. Encourage performance of activities of daily living (ADL) as much as possible to foster a sense of independence.
   3. Provide diversion/activity as tolerated.
   4. Give lots of positive reinforcement to enhance a sense of accomplishment.
   5. Provide realistic feedback on child's appearance; offer suggestions, such as a wig or cap to cover alopecia secondary to chemotherapy.
   6. Encourage early return to peers/school to avoid social isolation.
G. Goal: *prevent complications related to leukemia/ prolonged immobility/treatments which can exacerbate disease process.*
   1. Inspect skin for breakdown, especially over bony prominences, due to poor nutritional intake and limited mobility due to bone pain.
   2. Anticipate need for and provide (per MD order) multiple transfusions of platelets, packed red cells, etc.
   3. Check for hemorrhagic cystitis; *push fluids* (especially if *cyclophosphamide* is given).
   4. Check for constipation and/or peripheral neuropathy (especially if *vincristine* is given).
   5. Stress to parents and child that disease process has remissions and exacerbations. Loss of remission does *not* necessarily mean "the end."
H. Goal: **health teaching**. *Assist child and parents to cope with life-threatening illness and educate regarding disease process.*
   1. Teach rationale for: repeated hospitalizations, multiple invasive tests/ treatments, long-term follow-up care.
   2. Encourage compliance with all aspects of therapy, to increase chances of survival.
   3. Support family and their coping mechanisms.
   4. Offer factual information regarding ultimate prognosis ("80% cure" for acute lymphocytic leukemia [ALL]). Discuss bone marrow transplant.
   5. If death appears imminent, assist family to cope with dying and death.

V. **Evaluation/outcome criteria:**
   A. Child is maintained in infection-free state.
   B. Injuries are prevented or kept to a minimum.
   C. Adequate nutrition is maintained.
   D. Child is free from pain or can live with minimum level of pain.
   E. Energy is conserved and mobility maintained.
   F. Child's self-esteem is maintained; child is treated as living (not dying).
   G. Complications are prevented or kept to a minimum.
   H. Positive coping mechanisms are utilized by child and family to deal with illness.

Bone Tumors

I. *Introduction*: Less than 5% of all malignant neoplasms are malignant bone tumors; however, malignant bone tumors are more common in children than in adults. Before puberty, boys and girls are equally affected. After puberty, *boys* have an incidence two times *greater* than that for girls. The *peak* age for malignant bone tumors during childhood is 15–19 yr, during the growth spurt of adolescence.

The two most common types of malignant bone tumors are o*steogenic sarcoma* and *Ewing's sarcoma*. The prognosis for children with either type of tumor varies with the specific treatment protocol used and the site of the primary tumor and/or metastasis. Overall, the long-term survival rate is 60% or better.
   A. **Osteogenic sarcoma**: most common bone cancer in children. It is a tumor of the bone that arises from the *mesenchyme*. Primary sites are in long bones, e.g., femur, tibia and humerus (see also **Chapter 14, Table 14.1, p. 129**).
   B. **Ewing's sarcoma**: a tumor that arises in the *marrow*. Primary sites are in the shafts of long and trunk bones, affecting an arm or leg, rib, or pelvis.
II. **Assessment:**
   A. Most common initial symptoms: pain and swelling at the site of the tumor.
   B. *Pain*: localized; becomes increasingly severe and frequent; may be confused with "growing pains"; often relieved if child assumes a *flexed position*.
   C. Child's *behavior*: limits own activity; may limp or drop objects; cannot hold heavy objects.
   D. Examine affected area for: mass, functional status, lymph node involvement, inflammation.
   E. Examine for any evidence of metastasis, particularly in the lungs, which is the primary site of metastasis.
   F. *Diagnostic procedures and tests*: x-rays, scans, biopsy, bone marrow aspiration (*Ewing's sarcoma*).
III. **Analysis/nursing diagnosis:**
   A. *High risk for injury* related to malignancy and treatment.
   B. *High risk for infection* related to chemotherapy and depressed body defenses.
   C. *Risk for impaired skin integrity* related to chemotherapy, radiation therapy, immobility.
   D. *Altered family process* related to care of the child with a life-threatening illness.

E. *Body-image disturbance* related to amputation of affected limb.

F. *Knowledge deficit* related to the disease, its treatment, and prognosis.

IV. Nursing care plan/implementation:

A. Goal: *prevent complications related to chemotherapy.*

1. Administer chemotherapy according to guidelines.

2. D/C IV immediately if any signs of *infiltration* become evident.

3. Observe child carefully for at least 20–30 min after IV chemotherapy for possible *anaphylaxis.*

4. Have emergency drugs and equipment available to treat anaphylaxis promptly.

5. Monitor child for additional complications of chemotherapy: infection, bleeding tendencies, hemorrhagic cystitis, oral or rectal mucosal ulceration, nausea and vomiting, anorexia, peripheral neuropathy.

B. Goal: *prevent infection.*

1. Private room, with possible *reverse isolation.*

2. Good handwashing by all staff and visitors; screen all staff and visitors for possible infection.

3. Use *strict aseptic technique* for all invasive procedures.

4. Monitor possible sites of infection: needle punctures, mucosal ulcers, teeth and gums.

5. Monitor for signs and symptoms of infection, including temperature; report promptly and treat aggressively.

6. **No** live virus vaccines (i.e., measles, mumps, rubella, polio); give *only* inactivated immunizations.

C. Goal: *maintain skin integrity.*

1. Provide good skin care to all areas.

2. *Turn* and *position* frequently; monitor for: redness, irritation or signs of breakdown.

3. Have child wear loose-fitting clothes over irradiated skin.

4. Protect irradiated skin from sunlight or sudden changes in temperature.

D. Goal: *provide child and family with the support needed to cope with this situational crisis.*

1. Encourage verbalizations of feelings regarding illness and treatment.

2. Allow family to have periods of uninterrupted private time.

3. Discuss how to relate the diagnosis to the child, and other siblings.

4. Help the family interpret the child's reaction to this crisis.

5. Refer family to local chapter of American Cancer Society or other local cancer support group.

E. Goal: *assist the child and family to cope with potential loss of limb.*

1. Prepare child and family for limb salvage or amputation (*osteogenic sarcoma*); amputation if the results of radiation render the limb useless or deformed (*Ewing's sarcoma*).

2. Stress that this is the treatment of choice when other alternatives have been exhausted.

3. Answer questions honestly; be open and available to child and family.

4. Encourage child and family to discuss their questions or concerns.

F. Goal: **health teaching.** *Teach child and family understanding of the disease, treatment and prognosis.*

1. Explain all procedures and treatments to be done to the child.

2. Explain chemotherapy and/or radiation therapy.

3. Explain amputation accurately and honestly.

4. Explain long-term survival rates and factors that may influence long-term survival.

V. Evaluation/outcome criteria:

A. Child completes chemotherapy without complications.

B. Child remains infection free.

C. Skin integrity is maintained.

D. Family can cope with this crisis.

E. Child and family adjust to disability and change in body image.

F. Child and family verbalize understanding of disease, treatment, and prognosis.

Brain Tumors

I. *Introduction:* Brain tumors are the second most prevalent type of cancer in children. They are the most common cause of death from cancer in children. Most occur in children under 1 year of age or between 2 and 12 years of age. Prognosis varies based on the type and location of the tumor.

A. *Astrocytomas:* most common pediatric brain tumor; usually infiltrates brain *parenchyma*; can be *low* or *high* grade with low grade having the best survival rate of 75–85%.

B. *Medulloblastoma:* accounts for 20–25% of pediatric brain tumors; a primitive *neuroectodermal* tumor; fast growing and highly malignant; survival rate of 70%.

C. *Ependymoma:* accounts for 4% of pediatric brain tumors; most invade *ventricles* and obstruct flow of *cerebral spinal fluid*; survival rate of 45%.

D. *Glioma:* accounts for 15% of pediatric brain tumors; tumor locates in vital brain centers (especially *brain stem*); survival rate poor as surgical excision is difficult because of tumor location; tumor is highly resistant to therapy.

II. **Assessment:**

A. Headache and vomiting (unrelated to food consumption).

B. *Behavioral changes* (staring spells; involuntary movements; loss of previously attained developmental skills; ↓ in school performance).

C. Loss of *motor* control (ataxia; clumsiness; awkward gait; weakness; paralysis).

D. ↑*Intracranial pressure* (papilledema, hydrocephalus in infants; diplopia; seizures; changes in vital signs and level of consciousness).

E. *Diagnostic procedures and tests*: skull x-rays, brain scan, CT scan, MRI, cerebral angiography, lumbar puncture (spinal tap), tissue biopsy.

III. **Analysis/nursing diagnosis:**

A. *High risk for injury* related to loss of muscle control.

B. *Sensory-perceptual alterations* related to space-occupying lesion in brain.

IV. **Nursing care plan/implementation:**

A. Goal: *prevent injury.*

1. Keep side rails up.

2. Keep floors free of scatter rugs, cords, toys.

3. Have seizure precautions at bedside (oral airway, suction, oxygen, padded side rails).

B. Goal: *keep child oriented to reality.*

1. Call child by name before touching child; announce presence in room.

2. Describe surroundings, treatments, etc. to child.

3. Administer chemotherapy, radiation and prepare for surgical removal of tumor in effort to reduce ↑ ICP and prevent sensory-perceptual alterations.

V. **Evaluation/outcome criteria:**

A. Injury prevented.

B. Sensory-perceptual alterations are minimized.

Solid Tumor: Wilms' Tumor (nephroblastoma)

I. *Introduction*: Wilms' tumor is a malignant tumor of the kidney and is the most common form of renal cancer in children. *Peak* incidence occurs at 3 yr, with a slightly higher incidence in boys than in girls. Ninety percent of cases occur *unilaterally*; the treatment of choice is nephrectomy (and adrenalectomy) followed by chemotherapy and radiation.

II. **Assessment:**

A. Most common sign: abdominal mass (firm, nontender).

B. Most often first found by parent changing diaper; felt as a mass over the kidney area.

C. Intravenous pyelogram (IVP) confirms the diagnosis.

D. Metastasis occurs most frequently to the lungs: pain in chest, cough, dyspnea.

III. **Analysis/nursing diagnosis:**

A. *Altered urinary elimination* related to space occupying lesion in kidney.

B. *Knowledge deficit* related to diagnosis, treatment, prognosis.

IV. **Nursing care plan/implementation:**

A. Goal: *promote normal urinary function.*

1. Inform family that surgery is scheduled as soon as possible after confirmed diagnosis (within 24-48 h).

2. Explain to family that the preferred surgical approach is nephrectomy (and adrenalectomy).

3. *Preoperative*: **Do not palpate abdomen** because the tumor is highly friable, and palpation increases the risk of metastasis.

4. *Postoperative nursing care:* similar to care of adult with nephrectomy.

5. *Postoperative* care also includes long-term radiation therapy and chemotherapy (dactinomycin, vincristine, doxorubicin).

B. Goal: **health teaching**. *Discharge teaching to prepare parents to care for child at home.*

1. Teach parents need for long-term follow-up care with specialists: oncologist, urologist.

2. Answer questions regarding prognosis, offering realistic hope.

a. Child with localized tumor: *90%* survival rate.

b. Child with metastasis: *50%* survival rate.

V. **Evaluation/outcome criteria:**

A. Child is able to maintain normal urinary elimination.

B. Parents verbalize their understanding of home care for the child.

COMMONLY PRESCRIBED MEDICATIONS

Medication	Administration	Use/Action	⋈ Nursing Consideration
Alkylating Agents Cisplatin/*Platinol* Procarbazine/ *Matulane*	• Oral and parenteral • Calculate to child's weight in kilograms ⚠ • Use standard chemotherapy precautions • Administer in provided dropper or calibrated syringe • NEVER use household measuring spoon	Used in treatment of cancer Substitutes an alkyl group for a hydrogen atom leading to DNA replication Cell cycle non-specific (active in all stages of the cell cycle)	• *Avoid* foods *high* in tyramine (e.g., cheese, yogurt, chocolate) which elevate norepinephrine to toxic level • Monitor for renal toxicity • Encourage fluids with strict I&O • Do *not* use aluminum needle (↓ potency of drug)
Antibiotics Bleomycin/ *Blenoxane* Doxorubicin/ *Adriamycin*	• Parenteral • Calculate to child's weight in kilograms ⚠ • Use standard chemotherapy precautions	Used in treatment of cancer Interferes with nucleic acid Inhibits DNA and RNA synthesis Cell cycle non-specific (active in all stages of the cell cycle)	• Have vesicant kit nearby • Observe for changes in heart and/or respiratory rates or signs of failure • Have child on cardiac and apnea monitors • Pulmonary function tests as baseline, before and after therapy
Antimetabolites Cytosine arabinoside/ *Cytosar* Methotrexate/*MTX*	• Oral and parenteral • Calculate to child's weight in kilograms ⚠ • Use standard chemotherapy precautions • Administer in provided dropper or calibrated syringe • NEVER use household measuring spoon	Used in treatment of cancer Interferes with function of nucleic acid Inhibits DNA or RNA synthesis Cell cycle specific (active in synthesis phase)	• Administer with *steroid eye drops* to prevent conjunctivitis • Monitor renal and hepatic function • Use sun block • Mix with preservative-free diluent
Enzymes 1-Asparaginase/ *Elspar*	• Parenteral • Calculate to child's weight in kilograms ⚠ • Use standard chemotherapy precautions	Used in treatment of cancer Makes cell in G phase vulnerable to other agents Interferes with prosynthesis Cell cycle specific (active in G_1 phase)	• Observe for allergic reactions including anaphylactic shock • Have *emergency* drugs on hand
Hormones Hydrocortisone/ *Solu-Cortef* Methylprednisolone/ *Solu-Medrol*	• Oral, parenteral and intrathecal • Calculate to child's weight in kilograms ⚠ • Use standard chemotherapy precautions • Administer in provided dropper or calibrated syringe • NEVER use household measuring spoon	Used in treatment of cancer Makes cell in G phase vulnerable to other agents Interferes with prosynthesis Cell cycle specific (active in G_1 phase)	• Disguise bitter taste in chocolate syrup • Observe for expected side effect (hyperglycemia, weight gain, hirsutism, growth retardation, etc.) • Assess for infections • Test stools for occult blood
Nitrosoureas Carmustine/*BCNU*	• Parenteral • Calculate to child's weight in kilograms ⚠ • Use standard chemotherapy precautions	Used in treatment of cancer Causes breakage in DNA Crosses blood-brain barrier Cell cycle non-specific (active in all stages of the cell cycle)	• Observe for flushing and facial burning • Inform child and parents that contact with skin causes brown spots
Plant Alkaloids Vincristine/*Oncovin*	• Parenteral • Calculate to child's weight in kilograms ⚠ • Use standard chemotherapy precautions	Used in treatment of cancer Binds with cell proteins to inhibit nucleic acid and protein synthesis Cell cycle specific (active in mitosis phase)	• Have vesicant kit nearby • Assess for neurotoxicity • Tends to be constipating • Administer with *stool softener*

Study and Memory Aids

Leukemia—Incidence

Most common in *preschool boys*.
Most common cancer of childhood.

Leukemia—Early Sign

Repeated, lingering infections.

Leukemia—Diagnosis

Definitive *diagnostic test* for leukemia: bone marrow aspiration, which is typically hypercellular with primarily blast cells.

Leukemia—Lab Finding

Normal platelet count 150,000-300,000/MM³; usually *much lower* in children with leukemia, resulting in bleeding tendencies.

Leukemia—Vaccination Alert

Children who have been vaccinated within 2 wk before chemotherapy is started, or during chemotherapy, should be considered *not* immunized; the vaccines should be *repeated 3 mo after* chemotherapy is stopped.

Leukemia—Treatment

Chemotherapy is the single most important factor in the improved survival rate of children with leukemia.

Leukemia—Medication Alert

Viscous lidocaine is *not* recommended for younger children receiving chemotherapy as it may depress the gag reflex and increase the risk of aspiration. Viscous lidocaine is also *not* well liked by older children because it numbs the mouth and makes food taste bland. This medication is *no* longer widely used.

Common Bone Tumors— Treatment

Osteosarcoma: limb salvage or amputation and chemotherapy.
Ewing's sarcoma: surgery, chemotherapy, and radiation.

Osteosarcoma—Medication

Amitriptyline has been used successfully in children to decrease phantom limb pain.

Brain Tumors—Assessment/Prognosis

Prognosis varies based on type and location of tumor. Low grade tumors have the best survival rate.

Wilms' Tumor—Assessment

The child with Wilms' tumor is most often brought to the attention of the health care practitioner by a parent who palpated a mass over the kidney area when changing a diaper or dressing child.

Wilms' Tumor—Caution

The child with Wilms' tumor should have a sign that says "Do *Not* Palpate Abdomen" posted over the crib because of the high risk for metastasis.

Questions

1. An adolescent is admitted to the hospital pediatric unit with a suspected diagnosis of osteogenic sarcoma. The nurse should initially assess the teenager for pain in the:
   1. Rib cage.
   2. Abdomen.
   3. Small bones of the hands and feet.
   4. Long bones.

2. The nurse must be aware that a late finding in a child with Wilms' tumor is:
   1. An abdominal mass.
   2. Increasing abdominal girth.
   3. Weight loss.
   4. Shortness of breath.

3. Which assessment technique should the nurse *avoid* using when examining the abdomen of a child with Wilms' tumor?
   1. Inspection.
   2. Percussion.
   3. Auscultation.
   4. Palpation.

4. Following diagnosis, surgery for a Wilms' tumor is usually scheduled immediately. The nurse is faced with the challenge of directing the focus of the preoperative teaching toward:
   1. Simple, repeated explanations.
   2. Involving all family members in the plan of care.
   3. Experiences the child will actually have.
   4. Having the parents talk to another family with a child with a Wilms' tumor.

5. Which instruction must the nurse include in the discharge plan for a child who has undergone a unilateral nephrectomy secondary to Wilms' tumor?
   1. Resume activities as usual.
   2. Prevent urinary tract infections.
   3. Apply for a donor kidney.
   4. Await an at-home school teacher.

6. The RN observes an LPN/LVN offering viscous lidocaine to a 3-year-old child with oral mucosal ulceration (secondary to chemotherapy) when bringing in the child's lunch tray. The best action for the RN to take at this time is:
   1. Tell the LPN/LVN not to use viscous lidocaine, but rather to offer other mouthwashes or lozenges as ordered by the physician.
   2. Tell the LPN/LVN that viscous lidocaine should have been offered at least 15 minutes before the child's lunch.
   3. Check the nursing care plan to determine whether viscous lidocaine should be offered.
   4. Check if the child is allergic to viscous lidocaine.

7. When discontinuing the IV of a child whose platelet count is 86,000/mm³, the nurse should:
   1. Send the tip of the angiocath to the laboratory for culture.
   2. Apply direct pressure to the site for 5 minutes.
   3. Flush the line with heparin before pulling it.
   4. Observe for signs of clotting distal to the IV site.

8. The nurse notes that a child who is admitted for chemotherapy received immunizations 9 days before admission. Which statement by the nurse is most appropriate for the child's parents?
   1. "The immunizations will not be affected by the chemotherapy because the child received them 9 days ago."
   2. "The chemotherapy cannot be started until at least 2 weeks after the last immunization was given."
   3. "These immunizations will not be effective and the child should be revaccinated 3 months after the chemotherapy is stopped."
   4. "The chemotherapy should be started immediately, but there may be an increased risk of complications because the child was immunized recently."

9. The parents of a child with suspected leukemia ask the nurse when they will know "for sure" whether this is what their child has. The nurse should base a response on the knowledge that the definitive diagnostic test for leukemia is:
   1. Leukocyte count.
   2. Lumbar puncture.
   3. Bone marrow aspiration.
   4. Biopsy of the lymph glands.

10. The parents of a preschooler who is to have a bone marrow aspiration express their concern about pain their child may experience. The nurse is most correct in assuring them that their child will most likely receive which medication for pain?
    1. Ibuprofen.
    2. A local anesthetic.
    3. Conscious sedation.
    4. Demerol, phenergan, and thorazine.

11. Which medication should the nurse expect to be ordered for a child who is complaining of phantom limb pain following an amputation for osteosarcoma?
    1. Amitriptyline (*Elavil*).
    2. Meperidine (*Demerol*).
    3. Diazepam (*Valium*).
    4. Diphenhydramine (*Benadryl*).

12. The parents of a toddler who is newly diagnosed with Wilms' tumor ask the nurse why there is a sign on their child's bed that says "DO NOT PALPATE ABDOMEN." The nurse should inform the parents that palpating the area:
    1. Will cause pain.
    2. May cause hemorrhage.
    3. Can cause spread of cancer cells.

4. Is upsetting for children with a large tumor such as this one.

13. When caring for a child who has postoperative nephrectomy for Wilms' tumor, the nurse should:
    1. Institute pulmonary hygiene measures to prevent complications.
    2. Restrict fluids to avoid overloading the remaining kidney.
    3. Assist the patient to the bathroom to void.
    4. Encourage the patient to visit the playroom to interact with other children.

14. The clinic nurse is screening phone calls from parents of children who are being treated with chemotherapy for various cancers. Three of the following, if reported by the parents of a child receiving chemotherapy, would require referral to the MD for further evaluation. Which item is a normal side effect that, although troublesome, would not require medical evaluation?
    1. Mucosal ulceration.
    2. Hemorrhagic cystitis.
    3. Nausea and vomiting.
    4. Peripheral neuropathy.

15. The nurse is caring for a 15-year-old who has Ewing's sarcoma of the ulna and is being treated with radiation therapy. Which statement, if made by this teen, would indicate that the nurse's teaching regarding irradiation was effective?
    1. "I will wear loose-fitting clothes over my arm."
    2. "I will expose my arm to the sun for 1 hour daily."
    3. "I will use an ice pack on my arm when it aches."
    4. "I will keep my arm in a sling and avoid using it until the treatments are over."

16. Upon assessment of a child with newly diagnosed leukemia, which set of signs and symptoms should the nurse anticipate observing?
    1. Sore throat, draining ear, elevated blood pressure.
    2. Rash on lower extremities, lethargy, bone pain.
    3. Periorbital edema, bruising, ulceration of the mouth.
    4. Enlarged lymph nodes, pale skin, areas of bruising on the body.

17. When preparing a child for a bone marrow aspiration, the nurse should know that this test is usually performed over which area?
    1. Sternum.
    2. Lower lumber area.
    3. Femur.
    4. Posterior iliac crest.

18. Which nursing intervention is most effective in preventing the most common complication leading to death in children with leukemia?
    1. A nutritious diet.
    2. Frequent oral hygiene.
    3. Aseptic technique.
    4. Adequate hydration.

19. A child with leukemia is to have repeat blood studies drawn. The nurse should recall that a normal white blood cell count for a child is:
    1. 5000-10,000/mm^3.
    2. 1500-7500/mm^3.
    3. 2000-8000/mm^3.
    4. 15,000-20,000/mm^3.

Answers/Rationale

1. **(4)** During the time of bone growth spurts in adolescence, osteogenic sarcoma is seen predominantly in the long-bone areas that demonstrate rapid growth, such as the femur, tibia, and humerus. The initial symptom of osteogenic sarcoma is pain. *85%* of recurrences of osteogenic sarcoma are pulmonary in nature; pain in the rib cage (1) is a *late* symptom; The most likely cause of abdominal pain (2) in a teenager with osteogenic sarcoma is metastases to the liver, another *late* symptom. Osteogenic sarcoma is *not* associated with small-bone pain in the hands and feet (3). **AS, ANL, 3, PhI, Physiological adaptation**

2. **(4)** Shortness of breath is a late finding indicating that metastasis of the cancer to the lungs has occurred. Abdominal mass (1) is the most common *presenting* sign of Wilms' tumor. Often detected by a parent, increasing abdominal girth (2) and weight loss (3) are common *early* signs of an abdominal malignancy. **AS, APP, 6, PhI, Physiological adaptation**

3. **(4)** Palpation presents the possibility of rupturing the tumor and metastasizing the tumor contents throughout the abdomen. Inspection (1), percussion (2) and auscultation (3) do *not* present this risk. **AS, APP, 8, PhI, Reduction of risk potential**

4. **(3)** Because of the short time available, the nurse should direct preoperative teaching toward experiences the child will actually have to reduce anxiety and stress for the child and family. Simple, repeated explanations (1), involving all members of the family (2), and planning interactions with families with a similar diagnosis (4) are viable teaching strategies, but time may *not* permit them. **IMP, ANL, 1, HPM, Health promotion and maintenance**

5. **(2)** Because the child is left with only one remaining kidney, prompt detection and treatment of urinary tract infections is essential. Activities as usual (1), which may include contact sports or other high-risk play practices, are to be *avoided*. A donor kidney (3) is *not necessary* because the tumor was unilateral and the child still has one remaining functioning kidney. Awaiting an at-home school teacher (4) is *unnecessary* because the overall objective in discharge planning is to return the child to a normal, preoperative life-style. **PL, ANL, 8, HPM, Health promotion and maintenance**

6. **(1)** Viscous lidocaine is not recommended for use in younger children because it can depress the gag reflex and increase the risk of aspiration. In addition, seizures have been reported in children with oral ulcers who have used viscous lidocaine. Viscous lidocaine should not be used at all, irrespective of the time frame associated with meals (2). There is no need to check the nursing care plan (3) or if the client is allergic to viscous lidocaine (4) at this time. **IMP, COM, 1, SECE, Management of care**

7. **(2)** The normal platelet count is 150,000-300,000/mm^3; a count of 86,000/mm^3 is quite *low* and would likely cause bleeding tendencies. The nurse should therefore apply direct pressure to the site for a minimum of 5 minutes and treat the site as an arterial puncture. There is no reason to send the tip of the angiocath to the lab for a culture (1) because there is no undue concern regarding infection as indicated by this lab result. Flushing the line with heparin (3) would increase the risk of bleeding and is thus *contraindicated*. There is no reason to suspect clotting (4) with a decreased platelet count; the *opposite*, bleeding, is expected. **IMP, APP, 1, PhI, Reduction of risk potential**

8. **(3)** Children who have been vaccinated during the 2 weeks before chemotherapy is started, or during chemotherapy, should be considered unimmunized. They should be revaccinated (or receive a live-virus vaccine) 3 months after the chemotherapy has been stopped. It is untrue that the immunizations are not affected by chemotherapy (1), or that chemotherapy cannot be started until 2 weeks after the last immunization (2). There is no known increased risk of complications at this time (4). **IMP, COM, 1, HPM, Health promotion and maintenance**

9. **(3)** The definitive diagnostic procedure for leukemia is bone marrow aspiration, which typically is hypercellular with primarily blast cells. The leukocyte count (1) is evaluated but is *not* considered diagnostic, *only suspicious*; in leukemia, there are typically immature forms of leukocytes in combination with low blood counts. A lumbar puncture (2) might also be done to determine whether there is central nervous system involvement, but this is *not* considered diagnostic and is often *not* done until *after* the diagnosis has been determined. A biopsy of the lymph glands (4) might be done to determine whether there is metastasis to the lymph nodes, but this is *not* considered diagnostic and is often *not* done until *after* the diagnosis has been determined. **AN, ANL, 1, PhI, Reduction of risk potential**

10. **(3)** The nurse needs to consider the child's age (preschool), the fact that this is a painful procedure, and also the fact that it is highly likely the child will experience many more painful procedures if the diagnosis is positive for leukemia. Using medications that produce conscious sedation reduce the pain the child experiences and also induce amnesia, which makes the test less stressful and may make future

procedures less frightening. Ibuprofen (1) is *not* effective for this procedure in such a young child. A local anesthetic (2) would numb the skin, but when the needle enters the bone, the child would experience considerable pain. Demerol, phenergan, and thorazine (4) should *not* be used because of the risk of neurological side effects, including seizures. **AN, APP, 3, PhI, Pharmacological and parenteral therapies**

11. (1) Amitriptyline has been used successfully in children to decrease phantom limb pain. Meperidine (2) is *not* usually successful, although it is a narcotic analgesic. Diazepam (3) or Diphenhydramine (4) have no known therapeutic effect on phantom limb pain. **AN, COM, 3, PhI, Pharmacological and parenteral therapies**

12. (3) One of the most important preoperative concerns is to prevent the spread of the tumor, which is primarily accomplished by avoiding palpation of the tumor. Palpating the tumor can cause the spread of cancer cells to other sites such as the lungs, which are the primary site of metastasis. Palpation of a Wilms' tumor does *not* usually cause *pain* (1) *or* bleeding (2). Most toddlers are upset at simply being touched by strangers, but this is *not* because of the tumor itself (4). **IMP, COM, 1, PhI, Physiological adaptation**

13. (1) Following any major abdominal surgery, a routine of turning, coughing, and deep breathing should be instituted to prevent hypostatic pneumonia, particularly for the child who is postoperative after a nephrectomy for Wilms' tumor, because the child will also be receiving chemotherapy, which can induce myelosuppression and increase the risk of infection. Fluids are *not* generally restricted (2), but are given in normal amounts. The patient will be on bedrest in the immediate postoperative period, and should not be assisted out of bed to void (3); a catheter is usually in place. Going to the playroom (4) should be *delayed* until the patient can be ambulatory. **IMP, APP, 1, PhI, Physiological adaptation**

14. (3) The nurse who is screening calls from parents of children who are receiving chemotherapy must use judgment in recognizing which side effects are normal reactions and which could indicate toxicity. Nausea and vomiting are normal side effects that do *not* usually require medical evaluation, although the nurse should screen further to determine whether the child is dehydrated. Oral ulcers (1), hemorrhagic cystitis (2), and peripheral neuropathy (4) *do* require prompt medical evaluation either to prevent infection or to determine chemotherapy toxicity. **EV, APP, 1, SECE, Management of care**

15. (1) High-dose radiation can cause skin irritation, such as desquamation, and be followed by hyperpigmentation. The teen should wear loose-fitting clothes over the affected area to prevent further skin irritation. Because of increased sensitivity, the irradiated area should be *protected* from sunlight (2) and extremes of temperature (3). The teen should be encouraged to remain active and to use the extremity; there is no need to keep it in a sling (4); in fact, an exercise program may be instituted to preserve maximum function of the arm. **EV, APP, 1, PhI, Physiological adaptation**

16. (4) Enlarged lymph nodes are caused by infiltration of tissue with blast cells. Pale skin is caused by anemia, and bruising is caused by decreased latelets. All these signs and symptoms are consistent with newly diagnosed leukemia. **Options 1, 2, and 3** all contain some elements that are consistent with leukemia (such as lethargy, bone pain, ulceration of the mouth) but do *not* present the definitive picture of leukemia offered in **option 4**. **AS, ANL, 6, PhI, Physiological adaptation**

17. (4) In children, performing a bone marrow aspiration can be difficult because the size of the child can make finding an area of accessible marrow a challenge; for this reason, the posterior iliac crest is a preferred site in children. The sternum (1) is a site that may be used in *adults*. *Neither* the lower lumbar area (2) nor the femur (3) is an appropriate site for a bone marrow aspiration in children or adults. **AS, ANL, 6, PhI, Reduction of risk potential**

18. (3) Infection is the most common complication that leads to death in children with leukemia, and asepsis is the most effective nursing intervention in preventing infections. Nutrition (1), oral hygiene (2) to the buccal ulcerations that often result from chemotherapy, and adequate hydration (4) are appropriate nursing interventions for the child with leukemia, but *do not directly* help prevent infection. **IMP, ANL, 1, SECE, Safety and infection control**

19. (1) 5000-10,000/mm^3 is a normal value for a white blood cell count in a child. 1500 to 7500/mm^3 (2) and 2000 to 8000/mm^3 (3) are *too low* to be accepted as normal in a child. 15,000, to 20,000/mm^3 (4) is *too high* to be accepted as normal in a child. **AS, COM, 6, PhI, Reduction of risk potential**

Key to Codes

Nursing process: AS, assessment; **AN**, analysis; **PL**, planning; **IMP**, implementation; **EV**, evaluation. (See **Appendix L** for explanation of nursing process steps.)

Cognitive level: RE/KN, recall/knowledge; **COM**, comprehension; **APP**, application; **ANL**, analysis; **EVL**, evaluation; **SYN**, synthesis. (See **Appendix L** for explanation.)

Category of human function: 1, protective; 2, sensory-perceptual; 3, comfort, rest, activity, and mobility; 4, nutrition; 5, growth and development; 6, fluid-gas transport; 7, psychosocial-cultural; 8, elimination. (See **Appendix N** for explanation.)

Client need: SECE, safe, effective care environment; **HPM**, health promotion and maintenance; **PsI**, psychosocial integrity; **PhI**, physiological integrity. (See **Appendix O** for explanation.)

Client subneed: See **Appendix O** for explanation.

Central Nervous System Disorders

13

Chapter Outline

Key Words

ataxia defective muscular coordination, especially of voluntary muscles.

decerebrate posturing symptom of profound brain damage; extremities are stiff and rigid and head is retracted.

hyperventilation increase in the rate of respiration, which results in carbon dioxide depletion.

nuchal rigidity stiff neck associated with meningeal irritation.

opisthotonus position assumed by a patient with severe meningeal irritation; neck is hyperextended and back is arched.

petechiae small, purplish, pinpoint hemorrhages caused by ruptured blood vessels; can occur anywhere on the body.

photophobia unusual intolerance of light; occurs in meningitis, measles, or inflammation of the eye.

pica the nutritional habit of ingesting non-nutritive substances, such as flecks of lead-based paint.

tinnitus ringing sound the patient "hears" in the ears, without any external stimulus.

🔑 Summary of Key Points

1. *Bacterial meningitis* is an acute, life-threatening infection that requires *prompt, aggressive intervention* with high-dose *antibiotics*; the child should be isolated and prophylactic antibiotics should be given to members of the immediate family and close contacts of the child.

2. *Positioning* is important for the child with *bacterial meningitis*. The nurse should position the child with the head of the bed slightly *elevated* to decrease intracranial pressure; if the child assumes an opisthotonus position, the nurse should position the child in a *side-lying position*.

3. *Febrile seizures* are a common but *transient neurologic disorder* of childhood; treatment includes administering *antipyretics*, taking environmental measures, and monitoring closely as well as teaching the family about long-term care and possible recurrence.

4. *Seizures* are alterations in the firing of neurons in the brain resulting in sudden, involuntary alterations in: consciousness, motor activity, behavior, sensation or autonomic function; *epilepsy* is a chronic disorder characterized by recurrent seizures.

5. The primary system complication of *lead poisoning* is *permanent and irreversible neurologic* damage manifested by hyperactivity, learning disability, and seizures.

6. The treatment of *lead poisoning* is the administration of *chelating agents (EDTA, BAL)* by means of a series of repeated and painful IMs; *to reduce the trauma of this treatment*, the nurse should rotate the site of the injections, use a local anesthetic with the medication, apply warm soaks, and *avoid* pressure to the muscle.

7. The earliest sign of *salicylate poisoning* is hyperventilation; other signs and symptoms include: high fever, respiratory alkalosis, bleeding disorders, electrolyte disturbances, and liver/kidney failure.

8. The treatment of *salicylate poisoning* is to *induce vomiting* (if the child is *not* comatose), perform gastric lavage, and administer activated charcoal; additional treatment includes IV hydration, monitoring I&O, environmental measures to decrease fever, checking for bleeding, and administering *vitamin K*.

(continued)

9. *Attention-deficit hyperactivity* disorder is characterized by behaviors that are unusual in quality and appropriateness: motor activity is excessive and behavior is developmentally younger than chronologic age.

10. *Reye syndrome* is a fatty degeneration of the liver and acute metabolic encephalopathy that follows influenza, chickenpox, or other viral illness.

11. *Reye syndrome* has been linked to the administration of *aspirin* to a child with influenza, chickenpox, or any other viral illness; to prevent Reye syndrome, children with these illnesses should be treated with *acetaminophen.*

12. *Home care* for all children with central nervous system disorders: NEVER allow changes in level of consciousness (LOC) for more that 1 hour before seeking medical attention.

Selected Central Nervous System Disorders

See **Chapter 16** for *malformations* of the central nervous system (spina bifida and hydrocephalus).

Bacterial Meningitis

I. *Introduction*: Bacterial meningitis is an acute inflammation of the meningea and cerebral spinal fluid (CSF). It is caused by *multiple* agents (e.g., bacteria, viruses, otitis media, brain abscesses, penetrating head wounds, etc.); 90% of reported cases are between 1 month and 5 years of age.

II. **Assessment:**
   A. Abrupt onset: initial sign may be a seizure, following an episode of upper respiratory illness (URI), acute otitis media.
   B. Chills and fever.
   C. Vomiting; may complain of headache, neck pain.
   D. Photophobia.
   E. Alterations in level of consciousness: delirium, stupor, increased intracranial pressure. Bulging fontanel is the most significant finding in infants.
   F. Nuchal rigidity.
   G. *Opisthotonus position*: head is drawn backward into overextension.
   H. Hyperactive reflexes related to central nervous system (CNS) irritability.
   I. *Diagnostic tests*: lumbar puncture (LP)

III. **Analysis/nursing diagnosis:**
   A. *Risk for infection* related to communicability of meningitis.
   B. *Risk for injury* related to CNS irritability and seizures.
   C. *Altered nutrition, less than body requirements,* related to fever and poor oral intake.
   D. *Knowledge deficit* regarding prevention of disease.

IV. **Nursing care plan/implementation:**
   A. Goal: *prevent spread of infection.*
      1. Institute standard precautions.
      2. Enforce strict handwashing.
      3. Institute and maintain *respiratory isolation* for minimum of 24 h after starting IV antibiotics, at which time child is no longer considered to be infectious and can be removed from isolation.
      4. Supervise parents in isolation techniques.
      5. Identify family members and others at high risk: do cultures (*Haemophilus influenzae, E. coli,* etc.); possibly begin prophylactic antibiotics, e.g., *rifampin.*
      6. Treat with IV *antibiotics* (per MD order) as soon as possible after admission (after cultures are obtained); continue 10-14 d (until cerebrospinal-fluid culture is negative and child appears clinically improved).
      7. Anticipate large-dose IV medications only— administer *slowly* in *dilute* form to prevent phlebitis.
      8. Restrain as needed to maintain IV.
   B. Goal: *promote safety and prevent injury/seizures.*
      1. Maintain seizure precautions; administer *anticonvulsants* per MD order, e.g., *phenytoin.*
      2. Place child near nurses' station for maximal observation; provide private room for isolation.
      3. Minimize stimuli: quiet, calm environment.
      4. Restrict visitors to immediate family.
      5. *Position*: head of bed *slightly elevated* to decrease intracranial pressure. (If opisthotonus: *side-lying*, for comfort and safety.)
   C. Goal: *maintain adequate nutrition.*
      1. *NPO or clear liquids* initially; supplement with IVs, as child may be unable to coordinate sucking and swallowing.
      2. Offer diet for age, as tolerated—child may experience anorexia (due to disease) or vomiting (due to increased intracranial pressure).
      3. Monitor I&O, daily weights.
   D. Goal: **health teaching.** *Teach parents prevention of meningitis* for other children in family,
      1. Leading cause of meningitis in young children is *haemophilus influenzae.*
         Routine vaccination for H. flu type b is recommended for all children beginning at 2 months of age (See **Chapter 2**).

V. Evaluation/outcome criteria:
A. No spread of infection noted.
B. Safety maintained.
C. Adequate nutrition and fluid intake maintained.
D. Other children in family are immunized.

Febrile Seizures

I. *Introduction*: Febrile seizures are a *transient* neurologic disorder of childhood, affecting perhaps as many as 3% of all children. While the exact cause of febrile seizures remains uncertain, they seem to be a relatively transient problem that occurs *exclusively* in the presence of high, spiked fevers. Children in the infant and toddler stages (6 mo–3 yr) appear to be most susceptible to febrile seizures, and they are *twice* as common in *boys* as in girls. There also appears to be an increased susceptibility within families, suggesting a possible *genetic predisposition*.

II. Assessment:
A. History usually reveals presence of an upper respiratory infection or gastroenteritis.
B. Occurs with a sudden rise in fever: often spiked and quite *high* (102˚F or higher) versus prolonged temperature elevation.

III. Analysis/nursing diagnosis:
A. *Risk for injury* related to seizures.
B. *Knowledge deficit* related to prevention of future seizures, care of child having a seizure and possible long-term effects.

IV. Nursing care plan/implementation:
A. Goal: *reduce fever/prevent further increase in fever*.
1. Administer *antipyretics* per MD order: *acetaminophen* only (*not* aspirin).
2. Use cool, loose, cotton clothes to decrease heat retention.
3. Sponge with tepid water 20–30 min.
4. Encourage child to drink *cool fluids*.
5. Monitor temperature hourly.
6. Minimize stimulation, frustration for child.
B. Goal: **health teaching**. *Teach parents about care of child who experiences febrile seizure.*
1. Discuss how to prevent seizures from recurring: best method is to prevent temperature from rising over 102˚F (see Goal A).
2. Discuss how to handle seizures if they do recur: prevent injury, maintain airway, etc.
3. Answer questions simply and honestly:
a. 25% of children with one febrile seizure experience a recurrence.
b. 75% of recurrences occur within 1 yr.
c. Reassure parents of the benign nature of febrile seizures; 95-98% of children with febrile seizures do not develop epilepsy or neurologic damage.

V. **Evaluation/outcome criteria:**
A. Fever is kept below 102ºF; additional seizures are prevented.

B. Parents verbalize their understanding of how to care for child at home.

Seizures/Epilepsy

I. *Introduction*: Seizures are *alterations in the firing of neurons* in the brain, resulting in: sudden, involuntary alterations in consciousness, motor activity, behavior, sensation or autonomic function. Epilepsy is a *chronic* disorder characterized by *recurrent* seizures. Most seizure disorders in children are idiopathic while others can be caused by: injury, infection, lesions, toxins, etc.

II. Assessment:
A. Classified into 3 major categories:
1. *Generalized*: absence, atonic, myoclonic or tonic-clonic.
2. *Partial*: simple or complex.
3. *Unclassified*: neonatal, febrile or pseudoseizures.
B. May report aura (e.g., unusual tastes, feelings, odors) just before seizure onset.
C. *Diagnosis* determined by: history, EEG, MRI.

III. Analysis/nursing diagnosis:
A. *Risk for injury* related to type of seizure and possible loss of consciousness.
B. *Risk for aspiation* related to seizure activity.
C. *Knowledge deficit* related to care of child with seizure disorder.

IV. Nursing care plan/implementation:
A. Goal: *prevent injury*.
1. Do **not** attempt to stop seizure. Document activity during seizure (e.g., types of movements, duration of movements; onset aura; postictal level of consciousness and orientation).
2. Do **not** attempt to insert tongue blade into mouth during seizure (may break teeth).
3. Place child on side when seizure concludes; loosen constrictive clothing.
4. Administer *anticonvulsant* medication as ordered by pediatrician (e.g., diazepam, lorazepam, phenytoin).
B. Goal: *prevent aspiration*.
1. Have seizure precaution equipment at bedside (e.g., airway, suction, oxygen).
C. Goal: **health teaching**. *Teach parents care of a child with seizure disorder/epilepsy*.
1. Teach parent how to assess for possible seizure onset, care during and after seizure.
2. Correct administration of anticonvulsants medication; stress compliance with medication.
3. Purchase MedicAlert bracelet.
4. Notify school and other organizations that the child attends, and orient them to child's needs.

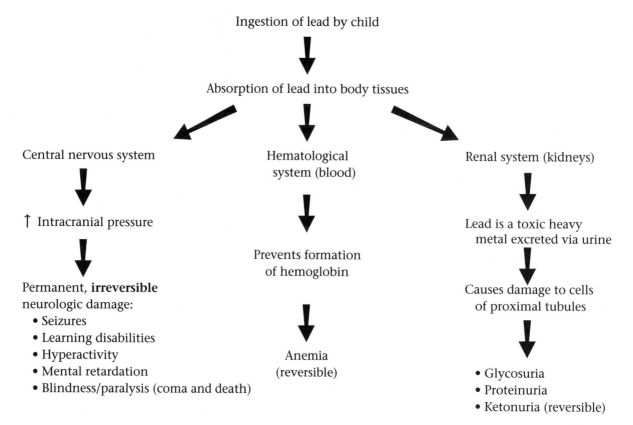

FIGURE 13.1 PATHOPHYSIOLOGIC EFFECTS OF LEAD POISONING

Source: ©Lagerquist, S. *Addison-Wesley's Nursing Examination Review.* Reading, MA: Addison-Wesley (out of print).

V. Evaluation/outcome criteria:
  A. Injury is prevented.
  B. Aspiration is prevented.
  C. Parents verbalize their understanding of how to care for child at home/school/outside activities.

Poisoning

See also general treatment for poisoning, **Chapter 17.**

I. **Lead Poisoning** (*plumbism*)
  A. *Introduction*: Lead poisoning is a heavy-metal poisoning that occurs as a result of the *ingestion* or *inhalation* of lead. In children, this is most common in the *toddler* age group (1–3 yr) and is usually a *chronic* type of poisoning that occurs as the result of *repeated* ingestions of lead. Children who engage in the practice of *pica*, the ingestion of non-nutritive substances, often ingest lead in flecks of lead-based paint from walls, furniture, or toys. In addition, research demonstrates that the parent-child relationship is a significant variable in lead poisoning; typically, there is a lack of adequate parental supervision that enables the child to engage in pica repeatedly over a fairly long period of time until symptoms of lead poisoning become evident (see **Figure 13.1** for pathophysiologic effects of lead poisoning).

B. **Assessment:**
  1. Investigate history of pica (ingestion of non-nutritive substance).
  2. Evaluate parent-child relationship.
  3. *Chronic lead poisoning*: vague, crampy abdominal pain; constipation; anorexia and vomiting; listlessness.
  4. Neurologic, renal, hematologic effects: see **Figure 13.1.**
  5. "Blood-lead line"—bluish black line seen in gums.
  6. X-rays: lead lines in long bones and flecks of lead in GI tract.
  7. Elevated serum blood lead levels: toxic ≥ 20 mcg/dL

C. **Analysis/nursing diagnosis:**
  1. *Risk for injury* (multisystem) related to retained lead.
  2. *Pain* related to lead poisoning and its treatment.
  3. *Knowledge deficit* related to etiology of lead poisoning.

D. **Nursing care plan/implementation:**
  1. Goal: *promote excretion of lead and prevent reingestion of lead.*
    a. Administer *chelating agents (EDTA, BAL)* per MD order: given via a series of painful, deep IMs (common dose: 6/d for 5 ds).

      b. Monitor kidney function carefully: the treatment itself is potentially nephrotoxic. Maintain adequate oral intake of fluids.

☞ c. *Institute seizure precautions.*

      d. In children with low lead levels,

⬭   *penicillamine* is given PO.

      e. Determine primary source of poisoning.

      f. Eliminate source from child's environment prior to discharge.

      g. Follow up with community health nurse referral.

          (1) Screen other siblings prn.

   〰 (2) Monitor blood-lead level of all children in the home.

  2. Goal: *assist child to cope with multiple painful injections*.

      a. Prepare child for treatment regimen.

      b. Stress that this is **not** a punishment.

      c. Rotate sites as much as possible.

⬭ d. May use a local anesthetic, e.g., *procaine*, injected simultaneously with chelating agent to decrease pain of injections.

☞ e. Apply warm soaks to injection sites; may help lessen pain.

      f. Encourage child to self-limit gross muscle activity (which increases pain).

      g. Offer child safe outlets for anger, fear, frustration—punching bag, pounding board, clay.

      h. Offer opportunity for medical play with empty syringes, etc.

🏠 3. Goal: **health teaching**.

      a. Stress (to child and parents) that removing the lead is the only way to prevent permanent, irreversible neurologic damage (irreversible damage may have *already* occurred).

      b. Teach that the action of the chelating agent is to bind with the lead and to promote its excretion via the kidneys.

✄ E. **Evaluation/outcome criteria:**

  1. Lead is successfully removed from child's body without permanent damage; no further episodes of lead poisoning.

  2. Pain is controlled.

  3. Family identifies and removes sources of lead in home.

II. Salicylate Poisoning

  A. *Introduction*: Aspirin is a common, multi-purpose, over-the-counter medication (analgesic, antipyretic, anti-inflammatory, etc.). The incidence of aspirin poisoning in children is declining since it is no longer recommended for fever reduction in children (Reye Syndrome). Aspirin poisoning can be acute or chronic in nature because aspirin is available separately or in common household remedies (e.g., Pepto Bismol, cold tablets, etc.).

✄ B. **Assessment:**

  1. Determine how much aspirin was ingested, when, which type.

  2. Evaluate salicylate levels: normal, 0; therapeutic range = 15–30 mg/dL; toxic, > 30 mg/dL.

  3. *Early* identification of *mild toxicity*:

      a. Tinnitus (ringing in the ears).

      b. Changes in vision, dizziness.

      c. Sweating.

      d. Nausea, vomiting, abdominal pain.

  4. *Immediate* recognition of salicylate *poisoning*:

      a. Hyperventilation (earliest sign).

      b. Fever—may be quite *high* (105°-106°F).

      c. *Respiratory alkalosis* and/or *metabolic acidosis.*

      d. *Late* signs: bleeding tendencies, severe electrolyte disturbances, liver and/or kidney failure.

✄ C. **Analysis/nursing diagnosis:**

  1. *Ineffective breathing patterns* related to hyperventilation/respiratory alkalosis.

  2. *Fluid volume deficit* (dehydration) related to increased insensible loss of fluids via hyperventilation, increased loss of fluids via vomiting and increased need for fluids due to hyperpyrexia (fever).

  3. *Risk for injury* related to bleeding.

  4. *Hyperpyrexia* related to dehydration, hyperventilation and aspirin ingestion.

  5. *Knowledge deficit* regarding accident prevention.

✄ D. **Nursing care plan/implementation:**

  1. Goal: *promote excretion of salicylates.*

⬭ a. If possible, induce vomiting using *syrup of ipecac* (save, bring to emergency room).

☞ b. Assist with gastric lavage, if appropriate.

⬭ c. Administer *activated charcoal* as early as possible.

      d. Assist with hemodialysis; as ordered, to promote excretion of salicylates and fluids.

⬭ e. Administer IV fluids, as ordered.

  2. Goal: *restore fluid and electrolyte balance.*

〰 a. Monitor I&O, *urinalysis, specific gravity*.

⬭ b. Prepare *sodium bicarbonate*, administer per MD order to correct metabolic acidosis.

〰 c. Monitor IV fluids and *electrolytes*.

      d. NPO initially (*nasogastric tube*).

  3. Goal: *prevent bleeding and possible hemorrhage.*

〰 a. Monitor urine and stools for *occult blood*.

☞ b. Insert NG tube to detect gastric bleeding.

      c. Observe for petechiae, bruising; monitor lab values for *hematocrit* and *hemoglobin*.

 d. Administer *vitamin K* per MD order to correct bleeding tendencies.

4. Goal: *reduce temperature.*

 a. No *aspirin* or *acetaminophen*, which might further complicate bleeding tendencies or lead to liver or kidney damage.

 b. Supportive measures: cool soaks, ice packs to armpits/groin, hypothermia blanket.

5. Goal: **health teaching.** *Prevent another accidental poisoning:*

 a. Teach principles of poison prevention.

 b. Stress need to avoid accidental overdose with over-the-counter medications or dosage mix-ups.

 c. Allow child/parents to verbalize guilt, but avoid blaming or scapegoating.

E. **Evaluation/outcome criteria:**

1. Aspirin is successfully removed from child's body without permanent damage and normal breathing pattern is restored.

2. Fluid and electrolyte balance is restored and maintained.

3. Bleeding is controlled, no hemorrhage occurs.

4. Child is afebrile.

5. No further episodes of poisoning occur.

Attention-Deficit Hyperactivity Disorder (ADHD); Behavioral Disorder (as defined by DSM-IV)

I. *Introduction*: As defined by the American Psychiatric Association, this diagnostic term includes a *persistent pattern* of inattention and/or hyperactivity-impulsivity. The exact cause and pathophysiology remain unknown. The major symptoms include a greatly shortened attention span and difficulty in integrating and synthesizing information. This disorder is *3 times* more common in *boys* than in girls, with onset before age 7; the diagnosis is based on the child's history rather than any specific diagnostic test.

II. **Assessment:**

A. The behaviors that are exhibited by children with ADHD are not unusual behaviors in children, but differ in both *quality* and *appropriateness*:

1. Motor activity is excessive.

2. Developmentally "younger" than chronologic age.

B. Inattention

1. Does *not* pay attention to detail.

2. Does *not* listen when spoken to.

3. Does *not* do what he or she is told to do.

C. Hyperactivity

1. Fidgets and squirms excessively.

2. Cannot sit quietly.

3. Has difficulty playing quietly.

4. Seems to be constantly in motion, moving or talking.

III. **Analysis/nursing diagnosis:**

A. *Altered thought processes* related to inattention and impulsiveness.

B. *Risk for injury* related to impulsivity.

C. *Impaired social interaction* related to hyperactivity and impulsivity.

D. *Knowledge deficit* related to behavioral modification program, medications, and follow-up care.

IV. **Nursing care plan/implementation:**

A. Goal: *reduce symptoms by means of prescribed medication.*

1. Medications: *methylphenidate* (*Ritalin*) and *pemoline*—both are CNS stimulants but have a paradoxical calming effect on the child's behavior.

2. **Health teaching** (child *and* parents).

 a. Need to take medication regularly, as ordered. *Avoid* taking medication late in the day as it may cause insomnia.

 b. Need for long-term administration, with decreased need as child nears adolescence.

B. Goal: *provide safe outlet for excess energy.*

1. Alternate planned periods of outdoor play with school work or quiet indoor play.

2. Channel energies toward safe, large-muscle activities: running track, swimming, bike riding, hiking.

C. Goal: *provide therapeutic environment* using principles of behavior modification.

1. Reduce extraneous or distracting stimuli.

2. Reduce stress by decreasing environmental expectations (home, school).

3. Provide firm, consistent limits.

4. Special education programs.

5. Special attention to safety needs.

D. Goal: **health teaching.** *Teach family and child about ADHD.*

1. Provide complete explanation about disorder, probable course, treatment, and prognosis.

2. Answer questions directly, simply.

3. Encourage family to verbalize; offer support.

V. **Evaluation/outcome criteria:**

A. Medication taken regularly, with behavioral improvements noted.

B. Excess energy directed appropriately and injury is prevented.

C. Therapeutic environment enhances socially acceptable behavior.

D. Family and child verbalize understanding of ADHD.

Reye Syndrome

I. *Introduction*: Reye syndrome, first described as a disease entity in the mid-1960s, is a *multisystem* disorder primarily affecting children from 6–12 yr. Although *not* a communicable disease, studies have confirmed a relationship between *aspirin* administration during a viral illness (e.g., chickenpox, influenza) and the onset of Reye syndrome. The exact cause remains unknown. Reye syndrome is characterized by *acute metabolic encephalopathy* and fatty degeneration of the visceral organs, particularly the *liver*. Earlier diagnosis, more sophisticated monitoring equipment, and more aggressive treatment have greatly improved the survival rate of children with Reye syndrome; recovery is generally rapid in those children who do survive.

II. **Assessment:**
   A. Onset typically follows a viral illness, just as child appears to be recovering.
   B. *Early signs and symptoms:*
      1. Rapidly progressing behavioral changes: irritability, agitation, combativeness, hostility, confusion, apathy, lethargy.
      2. Vomiting, which becomes progressively worse.
   C. Rapidly progressive neurologic deterioration:
      1. Cerebral edema and increased intracranial pressure.
      2. Alteration in level of consciousness from lethargy through coma, decerebrate posturing, and respiratory arrest.
   D. Liver dysfunction, necrosis and failure:
      1. *Elevated* ALT [SGOT], AST [SGPT], LDH, serum ammonia levels.
      2. Severe hypoglycemia.
      3. *Increased* prothrombin time, coagulation defects, and bleeding.

III. **Analysis/nursing diagnosis:**
   A. *Altered cerebral tissue perfusion* related to cerebral edema and increased intracranial pressure.
   B. *Altered hepatic tissue perfusion* related to fatty degeneration of the liver.
   C. *Risk for injury* related to coagulation defects and bleeding.
   D. *Knowledge deficit* related to diagnosis, course of disease, treatment, and prognosis.

IV. **Nursing care plan/implementation:**
   A. Goal: *reduce intracranial pressure.*
      1. Child is admitted to PICU for intensive nursing care, continuous observation and monitoring.
      2. Monitor *neurologic* status and *vital signs* continuously.
      3. Assist with/prepare for numerous invasive procedures, including *ET tube/mechanical ventilation* and intracranial pressure monitor.
      4. Monitor closely for the development of seizures; institute *seizure precautions.*
      5. *Position: elevate* head of bed 30-45 degrees.
      6. Administer medications as ordered:
         a. *Osmotic* diuretics (e.g., *mannitol*) to ↓ ICP.
         b. *Diuretics* (e.g., furosemide) to ↓ CSF production.
         c. *Anticonvulsants* (e.g., phenytoin, *phenobarbital*).
   B. Goal: *restore and maintain fluid and electrolyte balance, including perfusion of liver.*
      1. Administer IV fluids per MD order—usually 10% glucose.
      2. Strict I&O.
      3. Prepare for/assist with: Foley catheter placement, CVP, ICP monitor, NG tube, etc.
      4. Monitor serum electrolyte lab values.
   C. Goal: *prevent injury and possible bleeding.*
      1. Observe child for: petechiae, unusual bruising, oozing from body orifices or tubes, frank hemorrhage.
      2. Check all urine and stool for occult blood.
      3. Monitor lab values, including PT, PTT, platelets.
      4. Administer blood products per MD order.
   D. Goal: *provide parents with thorough understanding of Reye syndrome.*
      1. Primary nurse assigned to provide care and follow through with teaching.
      2. Encourage parents' presence, even in PICU—explain all equipment and procedures in simple, direct terms.
      3. Provide factual, honest and complete information re: disease, diagnosis, prognosis.

V. **Evaluation/outcome criteria:**
   A. Intracranial pressure is reduced and normal neurologic functioning is restored.
   B. Fluid and electrolyte balance is restored.
   C. No clinical evidence of bleeding is found.
   D. Parents express understanding of Reye syndrome.

COMMONLY PRESCRIBED MEDICATIONS

Medication	Administration	Use/Action	✉ Nursing Consideration
Anticonvulsants Clonazepam/*Klonopin* Diazepam/*Valium* Lorazepam/*Ativan* Phenobarbital/*Luminal* Phenytoin/*Dilantin* Valproic Acid/*Depakene*	• Oral or parenteral • Calculate to child's weight in kilograms • Administer in provided dropper or calibrated syringe • **NEVER** use household measuring spoon	Used in seizure disorders Depresses central nervous system (CNS) activity Depresses nerve transmission in motor cortex Suppresses abnormal electrical discharges and limits spread of seizure activity Stabilizes threshold against hyperexcitability	• Provide for child's safety (because of drowsiness) • Dosage adjusted by serum levels and degree of seizure activity • Limit caffeine (e.g. chocolate) intake • Do **not** abruptly withdraw • Dental care (especially for phenytoin → gingival hyperplasia).
Chelating Agents Dimercaprol/*BAL* Edetate calcium disodium/*EDTA; Versenate*	• Parenteral • Calculate to child's weight in kilograms • Administer deep IM	Used in treatment of lead poisoning Binds ions of lead, forming a non-ionizing soluble complex that is excreted in urine	• Assess renal and hematologic function studies • Add 1% lidocaine or procaine to solution to minimize pain at injection site
Psychostimulants Amphetamines Dextroamphetamine/*Dexedrine* Methylphenidate/*Ritalin* Pemoline/*Cylert*	• Oral • Calculate to child's weight in kilograms • Administer in provided dropper or calibrated syringe • **NEVER** use household measuring spoon	Used in attention deficit hyperactivity disorder Blocks reuptake mechanism of dopamine neurons Decreases motor restlessness Increases mental alertness	• Monitor weight and height, which may be slowed due to medication • Give medication in morning and at lunch to avoid interfering with sleep • Do **not** give after 4 pm • If dose is missed, do **not** "catch up" or give extra medication
Vitamins Phytonadione (Vitamin K)/*Mephyton*	• Oral or parenteral • Calculate to child's weight in kilograms • Administer in provided dropper or calibrated syringe • **NEVER** use household measuring spoon	Used in salicylate poisoning Synthesizes factors II, VII, IX and X (all of which are essential for blood clotting) Antagonizes anticoagulant effect of salicylate	• Monitor coagulation, liver and hematologic values • Eat foods *high* in Vitamin K (e.g., dairy, meat, green leafy vegetables)

☀ Study and Memory Aids

Bacterial Meningitis—Treatment

Antibiotic treatment must be prompt and aggressive; this infection is **life-threatening**.

Bacterial Meningitis—Treatment of Contacts

Prophylactic antibiotics are usually given to close contacts of child with bacterial meningitis.

Bacterial Meningitis—Monitor Lab Values

Normal therapeutic serum phenytoin levels = 10-20 mcg/mL.

Bacterial Meningitis—Positioning

Elevate head of bed, or place *side-lying* if in opisthotonus.

Febrile Seizures—Characteristics

Febrile seizures are generally benign; 95-98% of all children with febrile seizures do not sustain neurologic damage.

Seizures/Epilepsy—Assessment

All children with epilepsy have seizures but many children have seizure(s) that are not epilepsy.

⚡ Lead Poisoning—Hazards

Lead poisoning can result in permanent neurologic damage and cause:
Hyperactivity
Learning disability
Seizures

Lead Poisoning—Risk Factor

The parent-child relationship of children with lead poisoning is frequently abnormal, with lack of bonding or attachment.

Lead Poisoning—Treatment

The treatment of lead poisoning is the administration of ⊂◌ chelating agents such as EDTA, BAL, or *D-penicillamine*.

Lead Poisoning—Treatment Contraindications

Children with allergies to peanuts or penicillin *cannot* be ⊂◌ given BAL or *D-penicillamine* because of cross-sensitivity.

Salicylate Poisoning—Assessment

▸◂ The *earliest* sign of salicylate poisoning is hyperventilation.

Salicylate Poisoning—Medication

⊂◌ Vitamin **K** given to correct bleeding tendencies.

Attention-Deficit Hyperactivity Disorder— Assessment

In ADHD, the behaviors are not unusual; the *degree* of motor activity and of *developmentally inappropriate* behavior is unusual.

Attention-Deficit Hyperactivity Disorder—Treatment

The child with ADHD is frequently treated with stimulants, ⊂◌ such as *Ritalin*, which have a paradoxical calming effect on the child's behavior.

Reye Syndrome—Risk Factors

Antecedent factor to Reye syndrome: *aspirin* taken during viral illness (e.g., influenza, chickenpox).
⊂◌ *Acetaminophen* should be used instead during these illnesses.

Questions

1. A parent asks why a child with suspected meningitis must have a lumbar puncture. The nurse's best reply is:
   1. "It will allow the pediatrician to remove the infected fluid that is causing the meningitis."
   2. "It is part of the diagnostic workup for meningitis."
   3. "It allows the pediatrician to obtain a sample of the fluid that is infected. After the fluid is analyzed, the correct antibiotics needed to cure the infection can be prescribed."
   4. "It allows a way of administering needed antibiotics to your child."

2. A goal for an infant with meningitis is to prevent injury related to central nervous system irritability and seizures. This goal might be best operationalized by which nursing action?
   1. Tape a tongue blade at the head of the infant's crib.
   2. Place the infant in a room away from the nurses' station to minimize stimuli.
   3. Pad the side rails of the infant's crib.
   4. Place the infant in high-Fowler's position.

3. Which medication should the nurse anticipate administering to a child who has hypothrombinemia secondary to Reye syndrome?
   1. Vitamin K.
   2. Vitamin C.
   3. Vitamin D.
   4. Vitamin A.

4. Following a toxic ingestion of aspirin, a child demonstrates respiratory alkalosis. The nurse should expect the child to be:
   1. Hyperactive.
   2. Confused.
   3. Irritable.
   4. Without signs of behavioral change.

5. When caring for a child with plumbism, the primary goal is to:
   1. Assess for pica.
   2. Promote the excretion of lead via chelating agents.
   3. Correct the anemia.
   4. Reverse the neurological effect.

6. The nurse should instruct parents that the best method of preventing febrile seizures in a child is to:
   1. Dress the child in lightweight clothing.
   2. Encourage the child to drink plenty of cool fluids.
   3. Prevent the child's temperature from rising over 102°F.
   4. Begin antibiotic therapy at the onset of any illness.

7. Which is the safest nursing intervention to reduce fever in a young child?
   1. Sponge the child with cold water.
   2. Sponge the child with tepid water.
   3. Sponge the child with alcohol.
   4. Sponge the child in the bathtub.

8. Which medication should the nurse anticipate will be used to reduce fever in a young child who has a history of febrile seizures?
   1. Aspirin.
   2. Acetaminophen.
   3. Phenobarbital.
   4. Diazepam.

9. Following a febrile seizure, which route of administration is the safest method for a nurse to administer acetaminophen to a child?
   1. Liquid form.
   2. A tablet crushed and mixed with applesauce.
   3. Intravenously.
   4. Rectally.

10. When providing anticipatory guidance to the family of a child with attention deficit disorder, the nurse should emphasize the need:
    1. To have the child take medication prescribed for the disorder just before bedtime.
    2. To be lenient and understanding of the child's behavior.
    3. To help build up the child's self-esteem.
    4. To involve the child in structured play activities.

Answers/Rationale

1. (3) A lumbar puncture is the *definitive diagnostic test* for meningitis. The cerebrospinal fluid pressure is measured and cerebrospinal fluid samples are obtained for culture, Gram stain, blood cell count, and determination of glucose and protein content. Cerebrospinal fluid is the route by which infection spreads throughout the subarachnoid space. All infected cerebrospinal fluid (1) is not removed during a lumbar puncture, nor is it a method of administering antibiotics (4). It *is* part of the diagnostic workup for meningitis (2), but this response does *not fully* answer the parent's question. **IMP, COM, 1, PhI, Reduction of risk potential**

2. (3) Padding the side rails of the infant's crib reduces the possibility of injury during a seizure. Tongue blades (1) are no longer used because attempting to insert an object into the mouth of an infant who is having a seizure can result in oral trauma. Having an oral airway and oxygen readily available at the conclusion of a seizure are safer interventions. The infant *should be close* to the nurse's station for maximum observation (2). The infant's head should be *slightly elevated* to decrease intracranial pressure (4). **IMP, APP, 1, SECE, Safety and infection control**

3. (1) Vitamin K is administered to help correct clotting difficulties caused by hypothrombinemia as a result of liver dysfunction associated with Reye syndrome. Vitamin C (2), vitamin D (3), and vitamin A (4) are not used as therapy for clotting difficulties. Each

vitamin has a specific effect found to be useful in the general health of children—vitamin C aids in the utilization of iron; vitamin D aids in bone growth; vitamin A aids in visual processes. **IMP, COM, 1, PhI, Pharmacological and parenteral therapies**

4. (2) Confusion, loss of consciousness, and eventual respiratory failure are signs of respiratory alkalosis in a child. The symptoms result when stimulation of the respiratory center in the medulla cause hyperventilation, a fall in PCO_2, and respiratory alkalosis. Hyperactivity (1) and irritability (3) are *not* associated with respiratory alkalosis secondary to aspirin ingestion in a child. Behavioral signs (4) are expected, in the form of confusion. **AS, ANL, 6, PhI, Physiological adaptation**

5. (2) Plumbism is lead poisoning, and its treatment involves chelating agents (such as EDTA and BAL) to promote excretion of lead from the body. Small children usually ingest lead in the form of paint chips or putty containing lead because of *pica*, an appetite for unusual nonfood substances. Assessing for pica is important but *not* the primary goal (1) the anemia should resolve (3) with treatment, but is *not* the primary goal. Usually, neurological effects are *not* reversible (4). **PL, COM, 1, PhI, Physiological adaptation**

6. (3) Preventing the child's temperature from rising over 102°F is the best method of preventing febrile seizures in children. This involves beginning acetaminophen therapy at the onset of a temperature. Dressing the child in lightweight clothing (1) and encouraging fluid intake (2) also *assists* in reducing fevers, but the important goal is to *prevent* temperatures of over 102°F. Antibiotic therapy (4) should be reserved for *documented bacterial* infections. **IMP, APP, 2, PhI, Reduction of risk potential**

7. (2) Sponging the child with tepid water is recommended because tepid water does not cause the child to shiver, which re-elevates temperature. Cold water (1) should be avoided because extreme cooling causes shock to an immature nervous system. Alcohol (3) should be avoided because it can be absorbed by the skin or the fumes may be inhaled in toxic amounts, which compounds the child's problem. The bathtub (4) should *not* be used because it is easy for the child to slip under the water if a febrile seizure occurs. The hard surface of the bathtub also presents a source of injury if a seizure occurs. **IMP, APP, 2, SECE, Safety and infection control**

8. (2) Acetaminophen, an antipyretic, is used to safely reduce fever in children. The use of aspirin (1) to reduce fever in children should be avoided. Many childhood fevers are caused by viruses and there appears to be a relationship between the use of aspirin to control temperatures caused by viruses and Reye syndrome. Phenobarbital (3) is ineffective in reducing fever in children or in preventing

Key to Codes

Nursing process: AS, assessment; **AN**, analysis; **PL**, planning; **IMP**, implementation; **EV**, evaluation. (See **Appendix L** for explanation of nursing process steps.)

Cognitive level: RE/KN, recall/knowledge; **COM**, comprehension; **APP**, application; **ANL**, analysis; **EVL**, evaluation; **SYN**, synthesis. (See **Appendix L** for explanation.)

Category of human function: 1, protective; **2**, sensory-perceptual; **3**, comfort, rest, activity, and mobility; **4**, nutrition; **5**, growth and development; **6**, fluid-gas transport; **7**, psychosocial-cultural; **8**, elimination. (See **Appendix N** for explanation.)

Client need: SECE, safe, effective care environment; **HPM**, health promotion and maintenance; **PsI**, psychosocial integrity; **PhI**, physiological integrity. (See **Appendix O** for explanation.)

Client subneed: See **Appendix O** for explanation.

recurrences of febrile seizures. With prolonged use, it can also reduce cognitive function in children. Diazepam (**4**) can be given intravenously or rectally to control a lengthy or persistent seizure, but it has *no* effect on temperature. **IMP, APP, 2, PhI, Pharmacological and parenteral therapies**

9. (**4**) Rectal administration is the safest method of administering acetaminophen to a child who has just had a seizure. Any oral form of medication—liquid (**1**) or crushed tablets (**2**)—should be avoided because the child will be in a drowsy (postictal) state following the seizure and might aspirate the medicine. Acetaminophen is *not* available as an intravenous medication (**3**). **IMP, COM, 2, PhI, Pharmacological and parenteral therapies**

10. (**3**) A negative self-concept, often reinforced by the family and/or school, is a part of attention deficit disorder. These children need assistance in recovering from the time spent "not getting along." A side effect of the medication prescribed for attention deficit disorder is insomnia, so the drug should be administered early in the day, *not* at night (**1**). Children with attention deficit disorder benefit most from firm, consistent limits (**2**) and opportunities to channel energy into large-muscle activities such as running or bike riding, rather than structured activities (**4**). **PL, APP, 7, PsI, Psychosocial integrity**

Musculoskeletal Disorders

Chapter Outline

- Key Words
- Summary of Key Points
- Selected Musculoskeletal Disorders
  - Osteomyelitis
  - Legg-Calvé-Perthes Disease
  - Juvenile Idiopathic Arthritis
  - Scoliosis
- Common Orthopedic Conditions

  - Clubfoot
  - Developmental Dysplasia of the Hip
  - Osteosarcoma
- Commonly Prescribed Medications
- Study and Memory Aids
- Questions
- Answers/Rationale

Key Words

hepatosplenomegaly enlargement of the liver and spleen, often associated with disease.

iridocyclitis inflammation of the iris and the ciliary body of the eye.

myalgia tenderness or pain in the muscles.

orthotics making and fitting of orthopedic braces.

🔑 Summary of Key Points

1. *Osteomyelitis* is a bacterial infection of a bone; nursing care for a child with osteomyelitis includes IV antibiotics, immobilization, and pain relief.

2. *Legg-Calvé-Perthes* disease is the avascular necrosis of the head of the femur; nursing care for a child with Legg-Calvé-Perthes disease includes *teaching* the child and family about non-weight-bearing devices and/or traction.

3. *Juvenile idiopathic arthritis* is an *inflammatory multisystem* disorder of unknown cause. The primary nursing diagnosis is *impaired physical mobility* related to joint stiffness and pain; nursing interventions

directed towards *maintaining joint function* include maintaining proper alignment, range of motion exercises, and encouraging the child to be as active as possible.

4. *Scoliosis* is a lateral curvature of the spine; treatment generally includes *bracing* and/or surgery.

5. Routine screening for *scoliosis* is an important part of the adolescent's health care.

6. *Home care* for all children with musculoskeletal disorders: **NEVER** allow pain or inability/hesitation to bear weight for more than 48 hours before seeking medical attention.

Selected Musculoskeletal Disorders

Osteomyelitis

I. *Introduction*: Osteomyelitis is a *bacterial infection* of a bone that can be *acute or chronic*. Although it can occur at any age, it most frequently occurs in children from age 1–12 yr and is *four times* more common in *boys* than in girls. The most common bacteria causing osteomyelitis is *Staphylococcus aureus*. Although osteomyelitis can be difficult to treat, with proper treatment and long-term follow-up, the prognosis is good (see **Table 14.1, p. 129**).

II. Assessment:
   A. Onset: abrupt; most frequently preceded by trauma.
   B. Local: pain, warmth, swelling, erythema; refusal to use the extremity; decreased range of motion.
   C. General: fever, irritability, and restlessness; dehydration.
   D. *Diagnostic tests*: x-rays, CT scan, MRI; blood tests: *increased* white blood cells (WBCs), *increased* ESR, staph-positive cultures.

III. Analysis/nursing diagnosis:
   A. *Infection* related to bacterial organisms.
   B. *Pain* related to infection.
   C. *Knowledge deficit* related to diagnosis, treatment, and prognosis.

IV. Nursing care plan/implementation:

A. Goal: *treat the infection and prevent spread.*

1. Obtain all cultures *before* instituting antibiotic therapy per MD order.

   a. Monitor IV equipment and site; because treatment is often with long-term antibiotics, *central line* may be inserted.

   b. More than one *antibiotic* is usually ordered; check compatibility carefully and monitor for possible toxicities.

2. If wound is present, administer *wound care*: maintain *strict aseptic technique*; cleanse wound thoroughly; apply medications per MD order; apply dressing. Surgical drainage may be necessary if there is persistent soft tissue abscess or spread of infection to joint.

3. *Immobilize* the affected bone: position; apply orthotics per MD order (splint, traction).

4. *Diet*: *high* protein, *low* calorie, *extra* fluids; small, frequent, nutritious meals and snacks.

B. Goal: *relieve pain.*

1. Administer medications per MD order.
2. Allow child to assume position of comfort.
3. Handle affected limb gently and as little as possible.

C. Goal: **health teaching.** *Teach child and family about the condition, treatment and prognosis.*

1. Explain all diagnostic tests to family and child.
2. Explain all treatments to family and child:

   a. Child requires extended *bedrest* to prevent pathologic fractures as the infection clears.

   b. Following initial period of IV therapy, heparin lock may be used for antibiotics.

   c. Physical therapy should be instituted during the recovery phase.

   d. Discharge instructions usually include oral antibiotics and long-term, follow-up care.

V. Evaluation/outcome criteria:

A. Infection clears without complications.
B. Child is free of pain.
C. Family verbalizes understanding of disease, treatment, and prognosis.

Legg-Calvé-Perthes Disease

I. *Introduction*: Legg-Calvé-Perthes disease is the avascular necrosis of the head of the femur. This *self-limited* disorder is most common in children from 4–8 yr, with *boys* affected four or five times more frequently than girls. Caucasian children are affected ten times more frequently than African-American children. Although the disease is self-

limiting, two factors affect the child's ultimate prognosis: early diagnosis and treatment improves the prognosis; and younger children tend to make a more complete recovery than do older children. However, with full client compliance, the prognosis is generally considered to be excellent (see **Table 14.1, p. 129**).

II. Assessment:

A. Onset is insidious; an intermittent limp may be the first sign that brings the child to the attention of the health care practitioner.

B. *Pain*: hip soreness, ache, or stiffness; may be constant or intermittent; worse in early morning or late in the day; can extend along entire thigh and to the knee; pain is related to activity and is relieved by rest.

C. Joint dysfunction of the hip: limited range of motion; external hip rotation is a *later* sign.

D. *Diagnostic procedures*: x-rays, MRI scan.

III. Analysis/nursing diagnosis:

A. *Risk for injury* related to disease process and mobilization devices.

B. *Knowledge deficit* related to care of the child with Legg-Calvé-Perthes disease.

IV. Nursing care plan/implementation:

A. Goal: *prevent injury to the child.*

1. Instruct child in the use of mobilization devices: crutches, wheelchair, etc.
2. Evaluate environment for hazards and modify as needed.
3. Encourage appropriate diversion within acceptable safety limits.
4. Supervise application of non-weight bearing devices.
5. Provide traction care per MD order.

B. Goal: **health teaching.** *Teach child and family about the disease, treatment, and prognosis.*

1. Explain all diagnostic tests, treatments, and procedures to the child and family.
2. Discuss non-weight-bearing devices and mobilization devices to the child and family.
3. Discuss the need for compliance with treatment in order to improve client outcome. Conservation therapy must be continued for 2-4 years.
4. Discuss need for long-term follow-up care.

V. Evaluation/outcome criteria:

A. Child recovers without complications.
B. Family verbalizes understanding of the disease, treatment, and prognosis.

TABLE 14.1   COMMON PEDIATRIC ORTHOPEDIC CONDITIONS

Condition	Definition	Age at Onset/ Sex Difference	Treatment	► Nursing Considerations
Clubfoot	Downward, inward rotation of one or both feet: *talipes equinovarus* (95%).	Newborn (congenital); twice as common among *boys*.	Series of casts changed weekly, followed by *Denis Browne* splint and then corrective shoes (severe cases—surgery).	☞ Care of child in cast/brace: have cast cutters available. Stress need for follow-up.
Developmental Dysplasia of the Hip (DDH)	Abnormal development of hip joint (most frequently unilateral).	Newborn (congenital); more common among *girls*.	*Newborn*—Pavlic harness; *older infant or toddler*—possible surgery, spica cast.	☞ Early identification. Care of child in traction/cast: check circulation; turn every 2 hr while cast is damp. Encourage compliance. Check for other anomalies, e.g., spina bifida.
Juvenile Idiopathic Arthritis (JIA)	Chronic systemic inflammatory disease (cause unknown).	Peak: 1–3 yr and 8–10 yr; more common among *girls*.	Prevent joint deformity by exercise, splints, medications (NSAIDS, SAARDS, *corticosteroids*, *biologic* agents, *cytotoxic* agents); relieve symptoms (as per adult with arthritis).	☞ Care of child in brace/splint. Provide diversion. Encourage compliance.
Legg-Calvé-Perthes Disease	Aseptic necrosis of the head of the femur (cause unknown).	*Peak*: 4–8 yr; *range*: 3–12 yr; five times more common among *boys*; ten times more common among *Caucasians* than nonCaucasians.	Conservative therapy lasts 2–4 yr, usually begins with *bedrest* and traction, followed by non-weight-bearing devices such as brace, cast.	☞ Early identification. Care of child in traction/cast: check for frayed pulley ropes. Provide diversion for prolonged immobility.
Osteomyelitis	Most frequently occurring bone infection among children.	1–12 yr; four times as common among *boys*.	Blood cultures to diagnose causative organisms—select appropriate *antibiotic*; *bedrest*, *immobilization* with splint or cast.	☞ Care of child in splint/cast. Provide diversion. *Pain* medications/*antibiotics* per MD order.
Osteosarcoma	Most frequently occurring bone cancer among children.	Adolescence (10–25 yr); more common among *boys*.	Limb salvage or amputation → prosthesis; chemotherapy.	Prepare child for loss of limb. Help cope with prosthesis, **life-threatening** illness. Assist with grieving process.
Scoliosis	Lateral curvature of the spine (cause unknown).	Adolescence; more common among *girls*.	Brace fitted to specific type of curvature; surgical realignment of spine using a variety of techniques.	☞ Care of child in traction/cast/ brace. Teach that brace is worn 16–23 h/d, 7 d/wk for 6 mo-2 yr (**no** exceptions). Encourage compliance. Promote positive self-image.

See **Chapter 16** for other skeletal malformations (*congenital clubfoot* and *developmental dysplasia of the hip*).

TABLE 14.2   CHARACTERISTICS OF JUVENILE IDIOPATHIC ARTHRITIS RELATED TO MODE OF ONSET

	Systemic Onset	*Pauciarticular (Two or Three Subtypes)*	*Polyarticular (Two Subtypes)*
Percentage of clients	30%	45%	25%
Age at onset	Bimodal distribution: 　1–3 yr 　8–10 yr	Type I: < 10 yr Type II: > 10 yr	Throughout childhood and 　adolescence
Sex ratio (girls/boys)	1.5:1	Type I: Almost all girls Type II: 1:9	Mostly girls
Joints involved	Any Only 20% have joint 　involvement at time 　of diagnosis	Usually confined to lower 　extremities—knee; ankle; and 　eventually sacroiliac; sometimes 　elbow	Any joints: usually symmetric 　involvement of small joints Hip involvement in 50% Spine involvement in 50%
Extra-articular manifestations	Fever; malaise; myalgia; 　rash; pleuritis 　or pericarditis; 　adenomegaly; 　splenomegaly; 　hepatomegaly	Type I: Chronic iridocyclitis; 　mucocutaneous lesions Type II: Acute iridocyclitis; sacroiliitis 　common; eventual ankylosing 　spondylitis in many Type III: Arthritis only	Systemic signs minimal Possible low-grade fever; malaise; 　weight loss; rheumatoid 　nodules; and/or vasculitis
Laboratory tests	*Elevated* ESR; RF 　negative; ANA rarely 　positive; anemia; 　leukocytosis	*Elevated* ESR; CPR, ANA-positive Type I: HLA-DRW5-positive Type II: HLA-B27-positive Type III: HLA-TMO-positive	*Elevated* ESR Type I: RF positive Type II: RF negative
Long-term prognosis	Mortality—1–2% of all 　JIA clients Joint destruction in 　40%	Continuous disease; eventual 　remission in 60% Type I: Ocular damage; functional 　blindness in 10% Type II: Ankylosing spondylitis Type III: Best outlook for recovery	Longer duration; more crippling; 　remission in 25% Type I: High incidence of 　disabling arthritis Type II: Outlook good

CPR, C-reactive protein; **ESR,** erythrocyte sedimentation rate; **RF,** rheumatoid factor; **ANA,** antinuclear antibody; **HLA,** human leukocyte antigen

Adapted from Wong D. *Nursing Care of Infants and Children* (7th ed). St. Louis, Mosby.

Juvenile Idiopathic Arthritis

(*Formerly* known as *Juvenile Rheumatoid Arthritis* in USA; *Juvenile Chronic Arthritis* in Europe)

I. *Introduction*: Juvenile Idiopathic Arthritis (JIA) is an *inflammatory, multisystem* disorder that can follow one of three clinical courses: *systemic, pauciarticular* (involves few joints), or *polyarticular* (involves many joints simultaneously). *Girls* are affected more than boys, and the age of onset is 2–16 yr. Although the exact cause of JIA is unknown, it is generally believed to be *autoimmune* in nature. This chronic disease requires long-term follow-up care, but the prognosis is good, with 75% of children with JIA having long remissions without impaired function. The most common complications are severe hip involvement with loss of function, and possible blindness related to *iridocyclitis*. Refer to **Table 14.2** for characteristics of each type of JIA related to mode of onset. See also **Table 14.1, p. 129.**

II. **Assessment:**

A. Assess affected *joints*: stiffness that is worse in the morning on arising; swelling, decreased range of motion; joint warm to the touch and tender or painful.

B. Assess *systemic* signs and symptoms: fever, malaise, *myalgia, hepatosplenomegaly*, rash, pleuritis, or pericarditis.

C. *Diagnostic tests*: blood tests, including: *elevated* WBC, *elevated* ESR, negative latex fixation test in 90% of cases; rheumatoid factor may or may not be present; antinuclear antibodies present except in systemic-onset JIA.

D. X-rays: widening joint spaces, articular destruction.

III. **Analysis/nursing diagnosis:**

A. *Impaired physical mobility* related to joint stiffness and pain.

B. *Pain* related to inflammation of joints.

C. *Self-care deficit* related to pain and impaired joint mobility.

D. *Knowledge deficit* related to medications and treatments for JIA.

IV. **Nursing care plan/implementation:**

A. Goal: *maintain joint function.*

　1. Apply splints or sandbags as ordered.

　2. Perform range-of-motion exercises or assist with physical therapy as ordered.

3. *Position:* have client use firm mattress, lie *flat* in bed, and keep joints *extended*; alternate with *prone* position without a pillow.
4. Whenever possible, incorporate play into therapeutic exercises, e.g., throwing a ball, riding a tricycle.
5. Encourage child to be as active as possible without straining joints.
6. Assess joint function frequently and adjust treatment regimen as needed.

B. Goal: *provide relief from pain.*
1. Administer *nonsteroidal anti-inflammatory* drugs (NSAIDS) per MD order: acetaminophen (*Tylenol*), ibuprofen (*Motrin, Advil*), naproxen (*Naprosyn*), tolmetin sodium (*Tolectin*); slower-acting *antirheumatic* drugs (SAARDS); *corticosteroids*; *biologic* agents; *cytotoxic* agents may also be used.
2. Provide heat to painful joints with warm showers or baths (especially in morning), warm soaks, or moist pads.
3. *Avoid* overexercising painful or swollen joints.
4. *Avoid* excessive weight gain.
5. Use nonpharmacologic measures to relieve pain.

C. Goal: **health teaching.** *Prepare child to perform activities of daily living as independently as possible.*
1. Encourage child to be as independent as possible; do not perform activities which the child is capable of doing on his own.
2. Assist with activities of daily living only when child is truly unable to perform independently.
3. Select assistive devices that maximize the child's independence: clothes, utensils, grooming, toileting.
4. Teach child how to apply splints and encourage child to apply as appropriate.
5. Schedule regular rest periods and adequate sleep to conserve energy for activities of daily living.

D. Goal: *provide child and family with knowledge of medications and treatments.*
1. Encourage child and family to verbalize concerns about medications and treatments.
2. Teach child and family about medications and treatments, and also provide written information.
3. Involve the child and family with the administration of medications and treatments.
4. Prepare child and family for possible joint replacement when growth is complete.

V. **Evaluation/outcome criteria:**
A. Joint movement increases from the baseline; no contractures or flexion deformities develop.
B. Pain is either eliminated entirely or is relieved to a more tolerable level.
C. Activities of daily living are carried out independently to the best of the child's abilities.
D. Knowledge of medications and treatments is verbalized by the child and family.

Scoliosis

I. *Introduction:* Scoliosis is generally defined as a lateral curvature of the spine (see **Figure 14.1, p. 132**); it is the most common spinal deformity in children and adolescents. Scoliosis can be *congenital, neuromuscular,* or *idiopathic.* It is most common in adolescent *girls* who are experiencing a growth spurt (see also **Table 14.1, p. 129**).

II. **Assessment:**
A. Chief complaint: "ill-fitting" clothes, such as uneven skirt or pants hems.
B. Physical examination:
1. While child is standing erect and wearing only underwear, the nurse should view the child's back while standing behind the child. Observe for: uneven shoulder height, uneven scapula, uneven hips.
2. Ask child to bend forward at a 90-degree angle to the floor, with back parallel to the floor and arms hanging freely. Observe for asymmetry of ribs and flank. Use *scoliometer* to document the degree of curvature.
C. *Diagnostic tests:* assist with x-rays or possible MRI scan per MD order.

III. **Analysis/nursing diagnosis:**
A. *Risk for impaired skin integrity* related to Boston, thoracolumbosacral orthosis (TLSO), or Milwaukee Brace.
B. *Risk for injury* related to Boston, thoracolumbosacral orthosis (TLSO), or Milwaukee Brace.
C. *Body-image disturbance* related to scoliosis and wearing a brace.
D. *Knowledge deficit* regarding scoliosis, treatment, and prognosis.

IV. **Nursing care plan/implementation:**
A. Goal: *prevent skin irritation or breakdown.*
1. Daily examination of skin surfaces that come in contact with the brace for any signs of redness, irritation, or breakdown.
2. Teach child to wear cotton T-shirt under the brace to prevent rubbing or irritation.
3. Teach child to bathe or shower daily to keep skin clean, and to dry skin thoroughly.

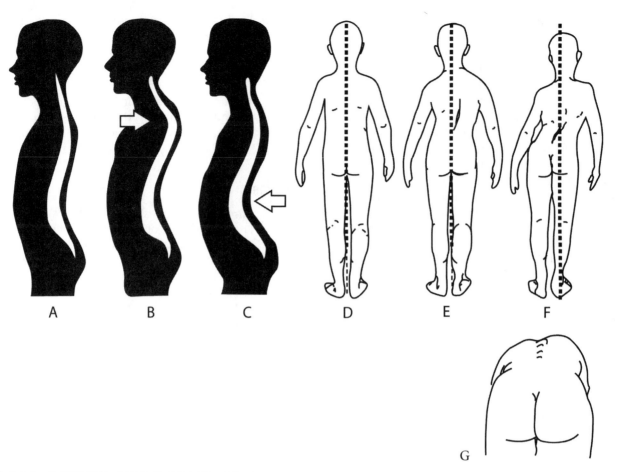

FIGURE 14.1 DEFECTS OF THE SPINAL COLUMN. A. *Normal* spine. B. *Kyphosis.* C. *Lordosis.* D. *Normal* spine in balance. E. *Mild* scoliosis in balance. F. *Severe* scoliosis *not* in balance. G. Rib, hump, and flank *asymmetry* seen in flexion caused by rotary component.

Wong D. *Nursing Care of Infants and Children*, 7th ed., St. Louis, Mosby.

B. Goal: *prevent injuries related to wearing a spinal brace.*
1. Assess environment for possible hazards and modify as needed.
2. Teach child safety precautions such as *avoiding* slippery surfaces and using handrail on stairs.
☞ 3. Demonstrate how to sit, and stand, or get into and out of bed while wearing the brace.
4. Discuss possible accidents likely to occur when spine and neck are immobilized, as well as preventative measures.
5. Suggest alternatives for activities that may be awkward or restricted.
🏠 C. Goal: **health teaching.** *Assist child to adjust to wearing the brace.*
1. Discuss child's feelings regarding the brace; stress positive long-term outcome with need for daily compliance.
2. Discuss activities that may be affected by the brace and suggest possible alternatives that do not require flexibility or movement.
3. Ask about any pain, discomfort, or irritation that may require adjustment of the brace; refer to *orthotist* as needed.

4. Discuss use of concealing clothes such as loose or baggy tops and pants that draw minimal attention to the brace.
5. Discuss possible reactions of peers and suggest appropriate responses.
6. Encourage socialization with peers.
7. Assist the child to feel as attractive as possible.
🏠 D. Goal: **health teaching.** *Teach child and family about the condition, treatment and prognosis.*
1. Discuss what scoliosis is and why this child seems to have it.
2. Discuss the need to wear the brace for 16–23 h/d for a prolonged period of time (6 mo–2 yr); stress the need for compliance to avoid surgery.
3. If curve is severe or the child does not comply with wearing the brace, surgery may be needed, although this is rare (risk of paralysis).
▶ V. **Evaluation/outcome criteria:**
A. Skin integrity is maintained.
B. No injuries occur.
C. Child complies with wearing the brace.
D. Child and family verbalize understanding of the disease, treatment and prognosis.

COMMONLY PRESCRIBED MEDICATIONS

Medication	Administration	Use/Action	Nursing Consideration
Antibiotics Clindamycin/*Cleocin* Nafcillin/*Nafcil*	• Oral and parenteral • Calculate to child's weight in kilograms • Administer in provided dropper or calibrated syringe • **NEVER** use household measuring spoon	Used in osteomyelitis if *Staphylococcus aureus* is causative agent (most common of all agents) Kills bacteria	• Assess for allergy prior to administration • Obtain specimen for culture and sensitivity prior to administration • Assess for drug-induced colitis (pain, tenderness, watery diarrhea) • Prepare child and family for length of treatment (minimum of 4 weeks)
Biologic agents/ Immunomodulator Etanercept/*Enbrel*	• SQ • Calculate to child's weight in kilograms	Used in juvenile idiopathic arthritis to provide symptomatic relief from inflammation Interrupts inflammatory process by blocking the cytokine tumor necrosis factor.	• Inform family that recent approval for use in children mandates that child be enrolled in a drug study to receive drug • Usually given in conjunction with other antirheumatoid drugs • Update all immunizations prior to beginning drug therapy • Teach home injection of drug
Nonsteroidal anti-inflammatory Drugs (NSAIDS) Acetaminophen/ *Tylenol* Ibuprofen/*Advil*; *Motrin* Naproxen/*Naprosyn* Tolmetin/*Tolectin*	• Oral and rectal • Calculate to child's weight in kilograms • Administer in provided dropper or calibrated syringe • **NEVER** use household measuring spoon	Used in treatment of juvenile idiopathic arthritis to provide symptomatic relief from pain/inflammation Inhibits mediators of inflammation (e.g., leukotrienes) Inhibits enzyme responsible for prostaglandin synthesis	• Assess for gastrointestinal disturbance • Take with milk or food • Evaluate for increase in joint mobility • Inform child and family that therapeutic effect will be noted in 1-3 weeks
Slower-acting Antirheumatic Drugs (SAARDS) Methotrexate/ *Rheumatrex* Sulfasalazine/ *Azulfidine*	• Oral and parenteral • Calculate to child's weight in kilograms • Administer in provided dropper or calibrated syringe • **NEVER** use household measuring spoon	Used in juvenile idiopathic arthritis to provide symptomatic relief from pain/inflammation Inhibits prostaglandin synthesis May inhibit cell replication in non-malignant conditions such as arthritis	• Assess hydration status and keep child well hydrated • May cause orange-yellow discoloration of urine • *Avoid* exposure to sunlight • Promote use of sunscreen • Warn regarding temporary, reversible alopecia • Sexually active adolescents need to use contraceptives

See also: **Chapter 7**: corticosteroids, **Chapter 10**: alkalyting agents

💡 Study and Memory Aids

Osteomyelitis (bacterial infection of the bone)—Treatment:

1. IV antibiotics
2. Immobilization
3. Pain relief

Osteomyelitis—Diet

The diet for a child with osteomyelitis should be *high* protein and *low* calorie, with *extra* fluids.

Legg-Calvé-Perthes Disease (avascular necrosis of the head of the femur)—Treatment:

1. Non-weight-bearing devices
2. Traction

Juvenile Idiopathic Arthritis (inflammatory disease of unknown cause)—Blood Tests Reveal:

1. *Elevated* WBC
2. *Elevated* ESR
3. *Negative* latex fixation (90%)
4. Rheumatoid factor (may not be present)
5. Antinuclear antibodies (except in systemic-onset JIA)

JIA—Priority Goal: Maintaining Joint Function

1. Range-of-motion exercises
2. Correct alignment and positioning
3. Activity

JIA—Treatment

Nonsteroidal anti-inflammatory drugs (NSAIDs) such as ibuprofen (*Motrin*) or naprosyn are used to treat JIA.

Scoliosis—Subjective Assessment

The most common complaint of a teenager with scoliosis: poor-fitting clothing.

Scoliosis—Objective Assessment

When screening teenagers for scoliosis, ask teenager to bend over at a 90-degree angle to the floor, with the back parallel to the floor and arms hanging freely.

Scoliosis—Treatment

The brace is worn 16-23 h/d for 6 mo-2 yr.

Questions

1. When planning care for a child with osteomyelitis, the nurse should know that the treatment modality that is most important for this child is:
   1. Diversional activities.
   2. Extremity immobilization with a splint.
   3. Temperature control.
   4. Antibiotic therapy.

2. Which nursing intervention is essential for a child suspected of having osteomyelitis?
   1. Assessing the affected area for heat, color, and edema.
   2. Applying heat to the affected area.
   3. Ambulating the child frequently.
   4. Performing active range-of-motion to the affected area.

3. A 7-year-old child develops Legg-Calvé-Perthes disease. The nurse anticipates that during the course of treatment the child will experience the most difficulty with:
   1. Immobility.
   2. Pain control.
   3. Skin integrity.
   4. Weight control.

4. The primary goal of treatment for the child with juvenile arthritis is to prevent:
   1. Loss of joint function.
   2. Excessive weight gain.
   3. Social isolation.
   4. Skin breakdown.

5. The nurse is caring for a school-aged child with juvenile arthritis. The nurse should schedule this child's bath:
   1. At bedtime.
   2. In the late afternoon.
   3. Just before lunch.
   4. Early in the morning.

6. Many children with juvenile arthritis experience increased fatigability. The nurse should know that the age group at greatest risk for failure to pace physical activities and rest time is:
   1. Toddlers.
   2. Preschoolers.
   3. Young school-aged children.
   4. Adolescents.

7. When taking an initial health history from an adolescent suspected of having scoliosis, the nurse would expect the adolescent to state that:
   1. "I always have a backache."
   2. "I become short of breath easily."
   3. "I can't find clothes that fit me properly."
   4. "I haven't grown much lately."

8. Noncompliance with brace therapy is common among adolescents with scoliosis. The nurse should recognize that this is primarily due to adolescent health beliefs that:
   1. Are oriented to the present, not the future.
   2. The brace will interfere with their sense of industry.
   3. The brace will interfere with their sense of initiative.
   4. The brace will interfere with their sense of autonomy.

9. An adolescent with scoliosis is fitted for a brace. Which statement made by the adolescent is most indicative of the success of the nurse's teaching regarding the brace?
   1. "I'll only have to wear the brace for a few months."
   2. "I can take the brace off for special occasions like the prom."
   3. "I can take the brace off for 1 hour a day while I bathe."
   4. "The brace will correct the curve."

10. A critical postoperative nursing assessment for an adolescent with scoliosis who has undergone a spinal fusion is:
    1. Urinary output.
    2. Bowel elimination.
    3. Sensation and movement of the lower extremities.
    4. Infection.

11. When working on an orthopedic unit, the nurse should be aware that the age group most negatively affected by being placed in traction is:
    1. Infant.
    2. Toddler.
    3. Preschool.
    4. School-age.

12. Which item should the nurse remove from the bedside table of a 4-year-old child who has just been placed in bilateral long leg casts?
    1. Legos.
    2. Etch-a-sketch.
    3. Fireman's hat.
    4. Coloring book.

13. A child is placed in traction and the nurse marks the side rails so that the child can play the game of monitoring his own position in bed. Which age group is most receptive to this nursing intervention?
    1. Toddler.
    2. Preschool.
    3. School-age.
    4. Adolescent.

14. An adolescent with a long leg cast is being prepared by the nurse to have the cast removed. The nurse informs the adolescent that the affected leg will temporarily appear smaller than before the cast was applied. This information is important to tell the adolescent because the adolescent:

1. Should be involved in all aspects of the health care .
2. If not properly prepared for the difference in shape, might become frightened that the change is permanent.
3. Is dealing with the critical developmental issue of body image.
4. Would be concerned that a difference in leg sizes might affect future career choices.

15. The nurse notes that a child in a long leg cast has an unexpected onset of discoloration, swelling, and pain in the casted extremity. The pedal pulse is also faint. After notifying the orthopedic surgeon, the nurse's next action should be to:
    1. Bring a cast cutter to the bedside.
    2. Note the findings on the child's chart.
    3. Place the child NPO.
    4. Reassess the child's neurovascular status in the extremity.

16. Which report about a child in traction, made by a nursing assistant to the nurse on a busy orthopedic unit, would require the nurse's immediate attention?
    1. "The child's toes are warm and pink."
    2. "Bilateral pedal pulses are equal and strong."
    3. "Pulleys remain in original position on the attachment bar."
    4. "Ropes are noted to be in center of pulleys and are frayed."

17. While a child's body cast is still damp, the nurse should:
    1. Turn the child every 2 hours.
    2. Attempt to dry the cast using a hair dryer.
    3. Refrain from placing pillows under the cast.
    4. Avoid using the palms of the hands on the cast when positioning the child.

18. A child returns from surgery in a hip spica cast. The nurse's first action is to:
    1. Circle and note the date and time of any drainage on the cast.
    2. Check the circulation to the toes.
    3. Note any rough edges on the cast.
    4. Assess the cast for areas of dampness.

Answers/Rationale

1. (4) Osteomyelitis is an infection of the bone caused by the hematogenous spread of a concurrent infection, such as otitis media. Antibiotic therapy is critical because the most common causative organism of osteomyelitis is *Staphylococcus aureus*. Diversional activities (1), extremity immobilization (2), and temperature control (3) are important but *secondary* treatment modalities. Infection control is the *main* goal of treatment. **PL, ANL, 3, PhI, Physiological adaptation**

2. (1) Increased warmth, redness, and diffuse swelling are signs and symptoms of osteomyelitis. The extremity is usually painful, especially on movement. Heat (2) is *never* applied to any infected area of the body because increased temperature can cause certain bacteria to multiply even more rapidly. Osteomyelitis frequently occurs in the femur or tibia, so ambulation (3) during active infection is *discouraged*. Active range-of-motion exercises (4) are *excluded* from the plan of treatment because the child experiences pain on movement. **IMP, APP, 3, PhI, Physiological adaptation**

3. (1) Prolonged immobility is prescribed for the child with Legg-Calvé-Perthes disease to help reduce inflammation and restore motion to the hip. Children affected with this disease are usually 4–8 years of age, and the prescribed bed rest interferes with their core developmental task—industry versus inferiority. Pain (2) is *lessened* by the child's non-weight-bearing status. Skin integrity (3) can be maintained by frequent repositioning and meticulous skin hygiene. Although a careful calorie count is suggested for the early part of the treatment regime to prevent unwanted weight gain, especially since eating may become the child's primary source of pleasure while immobile, weight control (4) is *not* likely to pose the *greatest* difficulty. **AN, ANL, 3, PhI, Basic care and comfort**

4. (1) Preventing loss of joint function and preserving mobility is the *primary goal* of treatment for the child with juvenile arthritis. The goal is usually achieved via a combination of drugs, physical therapy, and surgery. Excessive weight gain (2), social isolation (3), and skin breakdown (4) can all occur *when* the primary goal of preventing loss of joint function, and thus mobility, is achieved. **PL, ANL, 3, PhI, Basic care and comfort**

5. (4) Early morning stiffness may make normal activities and exercises extremely painful and difficult. A warm shower or soaking in warm water can help reduce early morning stiffness and relax muscles, thus enabling the child with juvenile arthritis to begin the activities of the day. Warm water therapy *can* be helpful at any time:

bedtime (1), late afternoon (2), or lunchtime (3), but it is *most* beneficial in assisting the child with juvenile arthritis to overcome *morning* stiffness after a night of bedrest. **IMP, APP, 3, PhI, Basic care and comfort**

6. (4) Adolescents tend to get caught up in peer activities and possible job responsibilities, and they need encouragement and guidance to allow themselves the needed rest time and pacing of activities. Rest, relaxation, leisure activities, and relief from emotional distress may relieve fatigue and avoid exacerbation; these factors are therefore important aspects in the management of juvenile arthritis. Toddlers (1), preschoolers (2), and young school-aged children (3) are still under parental control in terms of their physical activities and rest time, and therefore are *not* in the high-risk age group for failure to pace activities and avoid fatigue. **AS, COM, 3, PsI, Psychosocial integrity**

7. (3) Ill-fitting clothes, such as uneven pant lengths or uneven skirt hems, is an *early* sign of scoliosis because the back's curves begin to progress due to differential growth of the vertebrae. Back pain (1) and respiratory distress (2) do *not* usually appear until the deformity is *well established*. Most curves progress during periods of growth (4) and therefore become noticeable at the beginning of the *preadolescent growth* spurt. **AS, ANL, 3, PhI, Basic care and comfort**

8. (1) Adolescent health beliefs are oriented to the present, *not* the future, so not wearing the brace seems more important than preventing progression of the curve in the future. Industry (2) is the central task of school-aged children. Initiative (3) is the central task of preschool children. Autonomy (4) is the central task of toddlers. (The central task of adolescents is identity.) **AN, COM, 5, PsI, Psychosocial integrity**

9. (3) The brace may be removed for 1 hour a day without exception. Bracing has been shown to be effective in 85% of clients who are compliant. Braces are usually worn for 1-2 years (1) and special occasions (2) such as proms and birthdays do *not* justify removal. The brace can halt the *progression* of the curve, but it *will not correct* the curve (4). **EV, APP, 3, PhI, Basic care and comfort**

10. (3) If the spinal cord is injured or compressed by swelling, one of the greatest risks associated with spinal surgery is paralysis. The nurse must therefore assess the sensation and movement of the lower extremities every 2 hours for at least 24 hours postoperatively. The adolescent will have an indwelling catheter for the first 48 hours postoperatively, so urinary output (1) is easily calculated and the chance of urinary retention is *minimized*. The adolescent will be NPO for several days following surgery, and the resumption of bowel sounds and elimination (2) is *not* anticipated for the first 72 hours following surgery. The large

---

Key to Codes

Nursing process: AS, assessment; **AN**, analysis; **PL**, planning; **IMP**, implementation; **EV**, evaluation. (See **Appendix L** for explanation of nursing process steps.)

Cognitive level: RE/KN, recall/knowledge; **COM**, comprehension; **APP**, application; **ANL**, analysis; **EVL**, evaluation; **SYN**, synthesis. (See **Appendix L** for explanation.)

Category of human function: 1, protective; **2**, sensory-perceptual; **3**, comfort, rest, activity, and mobility; **4**, nutrition; **5**, growth and development; **6**, fluid-gas transport; **7**, psychosocial-cultural; **8**, elimination. (See **Appendix N** for explanation.)

Client need: SECE, safe, effective care environment; **HPM**, health promotion and maintenance; **PsI**, psychosocial integrity; **PhI**, physiological integrity. (See **Appendix O** for explanation.)

Client subneed: See **Appendix O** for explanation.

back incision will be covered with a bulky dressing, antibiotics will be administered and temperature monitored, so the risk of infection (**4**) is *minimized*. **AS, ANL, 1, PhI, Reduction of risk potential**

11. (**2**) Toddlers have the core developmental task of autonomy and the need to explore their environment. Being placed in traction interrupts the completion of this developmental task. Toddlers do not separate easily from parents, which is another disadvantage to placing a toddler in traction. Confinement is difficult for all age groups: infant (**1**), preschool (**3**), and school-age (**4**), but the special independence needs of toddlers make them even more vulnerable to the effects of confinement. **AN, APP, 5, HPM, Health promotion and maintenance**

12. (**1**) Legos, which are tiny pieces of interlocking plastic, should be removed because the young child might put the pieces inside the cast. Etch-a-sketch (**2**), a fireman's hat (**3**), and a coloring book (**4**) are larger toys that could *not* be inserted by the child into the cast. These toys are age-appropriate for a preschooler. **IMP, ANL, 5, SECE, Safety and infection control**

13. (**3**) School-aged children, with their strong sense of industry, work very hard to follow rules associated with games. This age group also tends to be competitive and is more compliant if there is a reward or winner at the conclusion of the game. Toddlers (**1**) and preschoolers (**2**) lack the cognitive abilities to cooperate with such games. Adolescents (**4**), who tend to resist authority, might view such a game as another attempt by an adult to control them. **AN, APP, 5, PsI, Psychosocial integrity**

14. (**3**) The adolescent is dealing with the critical developmental issue of body image as well as the need to be exactly like others in the same age-group. Physical differences and defects are poorly tolerated by adolescents. Involvement in health care (**1**), correcting false assumptions (**2**), and the effects of illness or injury on future career choices (**4**) *are appropriate* considerations on the nurse's part when instructing the adolescent, but *body image* should remain the nurse's *central focus*. **IMP, APP, 5, HPM, Health promotion and maintenance**

15. (**1**) The nurse needs to have a cast-cutter at the bedside as soon as possible because the orthopedic surgeon will immediately respond when notified of the child's neurovascular status. The surgeon will relieve the pressure by bivalving or cutting a large window in the cast. Making an entry on the chart (**2**) and reassessing the child's neurovascular status (**4**) can be done by the nurse *after* notifying the orthopedic surgeon and obtaining the cast cutter. There is no need to place the child NPO (**3**) at this point in time. **AN, ANL, 1, PhI, Physiological adaptation**

16. (**4**) Frayed ropes warrant the nurse's immediate attention. Pulleys and traction rope are used to maintain the correct line so that the traction can be effective. A frayed rope may break and cause loss of traction and correct alignment of the extremity. Warm, pink toes (**1**) and equal, strong pedal pulses (**2**) are signs of *adequate* tissue perfusion to the extremities. Pulleys should be in the original position (**3**) to ensure correct alignment. The attachment bar is often marked with tape so that the original site of the pulley can be documented. **AN, ANL, 3, SECE, Management of care**

17. (**1**) Turning the child every 2 hours helps to dry a body cast evenly and prevent complications related to immobility. Heated hair dryers or fans (**2**) should *not* be used because they cause the cast to dry on the outside and remain wet beneath, which causes mold. Pillows (**3**) covered in plastic placed under the child in the cast and using the palms of the hands (**4**) for turning purposes help to prevent indenting the cast and creating pressure areas; these actions should *not* be avoided. **IMP, APP, 3, PhI, Basic care and comfort**

18. (**2**) The key responsibility of the nurse in caring for a child with musculoskeletal problems is the assessment of neurovascular status to ensure that no change in neurologic or circulatory function has occurred. Noting drainage (**1**), which might indicate blood loss from the incision site, and assessing for rough edges on a cast (**3**), which could lead to skin breakdown, are also important for the nurse to note *after* the initial neurovascular assessment. The complete evaporation of water from a hip spica cast can take 24–48 hours, so some dampness (**4**) should initially be *expected*. **IMP, ANL, 1, PhI, Physiological adaptation**

Neuromuscular Disorders

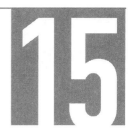

Chapter Outline

- Key Words
- Summary of Key Points
- Selected Neuromuscular Disorders
  - Cerebral Palsy
  - Duchenne Muscular Dystrophy
  - Guillain-Barré Syndrome

- Commonly Prescribed Medications
- Study and Memory Aids
- Questions
- Answers/Rationale

Key Words

atrophy wasting away of muscle tissue caused by disease or misuse.

contracture permanent contraction of a muscle, resulting in lack of function.

flaccid paralysis paralysis with loss of muscle tone, lack of reflexes, and atrophy of muscles.

paresthesia sensation of numbness or tingling in the extremities.

polyneuropathy any disease that affects many nerves.

Summary of Key Points

1. *Cerebral palsy*, which is caused by prenatal brain abnormalities, is the most common permanent physical disability of childhood.

2. The child with spastic *cerebral palsy* typically presents with delayed developmental milestones, tongue thrust, scissoring, and associated disabilities such as mental retardation or sensory impairment.

3. The *muscular dystrophies* are the most common muscle diseases in children; the most common and most severe type is *Duchenne muscular dystrophy*.

4. *Duchenne muscular dystrophy* has a gradual onset in boys between the ages of 3 and 5 yr; it is characterized by a generalized and progressive muscle weakness complicated by contracture deformities, disuse atrophy, infections, obesity, and cardiopulmonary problems.

5. The leading cause of death in *Duchenne muscular dystrophy* is respiratory tract infection or cardiac failure.

6. *Guillain-Barré* syndrome (GBS) is an acute postinfectious or idiopathic polyneuritis with progressive ascending paralysis. Death is rare; if mortality occurs, it is due to respiratory failure.

7. While caring for a child with GBS, the nurse must be acutely aware of *respiratory functioning*. A tracheostomy tray should be kept at the bedside along with suction, "ambu" bag, and emergency drugs; a ventilator should be on stand-by at all times.

8. *Home care* for all children with neuromuscular disorders: **NEVER** allow decline in fine and/or gross motor skills for more than 1 week before seeking medical attention.

Selected Neuromuscular Disorders

Cerebral Palsy

I. *Introduction*: Cerebral palsy (CP) is the most common *permanent* physical disability of childhood. It is a neuromuscular disorder of the *pyramidal motor system* resulting in the major problem of impaired voluntary muscle control. The damage appears to be *fixed* and *nonprogressive*, and the cause is unknown. However, although a variety of factors have been implicated in the etiology of CP, it is now known that CP results more commonly from *prenatal* brain abnormalities or *postnatal* injury.

II. Assessment:
   A. Most common type of cerebral palsy—spastic.
      1. Delayed developmental *milestones*.
      2. *Motor*: tongue thrust with difficulty swallowing and sucking (leading to poor weight gain). Aspiration may occur.
      3. Increased *muscle* tone: "scissoring" (legs crossed, toes pointed).

4. Persistent neonatal *reflexes*.
5. Associated problems:
   a. *Mental retardation* in 30% of children with cerebral palsy (70% are normal).
   b. *Sensory* impairment: vision, hearing.
   c. *Orthopedic* conditions: developmental dysplasia of hip, clubfoot.
   d. *Dental* problems: malocclusion.
   e. *Seizures*.

III. **Analysis/nursing diagnosis:**
A. *Ineffective airway clearance* related to hyperactive gag reflex and possible aspiration.
B. *Altered nutrition, less than body requirements*, related to difficulty sucking and swallowing.
C. *Impaired verbal communication* related to difficulty with speech.
D. *Risk for injury* related to difficulty controlling voluntary muscles.
E. *Sensory/perceptual alterations* related to potential vision and hearing defects.
F. *Impaired physical mobility* related to difficulty controlling movements.
G. *Self-esteem disturbance* related to disability.
Note: Because the level of disabilities with cerebral palsy can be varied, the nurse needs to select diagnoses that apply and clearly specify the individual child's limitations in any diagnostic statements.

IV. **Nursing care plan/implementation:**
A. Goal: *maintain patent airway.*
   1. Have suction and oxygen readily available.
   2. Use feeding and positioning techniques to maintain patent airway.
   3. Institute prompt, aggressive therapy for upper respiratory illnesses (URIs) to prevent the possible development of pneumonia.
B. Goal: *promote adequate nutrition.*
   1. *Diet*: *high* in calories (to meet extra energy demands).
   2. Assure balanced diet of basic foods that can be easily chewed.
   3. Provide feeding utensils that promote independence.
   4. Relaxed mealtimes, decreased emphasis on manners, cleanliness.
   5. Monitor I&O, weight gain.
C. Goal: *facilitate verbal communication.*
   1. Refer to speech therapist.
   2. Speak slowly, clearly to child.
   3. Use pictures or actual objects to reinforce speech.
D. Goal: *prevent injury.* (Refer to section on safety in chapters discussing *growth and development*).
   1. Utilize individually designed chairs with restraints for positioning and safety.
   2. Provide protective helmet to prevent head trauma.
   3. Implement seizure precautions.

E. Goal: *provide early detection of and correction for vision and bearing defects.*
   1. Arrange for screening tests.
   2. Assist family with obtaining corrective devices: eyeglasses, hearing aids.
F. Goal: *promote locomotion and encourage independence in activities of daily living (ADL).*
   1. Encourage "infant stimulation" program to assist infant in reaching developmental milestones.
   2. Refer to physical therapy for exercise program.
   3. Incorporate play into exercise routine.
   4. Use devices that promote locomotion: parallel bars, crutches, and braces.
   5. Surgical approach may be needed to relieve contractures.
   6. Adapt clothing, feeding utensils, etc. to facilitate self-help.
   7. Encourage child to perform ADL as much as possible; offer positive reinforcement.
   8. Assist parents to have realistic expectations for their child; *avoid* excessively high expectations that might increase frustration.
   9. Consider use of botulinum toxin type A (*Botox*) or *Baclofen* pump to relieve spasticity or *skeletal muscle relaxants*.
G. Goal: *promote self-esteem.*
   1. Praise child for each accomplishment or for sincere effort.
   2. Help child dress and groom self daily in an attractive normal manner for developmental level and age.
   3. Encourage child to form friendships with children with similar problems.
   4. Enroll child in "special ed" classes to meet his or her needs.
   5. Encourage parents to expose child to wide variety of experiences.

V. **Evaluation/outcome criteria:**
A. Patent airway and adequate oxygenation maintained.
B. Adequate nutrition maintained, and child begins to grow and gain weight.
C. Child has an acceptable means of verbal communication.
D. Safety is maintained.
E. Vision and hearing within normal limits, using corrective devices prn.
F. Child is as mobile as possible, given disabilities and engages in activities of daily living (ADL).
G. Child has positive self-image/self-esteem.

Duchenne Muscular Dystrophy

I. *Introduction*: The muscular dystrophies are the most common muscle diseases in children. The most severe and, unfortunately, the most common type of muscular dystrophy is Duchenne muscular dystrophy (DMD), an *inherited* disorder characterized by a generalized and progressive degeneration of *muscle fibers*, which causes weakness and muscle wasting. Because it is a *sex-linked* recessive disorder, *boys* are almost *exclusively* affected, with an incidence of 1:3500 male births. This chronic disease is ultimately *fatal*, and there is no known treatment.

II. **Assessment:**

A. Onset is gradual, occurring from ages 3–5 yr.

B. Assess for progressive muscle weakness: may be preceded by delay in motor development; usually appears by second year of life. Parents may note delayed walking, difficulty climbing stairs, or frequent falling. Progresses to abnormal gait, difficulty rising from the floor. Gait: waddling, with lordosis noted. Ambulation usually becomes impossible by age 12 yr.

C. Shoulder muscle involvement noted within 3–5 yr of onset, followed by pseudohypertrophy of the arms and calves.

D. Intellectual ability: mild mental retardation is common; IQ is often below 90.

E. *Complications:* contracture deformities, disuse atrophy, infections, obesity, cardiopulmonary problems. Death is generally due to *respiratory* tract infection or *cardiac* failure.

F. *Diagnostic tests:* prenatal diagnosis, genetic testing; elevated serum enzymes; muscle biopsy; EMG.

III. **Analysis/nursing diagnosis:**

A. *Impaired physical mobility* related to progressive muscle weakness.

B. *Self-care deficits* related to muscle weakness.

C. *Altered family process* related to having a child with a probably fatal disability.

IV. **Nursing care plan/implementation:**

A. Goal: *maintain function in unaffected muscles for as long as possible.*

　1. Assist child to remain as active as possible for as long as possible.

　2. Perform range-of-motion exercises.

　3. Assist with braces to maintain ambulation.

　4. Whenever possible, incorporate play into therapeutic exercises.

　5. Encourage socialization with peers.

B. Goal: *prepare child to perform ADLs as independently as possible.*

　1. Encourage the child to be as independent as possible; do not perform activities that child is capable of doing.

　2. Assist with ADLs only when child is truly unable to perform independently.

　3. Select assistive devices that maximize the child's independence: clothes, utensils, grooming, toiletry.

　4. Teach child how to apply splints and encourage child to apply them as appropriate.

　5. When child can no longer ambulate, assist child to use wheelchair. Discuss housing modifications that are necessary with parents and child.

　6. Schedule regular rest periods and adequate sleep to conserve energy for ADLs.

C. Goal: **health teaching.** *Support family and child.*

　1. Encourage family and child to discuss their concerns and issues related to diagnosis.

　2. Refer family to support group, supportive agencies.

　3. Discuss how parents will need to modify their social activities: e.g., specially trained babysitter to care for the child.

　4. Discuss with the parents long-term care needs and possible placement of the child.

　5. Allow family and child to discuss concerns related to death and dying.

V. **Evaluation/outcome criteria:**

A. Maximal independence is preserved as long as possible.

B. ADLs are carried out independently to the best of the child's abilities.

C. Family verbalizes perceived support.

Guillain-Barré Syndrome

I. *Introduction*: Guillain-Barré Syndrome (GBS) is an *acute postinfectious* or *idiopathic polyneuritis* with *progressive ascending paralysis*. Although it may affect children of any age and both sexes, children from ages 4–10 yr have the highest incidence of GBS. The exact cause of GBS is unknown, although its occurrence has been associated with upper *respiratory* or *gastrointestinal infections* as well as the administration of *immunizations* such as influenza vaccine. The younger child has a better prognosis; in addition, the greater the degree of paralysis, the longer recovery takes. If mortality occurs, death is usually due to respiratory failure (less than 5% of all cases of GBS).

II. **Assessment:**

A. History usually reveals an infection several days *before* the onset of the illness.

B. Onset: can be rapid and acute; or gradual over days or weeks.

C. *Neurologic signs and symptoms* include: generalized weakness and numbness or tingling in the feet and legs, which progresses to a flaccid, ascending, symmetrical paralysis (paresthesia). Paralysis usually *peaks* at 3 wk and then slowly resolves. Facial nerves are affected in as much as 75% of all cases of GBS. *Seventh* cranial nerve

〰️ (*facial nerve*) is usually affected; test by asking child to smile, make a funny face, or show teeth, to see symmetry in expression. If *intercostal or phrenic nerves are involved*, child may exhibit breathlessness in vocalizations and shallow, irregular respirations.

  D. *Elimination*: urinary incontinence or retention and constipation are likely.

〰️ E. *Diagnostic tests*: electromyography; cerebrospinal fluid reveals increased protein; all other lab work is within normal limits.

▶ III. **Analysis/nursing diagnosis:**

  A. *Ineffective breathing pattern* related to neuromuscular dysfunction.

  B. *Risk for injury* related to immobility.

▶ IV. **Nursing care plan/implementation:**

  A. Goal: *maintain adequate respirations.*

  ☞ 1. Maintain patent airway; suction prn. Assist child to cough to clear airway.

  2. *Position* for maximum lung expansion; organize care to decrease energy expenditure.

  3. Monitor respiratory status frequently; report any difficulty swallowing or breathing.

  ☞ 4. Monitor vital signs and level of consciousness; *cardiac monitor* should be used.

  5. *Respirator* should be available at all times, along with suction equipment and tracheostomy set.

  6. Reduce anxiety and stress. Encourage parents to remain with child. Nurse should remain nearby, especially if breathing difficulties arise.

  B. Goal: *prevent complications of immobility.*

  ☞ 1. *Turn and position* frequently; maintain good body alignment; perform passive range of motion exercises.

  ☞ 2. Provide bowel and bladder care.

  3. Monitor skin for signs of breakdown.

  4. Use sheepskin to prevent skin breakdown.

  ☞ 5. Assist with or implement physical therapy plan, including exercises to prevent contractures and assist with recovery.

▶ V. **Evaluation/outcome criteria:**

  A. Adequate respirations are maintained.

  B. No complications of immobility occur.

🔋 COMMONLY PRESCRIBED MEDICATIONS

Medication	Administration	Use/Action	▶ Nursing Consideration
Neuromuscular Conduction Blockers Botulinum toxin, Type A/*Botox*	• IM ONLY • Calculate to child's weight in kilograms • "Orphan drug" status in pediatrics • Must be administered by pediatrician	Used in cerebral palsy to relieve signs/symptoms of spasticity (especially of the lower extremities) Toxin blocks neuromuscular conduction by binding to receptor sites on motor nerve terminals, entering the nerve terminals, and inhibiting acetylcholine release	〰️ • Obtain electromyogram (EMG) first for guidance regarding involved muscles • Look for improvement within 2 weeks, with maximum benefit at 6 weeks post-injection • Injection needs to be repeated at 3–month intervals to retain effect
Skeletal Muscle Relaxants Baclofen/*Lioresal* Dantrolene/*Dantrium*	• Oral, parenteral or intrathecal • Calculate to child's weight in kilograms • Administer in provided dropper or calibrated syringe • **NEVER** use household measuring spoon • Intrathecal pump (Baclofen) must be surgically implanted and refilled every 4–6 weeks	Used in cerebral palsy to relieve signs/symptoms of spasticity (especially of the lower extremities) Inhibits transmission of reflexes of spinal cord level	• Begin with low dosage and gradually increase • Drowsiness diminishes with continued therapy • Evaluate therapeutic response 〰️ • Monitor liver function tests

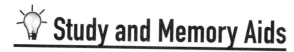

Study and Memory Aids

Cerebral Palsy—Cause

Cerebral palsy is caused by prenatal brain abnormalities.

Cerebral Palsy—Assessment

Delayed developmental milestones
Tongue thrust
Scissoring
Associated disabilities

Cerebral Palsy—Associated Problems

30% of children have mental retardation. 70% of children with cerebral palsy have normal intelligence, but they may have difficulty with testing.

Duchenne Muscular Dystrophy—Genetics

Duchenne muscular dystrophy is a sex-linked *recessive* disorder that occurs almost exclusively in *males*.

DMD— Typical Progression

1. Onset: at 3–5 yr
2. Wheelchair: at 9–11 yr
3. Death: usually at 15–25 yr
The leading causes of death in muscular dystrophy are *infection* (especially *respiratory*) and *cardiac failure*.

Guillain-Barré Syndrome is associated with:

Helicobacter pylori
Immunizations: influenza vaccines
Lyme disease
Measles
Mononucleosis
Mumps
Mycoplasma infections
Pneumocystis infections
Viral or bacterial infections

Adapted from Wong D. *Nursing Care of Infants and Children* (7th ed). St. Louis: Mosby.

Guillain-Barré Syndrome—Care

The priority goal in caring for a child with Guillain-Barré syndrome is maintaining adequate *respirations*; tracheostomy set, suction, and "ambu" bag should be kept at the bedside with a ventilator on stand-by at all times.

Questions

1. When assessing a child with cerebral palsy, which characteristic should the nurse expect to find?
   1. Progressive lower sensory neuron deficit.
   2. Well-controlled locomotion skills.
   3. Manifestation of some degree of mental retardation.
   4. Tendency to develop contractures.

2. The primary goal of nursing care for a child with cerebral palsy is to:
   1. Devise an individualized rehabilitation plan for the child.
   2. Assist the child in developing to maximum potential.
   3. Enroll the child in a special education program as soon as possible.
   4. Promote the child's sense of self-esteem.

3. The parent of a 7-year-old child hospitalized with cerebral palsy angrily confronts the nurse and asks, "Why isn't there some kind of medicine to help my child?" The nurse should inform the parent that:
   1. "There are many medications that can help control the symptoms of cerebral palsy."
   2. "Your physician is the best judge of whether your child would benefit from medication."
   3. "Children with cerebral palsy benefit most from an interdisciplinary team approach to their physical and social needs."
   4. "Younger children with cerebral palsy generally benefit the most from medication."

4. When preparing to feed a child with cerebral palsy, the nurse should first position the child:
   1. In semi-reclining position.
   2. In high-Fowler's position.
   3. In semi-Fowler's position.
   4. On the nurse's lap.

5. Which nursing measure best evaluates the response to the nutritional plan of care for a child with cerebral palsy?
   1. Daily intake and output.
   2. Weekly weight.
   3. Calorie count before each meal.
   4. Daily assessment of food items ordered for each meal.

6. When communicating with a child with cerebral palsy, the nurse should use:
   1. A picture board and allow a sufficient amount of time for the child to select letters or pictures.
   2. A computerized communication system.
   3. Language that is appropriate for the child's developmental level.
   4. Questions that require lengthy responses.

7. The nurse should be aware that the onset of muscular dystrophy most commonly occurs in which age group?
   1. Toddler.
   2. Preschool.
   3. School-age.
   4. Adolescent.

8. The parents of a boy with muscular dystrophy ask the nurse when they should expect that their son will need to be in a wheelchair. The nurse would be most correct in advising them that most children with muscular dystrophy generally lose the ability to walk on their own by age:
   1. 6–8 years.
   2. 9–11 years.
   3. 12–16 years.
   4. 17–24 years.

9. Which condition should the nurse recognize as a late complication that occurs in children with muscular dystrophy?
   1. Infection.
   2. Cardiac failure.
   3. Disuse atrophy.
   4. Contracture deformities.

10. While taking a history of a child with Guillain-Barré syndrome, the nurse should recognize that the condition most likely to be associated with the onset of this disease is:
    1. Mononucleosis.
    2. Strep throat.
    3. Chickenpox.
    4. Oral polio vaccine recently administered.

11. Because the seventh cranial nerve is usually affected by Guillain-Barré syndrome, the nurse should evaluate for the function of this nerve in a child suspected of having the syndrome by asking the child to:
    1. Follow a flashlight beam.
    2. Bite down hard and then open the jaw.
    3. Smile or make a funny face.
    4. Move the tongue in all directions.

12. When caring for a child with Guillain-Barré syndrome, which equipment should the nurse have at the bedside at all times?
    1. Tracheostomy tray.
    2. Mechanical ventilator.
    3. Nasogastric tube.
    4. Foley catheter.

Answers/Rationale

1. **(4)** Children with cerebral palsy have a neuromuscular disorder of the pyramidal motor system. This results in impaired voluntary muscle control, and places the child at high risk for the development of contractures. The damage caused by cerebral palsy is fixed and *nonprogressive* (**1**). The child with cerebral palsy *lacks* the coordination necessary to have well-controlled locomotion skills (**2**). This can be manifested by spastic, dyskinetic, ataxic, or mixed types of movements. Approximately 70% of children who are affected have a wide range of intelligence, all within normal limits; it is important not to interpret the child's speech difficulties as a sign of mental retardation (**3**). **AS, COM, 3, PhI, Physiological adaptation**

2. **(2)** The primary goal of nursing care for children with cerebral palsy is to assist children in developing to their maximum potential in light of their disability. The plan of care for a child with cerebral palsy is one of habilitation *not* rehabilitation (**1**). It is recognized that this child must learn to function as fully as possible despite limitations. Enrollment in special education programs (**3**), such as adaptive physical exercise and speech therapy, *contributes* to the primary goal of development, and is a *part* of the total habilitation program. Promotion of the child's sense of self-esteem (**4**) is essential to the primary goal, and it should be assessed on a *continual* basis throughout childhood. **PL, ANL, 3, HPM, Health promotion and maintenance**

3. **(3)** To date, drugs that decrease spasticity have had little usefulness in improving function in the child with cerebral palsy. The interdisciplinary approach remains the most successful treatment modality. There are *few* medications available with which to treat cerebral palsy (**1**). The primary drugs in use are skeletal muscle relaxants, and their use is largely restricted to *older* children and adolescents (**4**). Antiepileptic medications are used routinely for children who have seizures. The physician may be the best judge as to whether the child requires or would benefit from medication (**2**); but that is *not* the information the parent is seeking. **IMP, APP, 7, HPM, Health promotion and maintenance**

4. **(2)** High-Fowler's position minimizes the possibility of aspiration in a child with cerebral palsy. Tongue thrusting and difficulty sucking and swallowing increase the feeding difficulties in a child with cerebral palsy. Semi-reclining (**1**) and semi-Fowler's (**3**) positions make use of gravity flow to assist sucking and swallowing; these positions do *not* promote active swallowing, and neck hyper-extension may even interfere with swallowing. It is best to feed these children from the front or side of the face, which is difficult to accomplish with the child on the nurse's lap (**4**). **IMP, APP, 3, PhI, Basic care and comfort**

5. **(2)** Weekly weight is the best measurement to evaluate the response to the nutritional plan of care of a child with cerebral palsy. Because promoting adequate nutrition is critical for a child with cerebral palsy, weight gains or losses are an objective measure of dietary compliance and satisfaction. I & O (**1**) reveal important information about the child's

amount of fluid intake and output, but *not the calories consumed.* A calorie count before eating a meal (3) reveals how many *potential* calories the child can consume, rather than *actual* calories consumed after eating the meal. Assessing the types of food items ordered (4) reveals the child's likes and dislikes, *not* actual calories consumed. **EV, ANL, 4, PhI, Basic care and comfort**

6. (3) All forms of communication must be at the developmental level appropriate for the child. This is true for both children who are "normal" and disabled. Using a picture board (1) or a computerized communication system (2) are *not* necessary for all children with cerebral palsy; and even when using these systems, the principle of developmentally-appropriate communication remains the same. Questions that require lengthy responses (4) are difficult and exhausting for the child with cerebral palsy. Questions that can be answered with "yes" or "no" or with just a few words are easier for this child to respond to. **IMP, APP, 7, PsI, Psychosocial integrity**

7. (2) Muscular dystrophy is characterized by an early onset, frequently at 3–5 years. It most typically does *not* present either earlier (1) or later (3, 4). **AN, COM, 3, HPM, Health promotion and maintenance**

8. (2) Muscular dystrophy is evidenced by progressive muscle weakness; the loss of independent ambulation is generally experienced at 9–11 years of age, at which point the child needs a wheelchair. Loss of ambulation is generally *not* experienced earlier (1) or later (3, 4). **IMP, COM, 3, PhI, Basic care and comfort**

9. (2) Although all the complications listed are complications that can occur with muscular dystrophy, the major complication *that tends to occur later* as the disease progresses is a cardiac manifestation such as cardiac failure. This condition *should* be promptly treated with digoxin and diuretics, although it may be difficult to correct. The other complications (1, 3, 4) occur *earlier* in the course of the disease. **AN, ANL, 6, PhI, Physiological adaptation**

10. (1) Gullain-Barré syndrome (infectious polyneuritis) is often associated with an infection or the administration of an immunization; it has also been associated with mononucleosis (1), measles, mumps, Lyme disease, and influenza vaccine. It has *not* been associated with strep throat (2), chickenpox (3), or oral polio vaccine (4). **EV, COM, 1, HPM, Health promotion and maintenance**

11. (3) The *seventh* cranial nerve is the facial nerve that controls the muscles for facial expression. The nurse should evaluate for symmetry of expression by asking the child to smile, make a funny face, or show teeth. Following a flashlight beam (1) tests the *third* cranial nerve, the oculomotor nerve, which controls the extraocular muscles of the eye. Biting down hard and opening the jaw (2) tests the *fifth* cranial nerve, the trigeminal nerve, which controls the chewing muscles. Moving the tongue in all directions (4) tests the *twelfth* cranial nerve, the hypoglossal nerve, which controls the muscles of the tongue. **IMP, APP, 2, PhI, Reduction of risk potential**

12. (1) The emphasis of nursing care for a child with Guillain-Barré syndrome should be assessment of the child for progressive paralysis and associated complications, of which respiratory complications are the most significant; therefore, a tracheostomy tray should be kept at the bedside at all times in the event the paralysis affects the child's ability to breathe. A ventilator (2) should be kept on stand-by, but does *not* necessarily have to be kept at the bedside because as it may unnecessarily frighten the child. Although the child may have difficulty swallowing and may lose the gag reflex, an NG tube (3) does *not* need to be kept at the bedside; the nurse can secure one should it become necessary. A Foley catheter (4) is *not* generally required. **PL, ANL, 1, PhI, Reduction of risk potential**

Key to Codes

Nursing process: AS, assessment; **AN,** analysis; **PL,** planning; **IMP,** implementation; **EV,** evaluation. (See **Appendix L** for explanation of nursing process steps.)

Cognitive level: RE/KN, recall/knowledge; **COM,** comprehension; **APP,** application; **ANL,** analysis; **EVL,** evaluation; **SYN,** synthesis. (See **Appendix L** for explanation.)

Category of human function: 1, protective; 2, sensory-perceptual; 3, comfort, rest, activity, and mobility; 4, nutrition; 5, growth and development; 6, fluid-gas transport; 7, psychosocial-cultural; 8, elimination. (See **Appendix N** for explanation.)

Client need: SECE, safe, effective care environment; **HPM,** health promotion and maintenance; **PsI,** psychosocial integrity; **PhI,** physiological integrity. (See **Appendix O** for explanation.)

Client subneed: See **Appendix O** for explanation.

Problems of the Newborn (Birth Defects)

16

Chapter Outline

Key Words

abduction   movement of extremities away from the body.

meningocele   sac filled with spinal fluid (no nerves in sac) that protrudes through spinal canal opening; no motor-sensory deficit.

myelomeningocele   congenital defect in which spinal nerves protrude through spinal column in an enclosed saclike structure, resulting in sensory-motor loss below the site.

orthotic   an orthopedic brace.

polyhydramnios   excessive amniotic fluid during gestation.

Summary of Key Points

1. Congenital defects are the leading cause of death in infants from birth–1 mo.

2. The most common, and serious, type of spina bifida is *myelomeningocele*, which is manifest by a permanent, irreversible, and complete lack of motion or sensation below the level of the sac.

3. The infant with *spina bifida* should be closely observed for the development of hydrocephalus, which is present in 80-85% of all cases.

4. *Hydrocephalus* is an abnormal accumulation of cerebrospinal fluid (CSF) within the ventricles of the brain, resulting in increased intracranial pressure and possibly brain damage if not treated.

5. The treatment for *hydrocephalus* is a shunting procedure by which excessive fluid is shunted to the right atrium of the heart or the peritoneal cavity.

6. After a shunt procedure, *prevent subdural hematoma* caused by the too rapid draining of CSF, by keeping the infant flat in bed for 24 hr.

7. *Congenital clubfoot* is typically manifest with a downward and inward curvature of the newborn's foot; it is treated with a series of corrective casts.

8. *Developmental dysplasia of the hip* is a malformation of the hip that is present at birth; it is treated with a splint (*Pavlik harness*) or, in the older child, traction and/or surgery.

9. *Tracheoesophageal* fistula, an abnormal connection between the trachea and the esophagus, is considered a *surgical emergency* in the neonate.

10. The most common *short-term* complication of *tracheoesophageal fistula* is pneumonia; the most common *long-term* complication is stricture formation.

11. *Cleft lip and palate* are obvious facial defects that require surgery in the early months or years of the newborn's life; *two primary concerns of the nurse are*: feeding the infant safely and promoting bonding, or attachment, between the newborn and parents.

12. *Cleft lip* is always repaired *first*, when the infant is about 8-12 wk; *cleft palate* repair is delayed until 12-18 mo to allow growth of the bony structures of the mouth, but should be done before speech begins.

13. *Hypospadias*, a congenital anatomical defect of the male genitourinary tract, is readily detected at birth through simple visual inspection. The treatment is *staged surgical repair,* which should be completed *before* the child is 18 mo, *before body image is developed* or castration fears are evident.

14. *Home care* for all infants with birth defects: **NEVER** allow these defects to go unrepaired beyond the prescribed period of time. Compliance and follow-through are critical for the infant's survival.

Selected Birth Defects

Malformations of the Central Nervous System

I. Spina Bifida (Myelodysplasia)

    A. *Introduction*: There are three different types of spina bifida (see **Figure 16.1, p. 149**):

        1. **Spina bifida occulta**—a "hidden" bony defect *without* herniation of the meninges or cord; *not* visible externally; no symptoms are present, *no* treatment is needed.

        2. **Meningocele**—see **Table 16.1, p. 150**.

        3. **Myelomeningocele**—see **Table 16.1, p. 150**. Most serious type of spina bifida, and also most common. *The remainder of this section deals exclusively with myelomeningocele.*

    B. **Assessment:**

        1. Congenital defect.

        2. Readily detected by visual inspection in delivery room: round, bulging sac filled with fluid, usually in lumbosacral area.

        3. *Sensation and movement*: complete absence below the level of the lesion.

        4. *Urinary*: retention, with overflow incontinence.

        5. *Fecal*: constipation, fecal impaction, oozing of liquid stool around impaction.

        6. 90-95% develop signs and symptoms of *hydrocephalus*.

        7. May have associated *orthopedic* anomalies: clubfoot, developmental hip dysplasia.

    C. **Analysis/nursing diagnosis:**

        1. *Risk for injury/infection* related to rupture of the sac.

        2. *Altered urinary elimination* related to urinary retention and overflow incontinence.

        3. *Impaired skin integrity* related to immobility.

        4. *Constipation* related to fecal incontinence and impaired innervation.

        5. *High risk for sensory perceptual defect* related to possible postoperative development of hydrocephalus.

    D. **Nursing care plan/implementation:**

        1. Goal: *prevent rupture of the sac and possible infection (preoperative).*

            a. *Position*: *no* pressure on sac; *prone*, to prevent contamination with urine or stool.

            b. *No* clothing or diapers to *avoid* pressure on sac.

            c. Place in heated isolette or warmer to maintain body temperature. If overhead warmer is used, change dressing more frequently to prevent dehydrating → rupturing of sac.

            d. Keep sac covered with sterile moist nonadherent dressing (sterile normal saline) to prevent drying, cracking, and leakage of cerebrospinal fluid (CSF); change every 2–4 h; document appearance of sac each dressing change to note signs and symptoms of infection, leaks, abrasions, or irritation.

            e. Enforce strict *aseptic* technique to prevent infection (leading cause of morbidity/mortality in neonatal period).

        2. Goal: *prevent infection in postoperative period.*

            a. *Position*: prone, side-lying, or partial side-lying.

            b. Use *myelomeningocele apron* (specific type of dressing) to prevent urine or stool from contaminating suture line.

            c. Administer antibiotics as ordered.

            d. Use strict *aseptic* techniques in dressing changes; standard precautions to prevent infection.

        3. Goal: *prevent urinary retention and urinary tract infection.*

            a. Monitor I&O, offer *extra fluids* to flush kidneys.

            b. Keep urethral meatus clean of stool to prevent ascending bacterial infection.

            c. Monitor urinary output for retention.

            d. Administer *antibiotics/urinary tract antiseptics* per MD order.

            e. Teach parents clean intermittent catheterization (CIC); *avoid* use of latex products; prepare for future urinary diversion procedure.

        4. Goal: *prevent complications of prolonged immobility and/or associated orthopedic anomalies.*

            a. *Position*: hips *abducted*.

            b. Use positional devices, rotating pressure mattress/flotation mattress.

            c. Refer to physical therapy for ROM exercises.

            d. Make necessary referrals for care of possible club feet/developmental hip dysplasia.

        5. Goal: *prevent constipation*

            a. Begin early bowel program with diet modification, regular toilet habits, possible laxatives/enemas.

        6. Goal: *monitor for possible development of hydrocephalus.*

            a. Assess for ↑ head circumference. (occurs in 90-95% of infants born with myelomeningocele).

            b. May require shunting procedure soon after myelomeningocele repair.

    E. **Evaluation/outcome criteria:**

        1. Integrity of sac is maintained until surgery is done (preoperatively) and no infection occurs (postoperatively).

(continued on p. 150)

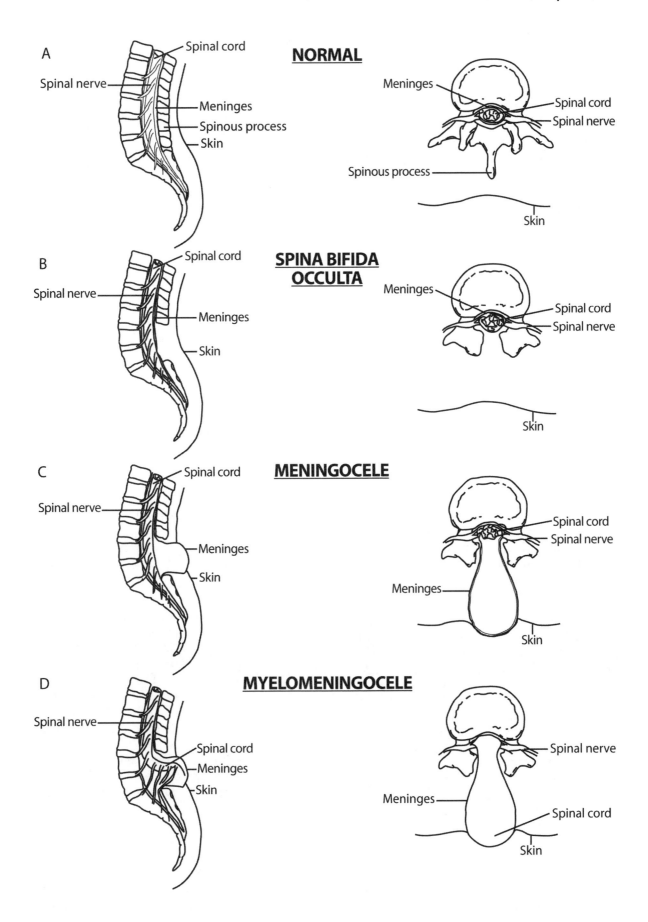

FIGURE 16.1 OSSEOUS SPINE DEFECTS IN MIDLINE. Varying degrees of neural herniations.

TABLE 16.1 COMPARISON OF TWO MAJOR TYPES OF SPINA BIFIDA

Dimension	Meningocele	Myelomeningocele
Contents of sac	Meninges and cerebrospinal fluid	Meninges, cerebrospinal fluid, spinal cord
Transillumination	Present	Absent
Percentage of total cases	25%	75%
Motor function	Present	Absent
Sensory function	Present	Absent
Urinary/fecal incontinence	Absent	Present
Associated orthopedic anomalies	Rare	Developmental dysplasia of the hip, clubfoot
Other anomalies	Rare	Hydrocephalus (80-85%)
Treatment	Surgery	Surgery
Major short-term complication	Infection (meningitis)	Infection (meningitis)
Major long-term complication	None	Chronic urinary tract infection renal disease/ failure
Prognosis	Excellent	Guarded

2. Adequate patterns of urinary elimination with necessary support.
3. Skin integrity is maintained.
4. Constipation is prevented.
5. Hydrocephaly is prevented via prompt surgical intervention.

II. Hydrocephalus

A. *Introduction*: Hydrocephalus, known to the lay person as "water on the brain," is actually a syndrome resulting from disturbances in the dynamics of *CSF*. The accumulation of the fluid causes enlargement and dilatation of the ventricles of the brain and increased intracranial pressure (ICP). If untreated, severe brain damage results; treatment is a surgical shunting procedure that allows drainage of CSF from the ventricles of the brain to another, less harmful area within the body: jugular vein, right atrium of the heart, or peritoneal cavity (**Figure 16.2, p. 151**). Hydrocephalus can develop as the result of a *congenital malformation* (e.g., *Arnold-Chiari* malformation), can be associated with *other* congenital defects (e.g., spina bifida), or can be *acquired secondary to infection* (e.g., meningitis), trauma, or neoplasm.

B. **Assessment:**
1. *Head*: increased circumference—earliest sign of hydrocephalus in the infant (> 1 inch/ mo).
2. *Fontanels*: tense and bulging without head enlargement.
3. *Veins*: dilated scalp veins.
4. *"Setting-sun" sign*: sclera visible above pupil; pupils are sluggish with unequal response to light.
5. *Cry*: shrill, high pitched.
6. *Developmental milestones*: delayed.

7. *Reflexes*: persistence of neonatal reflexes; hyperactive reflexes.
8. Feeds poorly.
9. **Signs of ↑ ICP:**
   a. Vomiting.
   b. Irritability.
   c. Seizures.
   d. ↓ Pulse.
   e. ↓ Respirations.
   f. ↑ Blood pressure.
   g. Widened pulse pressure.
10. History may reveal other CNS defects (e.g., spina bifida), infection (e.g., meningitis), trauma, or neoplasm.

C. **Analysis/nursing diagnosis:**
1. *Altered cerebral tissue perfusion* related to increased intracranial pressure.
2. *Impaired skin integrity* related to enlarged head size and lack of motor coordination.
3. *Altered nutrition, less than body requirements*, related to anorexia and vomiting.
4. *Anxiety* related to diagnosis and uncertain outcome.
5. *Knowledge deficit* related to care of the child with a shunt and follow-up care.

D. **Nursing care plan/implementation:**
1. Goal: *monitor neurologic status preoperatively*
   a. Measure head circumference daily and note any abnormal increase.
   b. Perform neurologic checks at least q 4 h to monitor for signs of ↑ ICP.
   c. Report signs of ↑ ICP **stat** to physician.
   d. Assist with *diagnostic procedures/ treatments*: ventricular tap, CAT scan, etc.

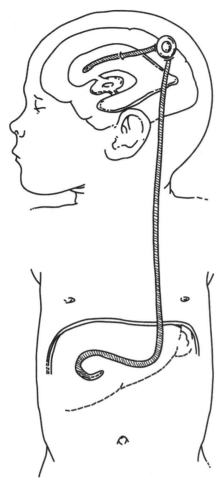

FIGURE 16.2 VENTRICULOPERITONEAL SHUNT. Catheter is threaded beneath the skin.

2. Goal: *monitor neurologic status* ***postoperatively***.

   a. *Position: flat* in bed for 24 hours to prevent subdural hematoma.

   b. Gradually increase the angle of elevation of head of bed, per MD order.

   c. *Position*: on *unoperative* side to prevent mechanical pressure and obstruction to shunt.

   d. Monitor head circumference daily to note any abnormal increase that might indicate malfunctioning shunt.

   e. Monitor vital signs; monitor for ↑ ICP.

   f. Monitor for complications: shunt malfunction; infection.

3. Goal: *maintain skin integrity*.

   a. Inspect skin frequently for pressure/irritation.

   b. Position: change frequently.

   c. Sheepskin/pressure reduction mattress to prevent pressure on prominent areas.

4. Goal: *maintain adequate nutrition*.

   a. NPO for first 24–48 hours postoperative, with IV coverage.

   b. Slowly resume feeding; small frequent feedings fed slowly to prevent vomiting; serve age-appropriate, easily swallowed, soft foods (e.g., jello, applesauce, etc.)

5. Goal: **health teaching**. *Reduce parental anxiety.*

   a. Do preoperative teaching regarding the shunt procedure: stress need to remove excessive CSF to relieve pressure on brain as soon as possible after diagnosis is established.

   b. Stress early diagnosis and prompt shunting procedure to minimize the risk of long-term neurologic complications.

   c. Offer realistic information regarding prognosis:

      (1) Surgically treated, with continued follow-up care = 80% survival rate.

      (2) Of these survivors, 50% are completely normal and 50% have some degree of neurologic disability such as inattentiveness or hyperactivity.

6. Goal: **health teaching**. *Provide discharge teaching to parents regarding home care of the child with a shunt.*

   a. Stress need for long-term follow-up care.

   b. Discuss feeding techniques, care of skin (especially scalp), need for stimulation.

   c. Prepare parents for shunt revisions to be done periodically as child grows.

d. Teach parents signs and symptoms of shunt malfunctioning (i.e., of ↑ ICP or infection) and to report these promptly to physician.

e. Encourage parents to enroll infant in "early infant stimulation" program to maximize developmental potential.

f. Stress need to monitor development at frequent intervals, make referrals prn.

E. Evaluation/outcome criteria:

1. Cerebral tissue perfusion and neurologic functioning is maintained or improved.

2. Skin integrity is maintained.

3. Adequate nutrition is maintained.

4. Parents' anxiety is relieved.

5. Parents verbalize understanding of how to care for child after discharge from hospital.

Skeletal Malformations

I. Congenital Clubfoot

A. *Introduction*: Congenital clubfoot is a broad term that describes a fairly common orthopedic *anomaly* in which the newborn's foot, or feet, are twisted from the usual shape or position. Although there are a variety of types of clubfoot, the most common type, which accounts for 95% of the cases of clubfoot, is *talipes equinovarus*— the foot is pointed downward and inward. Clubfoot can occur *alone* or in *conjunction* with other deformities such as spina bifida. It is twice as common in *boys* than in girls. (refer also to **Chapter 14, Table 14.1, p. 129**).

B. Assessment:

1. Observation of the newborn reveals a visible defect in the foot/feet (see **Figure 16.3**); it is possible to detect in the prenatal period through *ultrasound*.

2. Differentiate between *positional* deformities that can be moved to an overcorrected position and *true clubfoot*, which cannot be overcorrected.

C. Analysis/nursing diagnosis:

1. *Risk for injury* related to casts or corrective device.

2. *Knowledge deficit* related to care of the child with clubfoot.

D. Nursing care plan/implementation:

1. Goal: *prevent injury to the infant wearing cast(s) for clubfoot* (see **Figure 16.4, p. 153**).

a. Teach family how to hold and move infant with foot/feet in casts.

b. Teach family cast care (see **Table 16.2, p. 154**).

2. Goal: **health teaching**. *Provide family with understanding and knowledge of care of the infant with clubfoot.*

a. Teach family about the condition, treatment, and need for long-term follow-up.

(1) Treatment begins in the immediate neonatal period and continues for months or years.

(2) A successive series of casts is applied and reapplied to gradually move the foot/feet to an overcorrected position.

(3) Manipulation and casting will be repeated frequently during the early months of the infant's life.

(4) In some cases, surgical correction may be needed.

(5) After the casts, the infant may be placed in an orthotic device or orthotic shoes to maintain the correction.

b. Discuss the cast and cast care (see **Table 16.2, p. 154**).

(1) Stress signs and symptoms of circulatory impairment.

(2) Provide the family with emergency phone number for 24-hr use.

(3) Discuss good skin care and how to prevent breakdown.

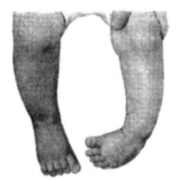 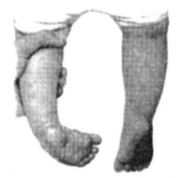 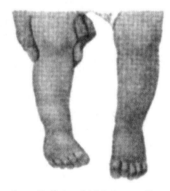

A   Unilateral Clubfoot (Talipes Equinovarus)   *B   Unilateral Metatarsus Varus*

FIGURE 16.3 FOOT ANOMALIES. A. Unilateral clubfoot (*talipes equinovarus*). B. Unilateral *metatarsus varus*.

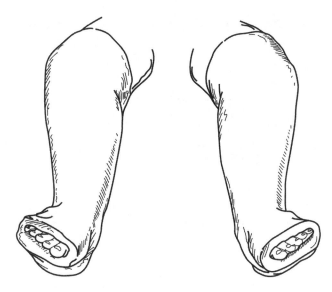

FIGURE 16.4 CASTS TO CORRECT BILATERAL CONGENITAL CLUBFOOT (TALIPES EQUINOVARUS).

    c. Discuss the need for long-term follow-up care to improve the infant's prognosis.

▶ **E. Evaluation/outcome criteria:**
1. No injury occurs to the infant wearing cast(s) for clubfoot.
2. Family demonstrates knowledge regarding clubfoot and complies with therapy.

II. Developmental Dysplasia of the Hip

  A. *Introduction*: Developmental dysplasia of the hip (DDH) was *formerly* known as *"congenital hip," "congenital hip dysplasia,"* or *"congenital dislocated hip."* The newer term refers to a variety of malformations of the hip that are *present at birth* and result in instability of the hip. DDH occurs more frequently in *girls* than in boys, and 80% of cases involve *only one hip*. The exact cause is unknown, although it is believed to be caused by *multifactors*, such as family history or intrauterine positioning which are thought to increase the risk of DDH. The overall goal of treatment is to stabilize the head of the femur within the acetabulum. Treatment involves wearing an abduction device or casting the hips in abduction; open reduction may occasionally be necessary. The earlier the treatment is begun, the greater the success rate (refer to **Chapter 14, Table 14.1, p. 129**).

▶ **B. Assessment:**
1. *Newborn*/infant:
   a. *Ortolani* and *Barlow* tests (see **Figure 16.5, p. 155**). Note: These tests should be performed only by a highly experienced practitioner, to avoid complications.
     (1) *Ortolani test*: the infant lies in a relaxed *supine position*, and the hips and knees are flexed. While the joint is stabilized manually, the examiner rotates the joint upward and outward. If the femoral head can be felt (or heard by a "clicking" sound) to slip forward into the acetabulum while the examiner exerts pressure from the rear, dislocation is present.
     (2) *Barlow test*: If the femoral head moves into or out of the back of the acetabulum while the examiner exerts pressure from the front, the hip is considered to be unstable or dislocatable.

   Note: These tests are most reliable from birth to 2–3 months.
   b. Shortening of the limb on the affected side.
   c. Limitation of abduction on the affected side.
   d. Additional thigh and gluteal fat folds on the affected side.
2. *Older* infant and child:
   a. Shortening of the affected leg.
   b. Delayed walking, walking with a significant limp on the affected side.
   c. *Trendelenburg sign*: when the child bears weight on the affected hip, the pelvis tilts downward on the unaffected side instead of upward as it normally should.
   d. Prominence of the trochanter on the affected side.
3. *Diagnostic tests*: ultrasound in younger infant, x-rays in older infant or child; CT scan; arthrography.

▶ **C. Analysis/nursing diagnosis:**
1. *Risk for injury* related to wearing a corrective device for DDH.

TABLE 16.2 🏠 FAMILY-CENTERED-TEACHING: HOME CARE OF CASTS AND SKIN

Instructions for Parents	*Instructions for Children*
The following points should be reviewed with parents before the child is discharged from care. 1. Cast must be kept dry; it can be protected with a plastic bag or plastic wrap during bathing if size permits. A sponge bath may be necessary. 2. Cast edges around the groin and perineum should be petaled with waterproof tape to protect the cast and padding from urine and stool. 3. Do *not* allow the child to poke pencils or other objects under the cast because this may injure the skin. 4. If skin under the cast itches, a hair dryer can be used to blow cool air under the cast. An antihistamine, such as *diphenhydramine (Benadryl) or hydroxyzine (Atarax)* may also be helpful if itching is severe. 5. Report any foul smell from the cast or any areas of drainage to the physician. This may indicate skin breakdown or infection. 6. Check sensation, color, and temperature. Swelling and pain are most acute the first days after injury or surgery. Any sudden increase in swelling or pain should be reported to the physician.	1. Do *not* bang or hit cast. 2. Do *not* let cast get wet. 3. Do *not* put anything inside cast. 4. Do *not* scratch underneath cast. 5. Tell parents or other adult if arm or leg hurts, feels numb, tingles, or looks puffy.

Source: Betz et al. *Family-Centered Nursing Care of Children*, Philadelphia: WB Saunders.

2. *Knowledge deficit* related to care of the infant/child with DDH.

🏠 D. **Nursing care plan/implementation:**

  1. Goal: *prevent injury to the infant/child wearing a corrective device for DDH.*

    a. Teach family how to hold and move the infant/child to prevent injury.

    b. Assist family to modify baby equipment (e.g., car seat, infant seat, stroller) to accommodate the corrective device.

    ☞ **c.** Teach family how to apply the corrective device appropriately, or teach family cast care as necessary (**Table 16.2**).

🏠 2. Goal: **health teaching**. *Provide family with knowledge of care of the infant/child with DDH.*

    a. Teach family about the DDH condition, treatment, and need for long-term follow-up.

      (1) *Infant* wears a corrective device (such as a *Pavlik harness*) continuously for 3-5 mo.

      (2) *Older infant or toddler* generally requires traction followed by application of a plaster cast.

      (3) *Older child* generally requires surgery, casting, and physical therapy.

    b. Demonstrate the corrective device, how to apply, signs and symptoms of pressure areas to look for (see also **Table 16.3, p. 156**).

      (1) Put cotton clothing on the infant under the corrective device: cotton T-shirt, cotton socks.

      (2) Check skin under straps several times daily for redness or breakdown.

      (3) Massage skin under straps gently to stimulate circulation; *avoid* powders or lotions.

      (4) Place diapers *under* the straps of the harness.

      (5) Shoulder straps may be padded.

      (6) Harness should *not* be adjusted without the supervision of the practitioner.

    c. Discuss alternative means of locomotion for the infant/child.

    d. Discuss the need for long-term follow-up care to improve the infant's prognosis.

🏁 E. **Evaluation/outcome criteria:**

  1. No injury occurs to the infant/child wearing a corrective device for DDH.

  2. Family demonstrates knowledge regarding DDH and complies with therapy.

Gastrointestinal Malformations

I. **Tracheoesophageal Fistula**

  A. *Introduction*: Tracheoesophageal fistula (TEF) is a congenital anomaly resulting from *faulty embryonic* development; although there are

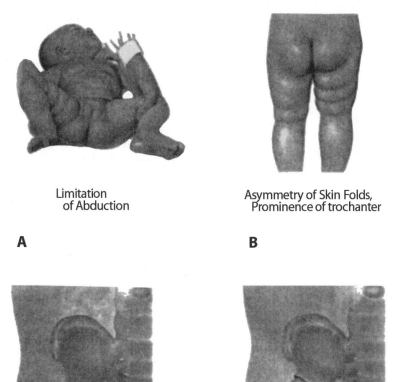

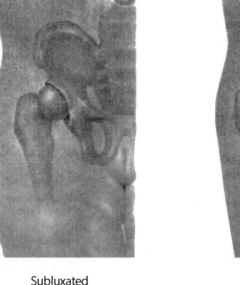

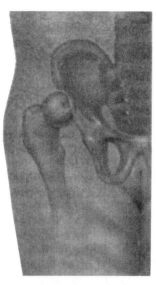

FIGURE 16.5 DEVELOPMENTAL DYSPLASIA OF THE HIP. A. Limitation of abduction. B. Asymmetry of skin folds, prominence of trochanter. C. Shortening of femur. D. Normal. E. Subluxated. F. Dislocated.

(From *Clinical Education Aid* No. 15. Colombus, OH: Ross Laboratories. Reproduced, with permission).

numerous types of TEF, the major problem is an anatomical defect that results in an abnormal connection between the trachea (respiratory tract) and the esophagus (GI system) (see **Figure 16.6, p. 157**). No specific cause has been identified; however, infants born with TEF are often *premature*, and there is a maternal history of *polyhydramnios*. Diagnosis should be made immediately, within hours after birth, and preferably before feeding (to avoid aspiration pneumonia). *Associated anomalies* include: congenital heart disease, anorectal malformations, and genitourinary anomalies.

✉ **B. Assessment:**
    1. Perinatal history: maternal polyhydramnios, premature birth.

2. *Most important system* affected is *respiratory*:
    a. Shortly after birth, infant has excessive amounts of mucus.
    b. Mucus bubbles or froths out of nose and mouth; infant literally "exhales" mucus.
    💡 **c.** *"3 C's": coughing, choking, cyanosis*—due to mucus accumulating in respiratory tract.
    d. Infant "pinks up" with suctioning, only to experience repeated respiratory distress within a short time as mucus builds up.
    e. Aspiration pneumonia occurs early.
    f. Respiratory arrest may occur.

TABLE 16.3 ⬛ GUIDELINES FOR BRACE WEAR

- Braces should be as comfortable as possible and child should have adequate mobility while wearing the brace.
- Have the child begin wearing the brace for periods of 1-2 h and then progress to 2-4 h.
- Check skin at 1-2-h intervals. If redness or breakdown is apparent, leave the brace off and allow the skin to clear. Reapply the brace when the skin returns to its normal color. If skin breakdown has occurred, the brace cannot be worn until skin integrity is restored. Assess brace frequently for rough edges and signs of "wear and tear."
- Always have the child wear a clean white sock, T-shirt, or other thin white liner beneath the brace. Be sure the liner is wrinkle-free under the brace. *Avoid* using powders or lotions that can cause skin to break down. Toughen any sensitive areas using alcohol wipes.
- Consult pediatrician or brace manufacturer/fitter if skin breakdown persists/brace becomes too small/needs repair or adjustment.

Adapted from Ball J. and Bindler R. *Pediatric Nursing: Caring for Children.* New Jersey, Prentice Hall.

3. *Second* system affected is *GI*:
   a. Abdominal distention because excessive air enters stomach with each breath infant takes.
   b. Inability to aspirate stomach contents when attempting to pass NG tube.
   c. If all signs are not correctly interpreted and feeding is attempted, infant takes 2–3 mouthfuls, coughs and gags, and forcefully "exhales" formula through nostrils.

⬛ C. **Analysis/nursing diagnosis:**
   1. *High risk for injury* related to excess mucus and difficulty maintaining patent airway.
   2. *Altered infant nutrition, less than body requirements*, related to inability to take fluids by mouth.
   3. *Anxiety* (parental), related to surgery, condition, premature delivery, and uncertain prognosis.
   4. *Knowledge deficit* related to discharge care of infant related to gastrostomy tube, feeding.

⬛ D. **Nursing care plan/implementation:**
   1. Goal: *prepare infant for immediate surgery.*
      a. Stress to parents that surgery is *only* possible treatment.
      b. Allow parents to see infant before surgery to promote bonding and attachment.
      c. Maintain NPO—provide IV fluids, monitor I&O, NG tube.
      d. *Position: elevate* head of bed (HOB) 20–30 degrees to prevent aspiration.

   e. Administer warmed, humidified oxygen per MD order to relieve hypoxia and to prevent cold stress.
   2. Goal (**postoperative**): *maintain patent airway.*
      a. *Position: elevate* HOB 20-30 degrees.
      b. Care of chest tubes (open-chest procedure).
      c. Care of endotracheal tube/ventilator (infant frequently requires ventilatory assistance for 24-48 h postoperatively).
      d. Monitor for symptoms and signs of pneumonia (most common postoperative complication):
         (1) Aspiration.
         (2) Hypostatic, secondary to anesthesia.
      e. Monitor for symptoms and signs of respiratory distress syndrome (RDS) (premature infant).
      f. **Use special precautions when suctioning**: suction with marked catheter to *avoid* exerting undue pressure on newly sutured trachea.
      g. Administer prophylactic/therapeutic *antibiotics*, per MD order.
      h. Administer warmed, humidified oxygen, per MD order; monitor arterial blood gases (ABGs).
   3. Goal: *maintain adequate nutrition.*
      a. Maintain NPO 10–14 d, until esophagus is fully healed (offer pacifier).
      b. 48-72 h after surgery: IV fluids only.
      c. When condition is stable: begin *gastrostomy tube* feedings per MD order.
         (1) Start with small amounts of clear liquids.
         (2) Gradually increase to full-strength formula.
         (3) *Postoperative*: leave G-tube open and elevated slightly *above* level of stomach to prevent aspiration if infant vomits.
         (4) Offer pacifier prn.
      d. Monitor weight, I&O.
      e. *10–14 postoperative day*: begin oral feedings.
         (1) Start with clear liquids.
         (2) Note ability to suck and swallow.
         (3) Offer small amounts at frequent intervals.
         (4) May need to supplement postop feeding with G-tube feeding prn.
   4. Goal: *encourage parents to express and control anxiety.*
      a. Provide opportunity for parents to express concerns.
      b. Support parents.
   5. Goal: **health teaching**. *Prepare parents to successfully care for the infant after discharge.*

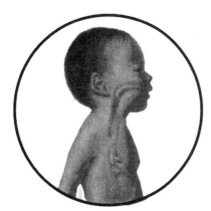

FIGURE 16.6 TRACHEOESOPHAGEAL FISTULA. In the most common type of esophageal atresia and tracheoesophageal fistula, the upper segment of the esophagus ends in a blind pouch connected to the trachea; a fistula connects the lower segment to the trachea.

(From *Clinical Education Aid* No. 4. Colombus, OH: Ross Laboratories. Reproduced with permission.)

TABLE 16.4 COMPARISON OF CLEFT LIP AND CLEFT PALATE

Dimension	Cleft Lip Only	Cleft Palate Only	Both Cleft Lip and Cleft Palate
Incidence	1/1000. More common among boys.	1/2500. More common among girls.	Most common facial malformation. More common among boys. More common among Caucasians than African-Americans.
Surgical repair	"Cheiloplasty" (Logan bow). Often done in a single stage. Timing: age 6–12 wk.	Palatoplasty. Often done in staged repairs. Timing: age 12–18 mo.	Lip always repaired before palate to enhance parent-infant attachment, bonding.
Position postoperatively	*Never* on abdomen.	*Always* on abdomen.	
Feeding postoperatively	*No* sucking. Use Breck feeder or Asepto syringe.	*No* sucking. Use wide-bowl spoon or plastic cup.	
⊠Nursing care postoperatively	Elbow restraints. Lessen crying. Croup tent.	Elbow restraints. Lessen crying. Croup tent.	OK to show parents pictures of "before" and "after" repair.
Long-term concerns	Bonding, attachment. Social adjustment—potential threat to self-image.	Defective speech—refer to speech therapist. Abnormal dentition—refer to orthodontist. Hearing loss—refer to pediatric eye, ear, nose, throat specialist/physician.	

a. Teach parents that infant will probably be discharged with G-tube in place; teach home care of G-tube.

b. Teach parents symptoms and signs of most common long-term problem, i.e., stricture formation:
   (1) Refusal to eat solids or swallow liquids.
   (2) Dysphagia.
   (3) Increased coughing or choking.

c. Stress need for long-term follow-up care.

d. Offer realistic encouragement; prognosis is generally good.

⊠ E. **Evaluation/outcome criteria:**

1. Infant survives immediate surgical repair without difficulties and patent airway is maintained.

2. Adequate nutrition is maintained; infant begins to gain weight and grow.

3. Anxiety is controlled

4. Parents verbalize confidence in ability to care for infant on discharge.

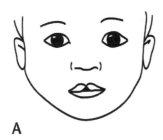 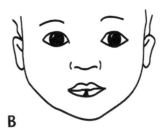

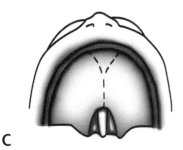 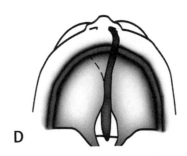 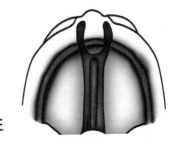

FIGURE 16.7 COMMON FORMS OF CLEFT LIP AND PALATE. A. Unilateral cleft lip. B. Bilateral cleft lip. C. Cleft hard and soft palate. D. Total unilateral cleft palate and cleft lip. E. Total bilateral cleft palate and cleft lip

II. Cleft Lip and Cleft Palate

A. *Introduction*: Cleft lip and cleft palate are congenital facial malformations resulting from faulty embryonic development; there appear to be *multiple factors* involved in the exact etiology: mutant genes, chromosomal abnormalities, teratogenic agents, etc. Infant may be born with cleft lip alone, cleft palate alone, or with both cleft lip and cleft palate (see **Table 16.4, p. 157** for a comparison of these conditions).

B. **Assessment:**
   1. *Cleft lip*—obvious facial defect, readily detectable at time of birth (see **Figure 16.7**).
   2. *Cleft palate*—need to feel inside infant's mouth to check for presence of palatal defect and to note extent of defect: soft palate only, or soft palate and hard palate.
   3. *Both cleft lip and cleft palate*—major problems with feeding: difficult to feed, noisy sucking, swallowing of excessive amounts of air, prone to aspiration.
   4. Parent-infant attachment (bonding) may be adversely affected due to "loss of perfect infant," multiple hospitalizations; note amount and quality of parent-infant interaction.

C. **Analysis/nursing diagnosis:**
   1. *Altered nutrition, less than body requirements,* related to physical defect.
   2. *Altered parenting* related to birth of child with obvious facial defect.
   3. *Knowledge deficit,* actual or potential, related to treatment and follow-up.

D. **Nursing care plan/implementation:**
   1. Goal: *maintain adequate nutrition.*
      a. *Preoperative*: first encourage parents to watch nurse feed infant, then teach parents proper feeding techniques:
         (1) Use Breck feeder or Asepto syringe.
         (2) Deposit formula on back of tongue to facilitate swallowing and prevent aspiration.
         (3) Rinse infant's mouth with sterile water after feedings, to prevent infection.
         (4) Feed slowly, with child in *sitting position*, to prevent aspiration.
         (5) Burp frequently; infant will swallow air along with formula due to the defect.
         (6) Monitor weight.
      b. *Postoperative*
         (1) Begin with *clear liquids* when child has fully recovered from anesthesia.
         (2) Monitor weight gain carefully, to assure adequate rate of growth.
         (3) *No* sucking for either cleft lip or cleft palate repair.
   2. Goal: *promote parent-infant attachment.*
      a. Show no discomfort handling infant; convey acceptance.
      b. Stay with parents the first time they see/hold infant.
      c. Offer positive comments about infant.

d. Give positive reinforcement to parents' initial attempts at parenting.

e. Encourage parents to assume increasing independence in care of their infant.

f. Allow rooming-in on subsequent hospitalizations.

3. Goal: **health teaching**. *Teach parents regarding feeding and need for long-term follow-up care.*

a. Teach parents regarding long-term concerns (see **Table 16.4, p. 157**).

b. Make necessary referrals before discharge:

(1) Specialists: speech, dentition, hearing.

(2) Community health nurse.

(3) Social service.

(4) Disabled children's services for financial assistance.

(5) Local facial-malformations support group.

c. Refer parents to genetic counseling services due to mixed genetic/ environmental etiology.

d. Encourage parents to promote self-esteem in infant/child as child grows and develops.

E. **Evaluation/outcome criteria:**

1. Adequate nutrition is provided, and infant grows at "normal" rate for age.

2. Parent-infant attachment is formed.

3. Parents verbalize confidence in their ability to care for infant.

Genitourinary Malformation

Hypospadias

I. *Introduction*: Hypospadias is a *congenital anatomical defect* of the male genitourinary tract, readily detected at birth through simple visual examination. In hypospadias, the urethral opening is located on the ventral surface of the penile shaft; this makes voiding in the standing position virtually impossible and has the potential to cause serious psychological difficulties. Ideally, staged surgical repair should be completed by 6–18 mo, before body image is developed or castration fears are evident.

II. **Assessment:**

A. Urethral opening is located on ventral surface of penis.

B. May be accompanied by "chordee"—ventral curvature of the penis due to a fibrous band of tissue.

C. (Rare) ambiguous genitalia, resulting in need for chromosomal studies to determine sex of infant.

III. **Analysis/nursing diagnosis:**

A. *Altered urinary elimination* related to congenital anatomical defect of penis.

B. *Self-esteem disturbance* related to anatomical defect in penis and resulting disturbance in ability to void standing up.

IV. **Nursing care plan/implementation:**

A. Goal: *promote normal urinary function.*

1. Teach family that surgery is done in several stages, beginning in early months of life and finishing by age 18 mo. Instruct parents *not* to circumcise infants as foreskin will be used to repair/reconstruct urethra.

2. Provide age-appropriate information to child regarding condition, surgery.

3. *Preoperative* teaching with child should include: simulated anticipated postoperative urinary drainage apparatus and dressings on dolls; allow child to handle and play with them, but stress need *not* to touch postoperatively.

4. *Postoperatively*: Monitor urinary drainage apparatus; note hourly urine output, color, appearance (should be clear yellow, *no* blood).

B. Goal: *promote self-esteem.*

1. Do *not* scold child if he exposes penis, dressings, catheters, etc.

2. Reassure parents that preoccupation with penis is normal and will pass.

3. Encourage calm, matter-of-fact acceptance of, and *avoid* strict discipline for, this behavior, which could negatively affect the child.

V. **Evaluation/outcome criteria:**

A. Child is able to void in normal male pattern.

B. Child does not experience disturbances in self-concept and has normal self-esteem.

Study and Memory Aids

Myelomeningocele—Assessment

Myelomeningocele is the most severe form of spina bifida;
► the resultant loss of motion and sensation (below level
of sac) is *irreversible*.
80-85% of infants with myelomeningocele also develop
hydrocephalus.

Myelomeningocele—Preoperative Care

Position: prone, to *avoid* pressure on sac.

Hydrocephalus—Treatment and Postoperative Care

Treatment is a shunt procedure.
Postoperative position for AV or VP shunt: *flat* for 24 h to
prevent subdural hematoma.

Congenital Clubfoot—Asssessment/Tx

► Assessment: *downward* and *inward* curve of foot.
Treatment: series of corrective casts.

► Developmental Dysplasia of the Hip—Assessment Manifestation in the Newborn

1. Positive *Ortolani* test
2. *Shortening* of the limb on affected side
3. *Limitation of abduction* on affected side
4. *Additional* thigh and gluteal fat folds on affected side

Tracheoesophageal Fistula—Major Symptoms: The 3 C's

Coughing
Choking
Cyanosis

Tracheoesophageal Fistula—Positioning

The infant with tracheoesophageal fistula should be
positioned with the head of the bed *elevated 20-30
degrees* both preoperatively and postoperatively.

Tracheoesophageal Fistula—Most Common Complications

Short-term:
  1. Preoperative: aspiration pneumonia
  2. Postoperative: hypostatic pneumonia
Long-term:
  The most common long-term complication of
  tracheoesophageal fistula is *stricture formation*.

Cleft Lip and Palate—Treatment: Surgical

1. Cleft lip is repaired *first*, when infant is 8–12 wk.
2. Cleft palate repair is delayed until 12–18 mo.
No sucking is allowed postoperatively for infants with cleft
  lip or palate repair.

Hypospadias—Definition, Treatment Result

Urethral opening is located on the ventral surface of penile
  shaft.
After hypospadias repair, the child's urine should be clear
  yellow.

Questions

1. The long-term plan of care for a child with a
   myelomeningocele must include:
   1. Speech therapy.
   2. Dietary counseling.
   3. Bowel and bladder training.
   4. Emotional guidance.

2. Which is the most critical nursing goal for an infant
   with an unrepaired myelomeningocele?
   1. Maintenance of hydration status.
   2. Maintenance of nutritional status.
   3. Prevention of contractures.
   4. Prevention of infection.

3. In which position should the nurse place an infant
   with an unrepaired myelomeningocele?
   1. Prone.
   2. Semi-Fowler's in an infant chair.
   3. On right side.
   4. On left side with head elevated.

4. What is the nurse's primary rationale for
   keeping the sac of an infant with an unrepaired
   myelomeningocele moist, via applications of sterile
   normal saline?
   1. To prevent the sac from rupturing.
   2. To aid in delivering additional fluids to the
      infant.
   3. To prepare the sac for surgical removal.
   4. To prevent cerebral spinal fluid from leaking
      onto the surgical incision site.

5. Which nursing assessment can be objectively
   measured in the postoperative nursing care required
   by an infant with myelomeningocele?
   1. Irritability.
   2. Lethargy.
   3. Changes in level of consciousness.
   4. Head circumference.

6. When assessing an infant during a "well-baby" check-up, the nurse notices that one of the infant's legs is slightly shorter than the other leg. The nurse's first action should be to:
   1. Ask the parents if they had noticed any discrepancy in leg lengths.
   2. Notify the pediatrician.
   3. Note this physical finding in the infant's chart.
   4. Alert the x-ray department.

7. The primary nursing goal of treating an infant with developmental dysplasia of the hip is to:
   1. Relocate the head of the femur within the acetabulum.
   2. Protect the blood vessels and nerves located on the exterior of the bone.
   3. Abduct the hips.
   4. Prevent adduction and extension of the hips.

8. When planning care for an infant in a Pavlik harness, the nurse should know that this infant is at high risk for:
   1. *Alteration in parenting* related to the presence of intimidating treatment modalities.
   2. *Impaired physical mobility* related to leg length discrepancy.
   3. *Pain* related to muscle spasm.
   4. *Skin impairment* related to the presence of the harness.

9. The parents of an infant with developmental dysplasia of the hip tell the nurse, "I know that the Pavlik harness is unbearable for our baby." The nurse should reply:
   1. "It's going to be worth it in the end when the baby doesn't have to have surgery."
   2. "There is no other choice for treating your baby."
   3. "Perhaps we can convince the pediatrician to release the baby from the harness for a few hours."
   4. "It is hard to see your baby like this, isn't it? Actually, babies adjust readily to the harness."

10. The parents of a newborn with clubfoot ask the nurse, "Why did this happen?" The nurse's best response is:
    1. "It was caused by a viral infection during the pregnancy."
    2. "It is related to the effects of smoking while pregnant."
    3. "It is unknown what causes clubfoot."
    4. "It is related to the age of the mother at the time of conception."

11. The most critical element to teach the parents of a newborn who has clubfoot and bilateral short leg casts is:
    1. Neurovascular assessment of the toes.
    2. General cast care.
    3. Cast removal before scheduled weekly orthopedic clinic appointments.
    4. Skin assessment on removal of the casts.

12. The mother of a newborn with a cleft lip asks "Why did this happen to me?" The nurse's best response is:
    1. "Did you have prenatal care?"
    2. "Did you follow your obstetrician's instructions while you were pregnant?"
    3. "Try to put this behind you. Cosmetic repairs have greatly advanced recently and your baby will look beautiful after the surgery."
    4. "This must be very difficult for you. How can I be of help to you?"

13. The nurse's primary preoperative goal for an infant with a cleft lip is to prevent:
    1. Infection at the site of the anomaly.
    2. The infant from crying, which places stress on the anomalous site.
    3. The infant from becoming malnourished.
    4. The infant from sucking on fingers or a pacifier.

14. During the postoperative recovery period for an infant with a repaired cleft lip, the nurse should:
    1. Provide the infant with toys for stimulation and play.
    2. Remove the restraints every 2 hours and comfort the infant.
    3. Keep the infant heavily sedated to prevent any touching of the incisional area.
    4. Prevent the parents from seeing the infant until the Logan's bow has been removed.

15. The parents of an infant with a newly repaired cleft lip question the nurse about the purpose of the Logan's bow. The nurse's best reply is:
    1. "It prevents aspiration during feedings."
    2. "It prevents trauma to the suture line."
    3. "It prevents the baby from sucking on his fingers or a pacifier."
    4. "It prevents the baby from vomiting."

16. The parents of an infant with a repaired cleft lip ask the nurse to explain what a Breck feeder is. The nurse's best response is:
    1. "It is a special type of spoon."
    2. "It is another name for a syringe."
    3. "It is a standard type of nipple."
    4. "It is a large syringe with soft rubber tubing."

17. In the postoperative period, in which position should the nurse place an infant with a cleft lip repair?
    1. On the abdomen, to allow drooling to occur.
    2. Side-lying, supported with rolled blankets.
    3. High-Fowler's position.
    4. Prone position with the head lower than the buttocks.

18. Which is a primary nursing concern when admitting an infant, who has undergone a cleft lip repair, to the pediatric unit from the recovery room?
    1. Preventing bleeding from the incision site.
    2. Maintaining a patent airway.
    3. Restraining the hands and feet.
    4. Obtaining the vital signs.

19. When planning preoperative care for a newborn with cleft lip and palate, the nurse's major concern is:
    1. Prevention of aspiration.
    2. Promotion of bonding.
    3. Prevention of malnutrition.
    4. Provisions for age-appropriate stimulation.

20. The parents of an infant with a cleft palate ask when the defect will be repaired. The nurse's best response is:
    1. "Before teeth erupt."
    2. "When the child is drinking from a cup."
    3. "Before speech develops."
    4. "When the child is able to separate easily from the parents."

21. The parents of an infant with an unrepaired cleft palate ask why their baby has frequent ear infections. The nurse's best response is:
    1. "The baby's poor nutrition predisposes her to infection."
    2. "The baby's eustachian tubes become clogged with formula."
    3. "The baby is in a high-risk age group for ear infections."
    4. "The cleft palate causes ineffective functioning of the eustachian tubes and improper drainage of the middle ear."

22. After a cleft palate repair, what should the nurse use to feed the child?
    1. The side of a plastic spoon.
    2. A flexible straw.
    3. A lamb's nipple.
    4. A Breck feeder.

23. Which food item should the nurse instruct the mother of a child with a newly repaired cleft palate to refrain from serving to the child?
    1. Applesauce.
    2. Oatmeal.
    3. Toast.
    4. Spaghetti.

24. Using the Denver Developmental Screening Test (DDST-II) on a 19-month-old toddler who underwent a cleft palate repair 1 month earlier, the nurse should anticipate that there would be a delay in the toddler's ability to:
    1. Remove own clothes.
    2. Build a tower with two cubes.
    3. Use a spoon without much spilling.
    4. Walk up steps.

25. Which would be contraindicated in the nursing care of an infant with an unrepaired tracheoesophageal fistula?
    1. Suctioning nose and mouth PRN.
    2. Maintaining NPO status.
    3. Small, frequent feedings of sterile water.
    4. Administering oxygen as ordered.

26. In planning preoperative care for a newborn with tracheoesophageal fistula, the nurse should anticipate positioning the newborn:
    1. Supine, with head turned to the side.
    2. Side-lying.
    3. Prone.
    4. Supine, with head elevated 20-30 degrees.

27. After surgery for a tracheoesophageal fistula, an infant has a gastrostomy tube in place. After feeding the infant via the gastrostomy tube, the nurse should:
    1. Clamp the gastrostomy tube.
    2. Leave the gastrostomy tube unclamped and level with the stomach.
    3. Flush the tube with 100 mL normal saline.
    4. Leave the gastrostomy tube unclamped and elevate the gastrostomy tube.

28. A preschooler who had a tracheoesophageal fistula repair at 24 hours of age comes to the clinic for a "well-child" check-up. During this visit, the nurse should remind the parents to avoid giving the child foods such as:
    1. Jello.
    2. Mashed potatoes.
    3. Hot dogs.
    4. Crackers.

29. A newborn is noted to have hypospadias. The newborn will be discharged and readmitted to the hospital at 6 months of age to begin multistaged surgeries for a period of several years. The nurse's discharge planning for the family at this time must include:
    1. Explanations of how to clamp off the indwelling catheter.
    2. Demonstrations of the Credé bladder-emptying technique.
    3. Instructions not to have the infant circumcised.
    4. Reassurance that the infant's penis will appear normal following the surgery.

30. A goal of treatment is to repair an infant with hypospadias during the toddler and preschool years. The nurse realizes that early intervention primarily accomplishes which goal?
    1. A decrease in separation anxiety.
    2. An interruption in maternal-infant bonding.
    3. Promotion of normal urinary function.
    4. Prevention of self-esteem and body image disturbances.

31. The nurse accompanies a 3-year-old child who has had a hypospadias repair to the hospital playroom. Which toy is contraindicated for this child?
    1. A rocking horse.
    2. Clay.
    3. A puzzle with large pieces.
    4. Stack-up blocks.

32. A 3-year-old with hypospadias is admitted to the hospital pediatric unit for the first of several staged repairs. The child is noted to touch his penis frequently. The nurse should:
    1. Restrain the child's hands because he may further damage his penis and cause a delay in the surgery.
    2. Inform the parents of their child's behavior.
    3. Avoid overreacting because this is a normal occurrence for this age group.
    4. Scold the child.

33. A newborn is noted to have an increasing head circumference. The diagnosis of hydrocephalus is confirmed. Which finding should the nurse anticipate?
    1. Tense, bulging fontanels.
    2. A soft, low-pitched cry.
    3. "On time" developmental milestones.
    4. Response to comforting.

34. An infant with a ventriculoperitoneal shunt has an elevated temperature postoperatively. The nurse's best assessment of this finding is that:
    1. This is to be expected in a child who is postoperative; no further action is required.
    2. This may be an early indication of a cerebrospinal fluid infection.
    3. This can be relieved by the administration of acetaminophen, which should be the next nursing action.
    4. The infant is also in need of additional fluids.

35. Which assessment must the nurse perform before feeding an infant who has had surgery for a ventriculoperitoneal shunt placement?
    1. Gag reflex.
    2. Bowel sounds.
    3. Urinary output.
    4. Incision site.

36. An infant with hydrocephalus receives a ventriculoperitoneal shunt. Postoperatively, in which position should the nurse place the infant?
    1. Prone with head down.
    2. Flat in bed on the unoperated side.
    3. Flat in bed on the operated side.
    4. Supine.

37. Which information should not be part of the discharge teaching for parents of an infant with a ventriculoperitoneal shunt?
    1. The shunt will probably require periodic revisions.
    2. Signs and symptoms of cerebrospinal fluid infection.
    3. Encouragement to avoid overprotecting the infant.
    4. An extra-firm mattress should be used on the infant's bed.

38. When using the Denver Developmental Screening Test (DDST-II) on a 4-month-old infant with hydrocephalus, the nurse should suspect a developmental delay when the infant:
    1. Laughs and squeals.
    2. Smiles socially.
    3. Reaches for objects but misses them.
    4. Has unsteady head control.

Answers/Rationale

1. **(3)** Varying degrees of bowel and bladder control are sacrificed in the repair of the myelomeningocele. In infants, the goal of treatment is to preserve renal function. Some degree of fecal continence is usually achieved in most children with this defect via diet modification, regular toilet habits, and prevention of constipation and impaction. The need for speech therapy (**1**) is *not* usually associated with a myelomeningocele. Dietary counseling (**2**) may *later* become a necessity as the child grows older and more sedentary, and weight gain due to inactivity may become an issue. The need for emotional guidance (**4**) is a possibility for *any* child with a serious, long-term disease process. **PL, APP, 8, PhI, Physiological adaptation**

2. **(4)** Great care must be taken to prevent rupturing the sac and exposing the infant with a myelomeningocele to potential infection. Maintenance of hydration status (**1**) and nutritional status (**2**) are important for *any* client before surgery; however, as the repair is usually done within 12-72 hours following birth, hydration and nutrition *rarely* become issues. Before surgery the infant usually is able to move extremities independently, thus prevention of contractures (**3**) is *not* a concern in the preoperative period. **PL, APP, 1, HPM, Health promotion and maintenance**

3. **(1)** One of the most challenging aspects of the preoperative care of an infant with a myelomeningocele is positioning; before surgery, the infant is kept in the prone position to minimize tension on the sac and the risk of trauma. The prone position also allows optimal positioning of the legs, especially in cases of associated developmental dysplasia of the hip. Semi-Fowler's position (**2**) allows direct tension to be placed on the sac. Right (**3**) or left (**4**) side positioning could present difficulty because of undue pressure on the sac from the mattress of the infant warmer. **IMP, ANL, 3, SECE, Safety and infection control**

4. **(1)** The infant with a myelomeningocele is usually placed in an incubator or warmer so that the temperature can be maintained without clothing or covers that might irritate the sac; when an overhead warmer is used, the dressings over the defect require more frequent moistening because of the dehydrating effect of the radiant heat. If the sac

ruptures due to dryness or cracking, the infant is at high risk for infection of the central nervous system. Moistening the sac (2) does *not* deliver additional fluids to the infant because the application of moisture is *topical*. Application of moisture to the sac does *not* directly prepare the site for surgery (3). Moisture is applied to the sac in the *preoperative* period because no surgical incision (4) has yet been created. **PL, APP, 1, PhI, Physiological adaptation**

5. (4) Daily head circumference is an objective nursing assessment. The reason for this assessment is early detection of increased intracranial pressure and developing hydrocephalus. Irritability (1), lethargy (2), and changes in level of consciousness (3) are also important nursing assessments to detect increased intracranial pressure and developing hydrocephalus; however, they are *subjective* assessments and may thus vary from nurse to nurse. **AN, ANL, 3, PhI, Physiological adaptation**

6. (2) The nurse's first action in this case is to alert the pediatrician. The pediatrician will further evaluate the infant for unequal skin folds, limitation of abduction, and unequal knee height to establish the diagnosis of developmental dysplasia of the hip. The infant will probably undergo additional maneuvers (Barlow, Ortolani) to assess hip stability and procedures (CT, MRI, arthrogram) to determine the shape and structure of the joint. Questioning the parents about their observations (1), noting the finding in the infant's chart (3), and alerting the x-ray department (4) are all appropriate *secondary* nursing interventions. **IMP, ANL, 3, HPM, Health promotion and maintenance**

7. (1) Relocating the head of the femur within the acetabulum is the primary nursing goal for an infant with developmental dysplasia of the hip. The femoral head and acetabulum develop synergistically and must be in contact with each other for proper growth and development to occur. Protecting blood supply (2), keeping the hips abducted (3) and preventing adduction and extension of the hips (4) are all important *secondary* goals of treatment. **AN, ANL, 3, PhI, Physiological adaptation**

Key to Codes

Nursing process: AS, assessment; **AN**, analysis; **PL**, planning; **IMP**, implementation; **EV**, evaluation. (See **Appendix L** for explanation of nursing process steps.)

Cognitive level: RE/KN, recall/knowledge; **COM**, comprehension; **APP**, application; **ANL**, analysis; **EVL**, evaluation; **SYN**, synthesis. (See **Appendix L** for explanation.)

Category of human function: 1, protective; 2, sensory-perceptual; 3, comfort, rest, activity, and mobility; 4, nutrition; 5, growth and development; 6, fluid-gas transport; 7, psychosocial-cultural; 8, elimination. (See **Appendix N** for explanation.)

Client need: SECE, safe, effective care environment; **HPM**, health promotion and maintenance; **PsI**, psychosocial integrity; **PhI**, physiological integrity. (See **Appendix O** for explanation.)

Client subneed: See **Appendix O** for explanation.

8. (4) Skin impairment is a concern for an infant in a Pavlik harness because skin-to-skin contact occurs behind the knees. The infant should wear cotton clothing and long socks to protect areas of the body from pressure due to skin-to-skin contact or the straps of the harness. Alterations in parenting (1) should *not* occur when adequate instructions regarding the harness have been given. Impaired physical mobility (2) is *alleviated* by the correction of the anomaly; moreover, infants treated with a Pavlik harness are usually under 6 months of age, so physical mobility is not yet a major issue. Pain due to muscle spasm (3) is *not* associated with the use of the Pavlik harness. **AN, ANL, 1, PhI, Reduction of risk potential**

9. (4) Infants adjust readily to the Pavlik harness because they are used to the knee-chest position which the harness maintains. It is usually more difficult for the parents to learn to manage care without removing the harness than it is for the infant to adjust to wearing the harness 24 hours a day. Supporting the entire family is critical during this period of time. Pointing out the potential benefits of the harness (1) or offering false hope (3) gives the parent unrealistic expectations. Becoming authoritarian (2) cuts off communication between parent and nurse. **IMP, APP, 3, PsI, Psychosocial integrity**

10. (3) The cause of clubfoot is unknown. Suggested possible causes include intrauterine compression and distal tibial growth arrest. The incidence of clubfoot is increased among first-degree relatives and infants with neuromuscular abnormalities, such as myelomeningocele. Viral infections (1), smoking (2), and maternal age (4) are *not* known causes of clubfoot in newborns. **IMP, COM, 3, HPM, Health promotion and maintenance**

11. (1) Instructions regarding neurovascular assessment of the toes is critical because small babies grow rapidly and may quickly outgrow the casts. A cast that is too tight can put pressure on neurovascular structures. For this reason, casts on babies with clubfoot are usually changed every week. General cast care (2) such as hygiene measures and checking for broken spots in the cast, cast removal (3) by soaking the casts to remove them, and skin assessment (4) on cast removal are all appropriate care measures to teach the parents of an infant with clubfoot who is newly casted; however, none of these three interventions carries the *potential for injury* to the infant as does failing to recognize pressure on a neurovascular structure. **IMP, ANL, 3, PhI, Reduction of risk potential**

12. (4) "This must be very difficult for you" is a compassionate, supportive statement that provides the mother with a way of expressing her feelings and concerns. The exact cause of cleft lip is unknown; it is probably multifactoral in nature. Questioning the mother regarding prenatal care (1) and compliance (2) does *not* provide the mother

with an opportunity to ventilate her feelings because these responses are "closed" rather than open-ended and may also cause the mother to feel guilty about doing something while pregnant to cause the condition. Suggesting that the baby will be beautiful after surgery and that the mother "put this behind you" (3) is patronizing and offers unrealistic expectations. **IMP, APP, 7, PsI, Psychosocial integrity**

13. (3) The primary *preoperative* goal is to establish a feeding method that can be continued postoperatively. This prevents malnutrition from occurring during all stages of the operative experience. Preventing infection (1) via meticulous oral hygiene and careful cleansing of the suture line, preventing crying, which places tension on the suture line (2), and preventing sucking, which might traumatize the incision site (4), are all *post*operative concerns. **PL, ANL, 1, PhI, Reduction of risk potential**

14. (2) The restraints *should* be removed every 2 hours to allow for exercising the extremities and to observe the skin for irritation. It also provides an opportunity for needed cuddling and body contact. Toys (1) for play purposes are of limited value because the repair is usually done when the infant is 6–12 weeks of age. Toys may also be a source of trauma or infection to the suture line. Sedation (3) *may* be necessary for an infant who is *restless* and anxious; it must be used *cautiously* to prevent respiratory complications. Parents (4) *should* be actively involved in the infant's care throughout the hospitalization. **PL, APP, 1, PhI, Reduction of risk potential**

15. (2) The Logan's bow and a butterfly bandage strip are examples of the many devices surgeons use to prevent trauma from occurring to the suture line after a cleft lip repair. Preventing aspiration (1) is best achieved by *positioning* the infant in an upright or side-lying position. Preventing objects such as fingers or pacifiers (3) from being placed in the mouth is best achieved by applying *elbow restraints*. Preventing vomiting (4) is best achieved by resuming feedings very *slowly* during the postoperative period. **PL, ANL, 4, PhI, Reduction of risk potential**

16. (4) The Breck feeder is a large syringe with soft rubber tubing. The rubber tip should be placed inside the oral cavity from the side of the mouth to avoid the operative area. The formula is deposited on the tongue and flow is controlled by syringe compression. The Breck feeder is *not* a spoon (1); spoons are generally not used immediately after surgical repair of the cleft lip. A syringe (2) is *another* type of acceptable feeding device for an infant with a cleft lip. The same precautions are used as those for a Breck feeder. The Breck feeder is *not* a nipple (3), and standard nipples are *unsuitable* for these infants because they are unable to generate the required suction. **IMP, COM, 4, PhI, Basic care and comfort**

17. (2) The side-lying position supported with rolled blankets prevents the infant from rolling onto the stomach. Infants in this age group (6–12 weeks of age) can usually roll only from stomach to back, *not* vice versa. Abdominal (1) or prone (4) positions must be *avoided* because the infant might rub the face on the bed and traumatize the suture line. High-Fowler's position (3) *is impossible* for an infant in this age group because of inadequate gross motor skills and neuromuscular development. **IMP, APP, 1, PhI, Basic care and comfort**

18. (2) Maintaining an airway is *always* the primary concern for any patient recovering from anesthesia. It is even more important for an infant with a facial deformity. Preventing bleeding (1), restraining the hands and feet (3), and obtaining vital signs (4) are all appropriate *secondary* postoperative nursing concerns. **PL, ANL, 1, PhI, Reduction of risk potential**

19. (1) Aspiration is a major concern for an infant with oral-facial anomalies. Promoting bonding (2), preventing malnutrition (3), and providing for age-appropriate stimulation (4) are all appropriate *secondary* goals for an infant with cleft lip and palate. **PL, ANL, 1, PhI, Reduction of risk potential**

20. (3) Cleft palate repair is usually performed when the infant is 12–18 months of age. Most surgeons prefer to close the cleft before the child develops faulty speech habits. Teeth (1) generally begin to appear at 6 months in the average infant. Drinking from a cup (2) generally occurs at 10–12 months. The ability to drink from a cup is highly desirable in the postoperative period for a child with a cleft palate, but ensuring correct speech habits is the *primary* rationale for the age of the child at the time of the surgery. Throughout childhood there is no easy separation from parents (4). Rooming-in policies help to alleviate many separation anxiety issues. **IMP, ANL, 5, HPM, Health promotion and maintenance**

21. (4) Improper drainage of the middle ear, as a result of inefficient functioning of the eustachian tube, causes increased pressure in the middle ear and contributes to recurrent infections. Because ear infections are easily overlooked in young children, hearing impairment can occur in some children with cleft palate. Preventing poor nutrition (1) is a major goal in the care of an infant with cleft palate, so nursing interventions to prevent poor nutrition would have been implemented at *birth*. Infants with cleft palate are always fed in an *upright* position, *not* propped with a bottle, so that formula does not drain into the ear (2). Ear infections are most prevalent in children under 3 years of age (3), but this response does *not* specifically address the *relationship* between cleft palate and ear infections. **IMP, ANL, 5, PhI, Physiological adaptation**

22. (1) The side of a plastic spoon may be brought up to the child's lips for feeding purposes (as may a cup). The feeding utensil must not enter the child's

mouth, where it might accidentally traumatize the suture line. A flexible straw (2), a lamb's nipple (3), and a Breck feeder (4) are all *inappropriate* feeding utensils for a child after a cleft palate repair. Because each item is placed directly into the oral cavity, each is capable of producing trauma. **IMP, APP, 4, PhI, Basic care and comfort**

23. (3) Toast, potato chips, crackers, and other hard food items should be discouraged because they could damage the newly repaired palate. Applesauce (1), oatmeal (2), and spaghetti (4) are *soft* in texture and pose *no threat of injury* to the palate. They are also *age-appropriate* and usually liked by toddlers, who tend to be finicky eaters. **IMP, APP, 4, PhI, Basic care and comfort**

24. (3) The toddler with a cleft palate is usually fed with a special device such as the Breck feeder preoperatively, and with a cup or the side of a wide-bowl spoon postoperatively until healing is completed. This toddler would therefore have limited experience in the use of a spoon and could demonstrate a developmental lag in the task, which is usually achieved between 12 and 18 months of age. Removing clothes (1), stacking cubes (2), and walking up steps (4) are behaviors expected of a toddler 12–18 months of age, and *should* definitely be demonstrated by 19 months of age, *regardless* of the cleft palate repair. **EV, APP, 5, HPM, Health promotion and maintenance**

25. (3) Tracheoesophageal fistula is a failure of the trachea and esophagus to separate into distinct structures. As a result, liquids taken by mouth are aspirated into the trachea or bronchus and can lead to pneumonia. Infants with tracheoesophageal fistula exhibit the *3 C's*—coughing, choking, cyanosis—as excessive mucus accumulates in the respiratory track; therefore, the infant should be kept NPO (2), suctioned frequently (1), and given oxygen to prevent hypoxia (4). **IMP, ANL, 4, PhI, Reduction of risk potential**

26. (4) The supine position with head elevated 20–30 degrees *prevents* aspiration in the newborn with tracheoesophageal fistula. Supine, with head turned to the side (1), leaves the newborn free to return his head to the midline position, and thus be flat on his back and at risk for aspiration. Side-lying (2) or prone (3) without the head elevated also poses the risk of aspiration. **IMP, APP, 1, PhI, Reduction of risk potential**

27. (4) The nurse should leave the gastrostomy tube unclamped and elevate the gastrostomy tube slightly above the stomach to prevent aspiration in case the infant vomits. Clamping the gastrostomy tube (1) could promote aspiration if the infant vomits. Leaving the gastrostomy tube unclamped and level with the stomach (2) would allow the feeding to leak out of the tube. Maintaining the patency of the gastrostomy tube (3) is a nursing function, but 100 mL normal saline is an *excessive* amount of flushing

solution—5-10 mL should suffice for a newborn. **IMP, APP, 4, PhI, Reduction of risk potential**

28. (3) Foods such as hot dogs or large pieces of meat can easily become lodged in the esophagus and should be *avoided*. This child remains at high risk for aspiration; the parents should be instructed to teach the child to chew thoroughly and to cut solid foods into small pieces. Signs of constriction of the esophagus include: poor feeding, dysphagia, drooling, or regurgitating undigested food. Jello (1), mashed potatoes (2), and crackers (4) *are safe* as well as *age-appropriate* foods for a preschooler who has had tracheoesophageal fistula repair. **IMP, APP, 4, PhI, Basic care and comfort**

29. (3) Circumcision is usually delayed to save the foreskin for the proposed urethral repair. A catheter (1) is inserted when the infant is readmitted to the hospital for surgery, and it is *never* clamped off. The Credé bladder-emptying technique (2) is *not* necessary at this time because the newborn is voiding spontaneously. The parents must be advised that the urethral defect can be surgically corrected but the penis will be physically imperfect despite the repair (4). **PL, APP, 8, HPM, Health promotion and maintenance**

30. (3) The primary goal of early treatment is to promote normal urinary function and prevent complications. Separation anxiety (1) is *highest* in the toddler years, when the staged repairs begin. Maternal-infant bonding (2) has *already* taken place. Completing the surgeries before the child enters kindergarten helps prevent self-esteem and body image issues (4), but this is *not* the *primary* reason for early intervention. **PL, APP, 8, PhI, Basic care and comfort**

31. (1) To prevent trauma to the incision site, a rocking horse or any type of "straddle" toy must be avoided until the pediatric surgeon allows this type of toy. Clay (2), puzzles (3), and blocks (4) are age-appropriate and *safe* for this child. **IMP, APP, 5, HPM, Health promotion and maintenance**

32. (3) Masturbation is a common behavior for preschool children. Freud calls this the phallic stage, when the child learns sexual identity through awareness of the genital area. The nurse should refrain from overreacting. Restraining the child's hands (1) is *unnecessary* in the *preoperative* period but may be necessary immediately after surgery to avoid trauma to the suture line. Informing the parents (2) is of value only in that they should know that this is a normal behavior for this age group. Scolding the child (4) could have a *negative* long-term emotional effect. **IMP, COM, 5, PsI, Psychosocial integrity**

33. (1) In infants with hydrocephalus, an imbalance between secretion and absorption of cerebrospinal fluid, causes an increased accumulation of cerebrospinal fluid in the ventricles, which become dilated. This is reflected by tense, bulging fontanels. Infants with hydrocephalus have shrill, *high*-pitched cries (2), *delayed* developmental milestones

(3) and irritability, which causes them to be *difficult* to comfort (4). **EV, APP, 5, PhI, Physiological adaptation**

34. (2) Elevated temperature, poor feeding, vomiting, decreased responsiveness, and seizure activity signal the onset of a cerebrospinal fluid infection—the greatest hazard in the postoperative period for an infant with a ventriculoperitoneal shunt. Many children do have an elevated temperature postoperatively (1), but its cause *must* always be determined. Acetaminophen is used to reduce postoperative fevers (3) in children *after* appropriate cultures have been obtained and in conjunction with antibiotic therapy. This infant would have been carefully monitored while on intravenous infusions postoperatively, so fluid *deficit* is an *unlikely* cause of the elevated temperature (4). **AN, APP, 1, PhI, Physiological adaptation**

35. (2) The infant is usually NPO for the first 24–48 hours following surgery. Routine feeding is resumed after the prescribed NPO period, but the presence of bowel sounds is determined before feeding infants with ventriculoperitoneal shunts because the bowel has been manipulated during the surgery. The gag reflex (1) would have been well established postoperatively by the time feedings are reinstituted. Assessment of urinary output (3) and the incision site (4) are part of routine postoperative care for *any* surgical client and are *not specific* to the feeding of this infant. **AS, ANL, 4, PhI, Reduction of risk potential**

36. (2) Flat in bed on the unoperated side helps avert complications resulting from too rapid reduction of intracranial fluid, and prevents pressure on the shunt valve. Prone with the head down (1) interferes with unobstructed flow of cerebrospinal fluid. Lying on the operated side (3) may place unnecessary pressure on the shunt valve. Supine (4) presents the danger of aspiration because the infant lacks head control as a result of the enlarged head size. **IMP, APP, 1, PhI, Reduction of risk potential**

37. (4) The infant with hydrocephalus, despite placement of a ventriculoperitoneal shunt, has an enlarged head with prominent areas. Pressure-reducing mattresses or beds, such as water beds, are preferred to prevent pressure on the prominent areas, which can lead to skin breakdown. Periodic revisions of the shunt (1) and cerebrospinal fluid infections (2) *are* anticipated complications of a ventriculo-peritoneal shunt. The purpose in shunting the infant is to enable the infant to live as normal a life as possible; therefore overprotection *is* to be avoided (3). **IMP, APP, 3, PhI, Reduction of risk potential**

38. (4) Steady head control is achieved between birth and 3 months of age. The size of the infant's head may account for gross motor lag. Laughing and squealing (1), a social smile (2), and reaching for objects but missing them (3) *are expected* behaviors for an infant between birth and 3 months of age. **EV, APP, 5, HPM, Health promotion and maintenance**

Nursing Care for Children's Unique Needs

17

Chapter Outline

Key Words

antecubital   the space in front of the elbow.
brachycephalic   characterized by a small, round head.
clinodactyly   in-curved little finger seen in Down sydrome.

coryza   acute inflammation of the nasal mucus membrane accompanied by a profuse nasal discharge.
pruritus   severe itching.
rhinorrhea   thin, watery nasal discharge.

🔑 Summary of Key Points

1. *Acute otitis media* can precede the development of bacterial meningitis; the administration of all antibiotics ordered is essential to prevent this complication.

2. *Eczema* is an allergic skin reaction to allergens; most common is cow's milk.

3. Most childhood communicable diseases can be *prevented* with immunizations.

4. *Basic principles* of care for a child with a childhood *communicable disease* include: standard precautions, fever control, extra fluids for hydration, and home care.

5. For a child who has ingested a poison, vomiting can be induced by administering *syrup of ipecac*; if indicated (need pediatrician's approval in children under 1 year of age); vomiting is *contraindicated*: if the child is comatose, having seizures, is in severe shock, has lost the gag reflex, or if the poison is a corrosive substance or petroleum distillate.

6. *Acetaminophen poisoning* can result in potentially fatal liver damage; it is treated with the antidote *acetylcysteine*.

7. The child with *lice* can be seen constantly scratching the scalp; a simple visual examination reveals the infestation. Lice are treated with an anti-louse shampoo along with *household measures* to prevent *re-infestation* or spread.

8. The child with *pinworms* experiences intense perianal itching; visible worms are present in the stool. Pinworms are treated with an *antiparasitic* agent such as pyrantel pamoate or mebendazole.

9. Hemorrhage is the most frequent complication of *tonsillectomy*; signs and symptoms of hemorrhage include: frequent swallowing, emesis of bright red blood, and shock.

10. *Down syndrome* is the most common chromosomal abnormality; it is characterized by: brachycephaly (small, round head), epicanthal fold, *Brushfield spots* (speckling of iris), saddle nose, small, low-set ears, and a *simian* crease across the palms of the hands and varying degrees of mental retardation.

11. The leading cause of death in a child or adult with Down syndrome is usually related to *respiratory* complications such as pneumonia or lung disease.

(continued)

12. All 50 states in the U.S. require health professionals, by law, to report all forms of *child abuse*.

13. When caring for a child at *end-of-life*, the nurse must meet the physical and emotional needs of the child and family.

14. The *administration of medications* to children is based on 3 guiding principles: 1) calculate child's weight in kilograms; 2) administer in provided dropper or calibrated syringe (**NEVER** in household measuring spoon); 3) use age-appropriate technique.

Selected Disorders/Conditions of Childhood

Acute Otitis Media

I. *Introduction*: Acute *bacterial* ear infection (*acute otitis media*) is common in young children, primarily because their eustachian tube is shorter and straighter than that of the adult, which allows ready drainage of infected mucus from *upper* respiratory illnesses (URIs) directly *into the middle* ear. In *some* cases, acute otitis media precedes the onset of *bacterial meningitis*, an extremely serious and potentially fatal disease (see **Chapter 13**). Bacterial meningitis is a *medical emergency*, requiring early detection and prompt, aggressive therapy to prevent permanent neurologic damage or death (see **Chapter 16**, on hydrocephalus). *Serous otitis (chronic)* may result in hearing impairment or loss but is not likely to result in meningitis (see **Myringotomy, Table 17.2 p. 181.**)

II. **Assessment:**
   A. Fever.
   B. Pain in affected ear. Infant may not complain of pain but may tug at ear, cry, shake head, refuse to lie down.
   C. Malaise, irritability, anorexia (possibly vomiting).
   D. May have symptoms and signs of URI: rhinorrhea, coryza, cough.

III. **Analysis/nursing diagnosis:**
   A. *Infection* related to bacteria in middle ear.
   B. *Pain* related to pressure of pus/purulent material on eardrum.
   C. *Risk for injury* related to complication of meningitis.

IV. **Nursing care plan/implementation**
   A. Goal: *eradicate infection and prevent further complications (meningitis).*
      1. Administer *antibiotics* per MD order.
   B. Goal: *relieve pain and promote comfort.*
      1. Administer *decongestants* per MD order.
      2. Offer *analgesics/antipyretics* to provide symptomatic relief and to decrease fever.
   C. Goal: **health teaching.** *Prevent future injury.*
      1. Teach parents that the child needs to finish all medication, even though child will seem clinically better within 24–48 h.

   2. Review appropriate home care measures to control fever: antipyretics, cool sponges.
   3. Stress smoking in home and going to sleep with a bottle (favors pooling of fluid in pharyngeal cavity) play in development of otitis media.

V. **Evaluation/outcome criteria:**
   A. Infection is eradicated, no complications.
   B. Child appears to be comfortable.
   C. Child does not have recurrence of otitis media.

Infantile Eczema (Atopic Dermatitis)

I. *Introduction*: Eczema is an *allergic* skin reaction, most typically to foods, e.g., cow's milk or eggs. It is most common in infants and young children (< age 2 yr). Infantile eczema generally undergoes permanent, spontaneous remission by age 3 yr; however, approximately 50% of children who have had infantile eczema develop *asthma* during the preschool or school-age years.

II. **Assessment:**
   A. Erythematous lesions, beginning on cheeks and spreading to rest of face and scalp.
   B. Lesions may spread to rest of body, especially in flexor surfaces, e.g., antecubital space.
   C. Lesions may ooze or crust over.
   D. Severe pruritus, which may lead to secondary infection.
   E. Lymphadenopathy near site of rash.
   F. Unaffected skin tends to be dry and rough.
   G. Systemic manifestations are rare—but child may be irritable, cranky.

III. **Analysis/nursing diagnosis:**
   A. *Impaired tissue integrity* related to lesions.
   B. *Pain* related to pruritus.
   C. *Knowledge deficit* related to care of child with eczema, prognosis, how to prevent exacerbations.

IV. **Nursing care plan/implementation:**
   A. Goal: *promote healing of lesions.*
      1. Give frequent baths in tepid water or mild soap (e.g. Dove, Neutrogena), to relieve pruritus, but with **no soap**—apply light coat of *emollient* (e.g. Cetaphil, Eucerin) after bath while skin is still wet.
      2. Apply light coat of topical *anti-inflammatory* agent and wrap child in cool, wet towels for 10 minutes.

3. Protect child from possible sources of infection; *standard precautions* to prevent infection.

4. Give absolutely **no immunizations** during acute exacerbations of eczema because of the possibility of an overwhelming dermatitis, allergic reaction, shock, or death.

5. Apply topical creams/ointments per MD order: lanolin/petroleum ointment, *hydrocortisone* cream to promote healing.

B. Goal: *provide relief from itching/keep child from itching*.

1. Administer systemic medications as ordered, e.g., diphenhydramine hydrochloride (*Benadryl*) or hydroxyzine hydrochloride (*Atarax*).

2. Keep child's nails trimmed short—may need mittens (preferable *not* to use elbow restraints since the antecubital space is a common site for eczema).

3. Use clothes and bed-linens that are nonirritating, i.e., pure cotton (**no** wool or blends).

4. Institute *elimination/hypoallergenic diet*:
   a. *No* milk or milk products.
   b. Change to *lactose-free* formula.
   c. *Avoid: eggs*, wheat, nuts, beans, chocolate.

5. Do *not* allow stuffed animals or hairy dolls.

C. Goal: **health teaching**. *Provide discharge planning/ teaching for parents and child*.

1. Include all information listed above.

2. Include information on course of disease: characterized by exacerbations and remissions throughout early years.

3. Include information on prognosis: 50-60% go into spontaneous (and permanent) remission during preschool years; 40-50% develop asthma/hayfever during school-age years.

V. **Evaluation/outcome criteria:**

A. Lesions heal well, without secondary infection.

B. Adequate relief from itching is achieved.

C. Parents verbalize understanding of eczema, prognosis, and how to prevent exacerbations.

Childhood Communicable Diseases

I. See specific diseases, **Table 17.1 p. 172-178.**

II. *Basic principles of care*:

A. Standard precautions to prevent communicability/infection.

B. Fever control.

C. *Extra fluids* for hydration.

D. General home care procedures aimed at symptomatic relief and supportive care.

III. *Immunizations*—see **Chapter 2.**

Accidents: Ingestions and Poisonings

See **Chapter 13** for *lead poisoning* and *salicylate poisoning*.

I. **General principles** of treatment for ingestions and poisonings:

A. *Prevention*: see **Chapter 3**, section on toddler safety.

B. How to induce vomiting:

1. Drug of choice—*syrup of ipecac* (available over the counter; does not require MD order) if indicated and approved by pediatrician. Families with young children should keep this medication on hand in case of accidental poisoning.

2. Dose:
   a. 30 mL for adolescents (> 12 yr).
   b. 15 mL for children (1 yr-12 yr).
   Note: do *not* administer to infants less than 1 yr without MD order.
   c. Repeat dose once if vomiting does not occur within 20 min.

3. Follow dose of *ipecac* with 4–8 oz tap water or as much water as child will drink. In young children, give water first—child may refuse to drink anything else after tasting the *ipecac*.

4. The child *must* vomit the *syrup of ipecac* to avoid it being absorbed and causing potentially *fatal cardiotoxicity*, i.e., cardiac arrhythmias, atrial fibrillation, severe heart block. If child does not vomit within 20 min of second dose, obtain **immediate emergency care**.

C. Do **not** induce vomiting when:
1. Child is stuporous or comatose.
2. Poison ingested is a corrosive substance or petroleum distillate.
3. Child is having seizures.
4. Child is in severe shock.
5. Child has lost gag reflex.

II. **Acetaminophen Poisoning**

A. **Assessment:**

1. Determine how much acetaminophen (*Tylenol*) was ingested, when, and which type.

2. Evaluate acetaminophen levels: normal = 0; therapeutic range = 15-30 mcg/mL; toxic = 150 mcg/mL 4 h after ingestion.

3. *Initial period* (2–4 h after ingestion): malaise, nausea, vomiting, anorexia, diaphoresis, pallor.

4. *Latent period* (1–3 d after ingestion): clinical improvement with asymptomatic rise in liver enzymes.

5. Hepatic involvement (may last 7 d or may be permanent): pain in right upper quadrant (RUQ), jaundice, confusion, hepatic encephalopathy, clotting abnormalities.

6. Gradual recuperation.

(continued on p. 179)

TABLE 17.1 COMMUNICABLE DISEASES OF CHILDHOOD

Disease	◄ Assessment: Clinical Manifestations	Therapeutic Management/Complications	◄ Nursing Considerations

CHICKENPOX (VARICELLA)

Agent: Varicella zoster virus (VZV)

Source: Primary secretions of respiratory tract of infected persons; to a lesser degree skin lesions (scabs *not* infectious)

Transmission: Direct contact, droplet (airborne) spread, and contaminated objects

Incubation period: 2–3 wk, usually 13–17 d

Period of communicability: Probably 1 d *before* eruption of lesions (prodromal period) to 6 d *after* first crop of vesicles when crusts have formed

Prodromal stage: Slight fever, malaise, and anorexia for first 24 h; rash highly pruritic; begins as macule, rapidly progresses to papule and then vesicle (surrounded by erythematous base, becomes umbilicated and cloudy, breaks easily and forms crusts); all three stages (*papule, vesicle, crust*) present in varying degrees at one time

Distribution: Centripetal, spreading to face and proximal extremities, but sparse on distal limbs and less on areas not exposed to heat (i.e., from clothing or sun)

Constitutional signs and symptoms: Elevated temperature from lymphadenopathy; irritability from pruritus

Treatment:
- **Specific:** antiviral agent **acyclovir (Zovirax)**; *varicella-zoster immune globulin* (VZIG) after exposure in high-risk children
- **Supportive:** *diphenhydramine hydrochloride or antihistamines* to relieve itching; skin care to prevent secondary bacterial infection

Complications:
Bacterial infections, secondary (abscesses, cellulitis, pneumonia, sepsis)
Encephalitis
Hemorrhagic varicella (tiny hemorrhages in vesicles and numerous petechiae in skin)
Thrombocytopenia (chronic or transient)
Varicella pneumonia

⚠ Maintain strict *isolation* in hospital; isolate child in home until vesicles have dried (usually 1 wk after onset of disease), and isolate high-risk children from infected children

☞ Administer skin care, give bath and change clothes and linens daily

Keep child's fingernails short and clean; apply mittens if child scratches

Keep child cool (may decrease number of lesions)

Lessen pruritus; keep child occupied

☞ Remove loose crusts that rub and irritate skin

Teach child to apply pressure to pruritic area rather than scratching it

If older child, reason with child regarding danger of scar formation from scratching

- *Avoid* use of aspirin; use of *acetaminophen* controversial

(continued)

TABLE 17.1 COMMUNICABLE DISEASES OF CHILDHOOD *(continued)*

Disease	◄ Assessment: Clinical Manifestations	Therapeutic Management/Complications	◄ Nursing Considerations

DIPHTHERIA

Agent: *Corynebacterium diphtheriae*

Source: Discharges from mucous membranes of nose and nasopharynx, skin, and other lesions of infected person

Transmission: Direct contact with infected person, a carrier, or contaminated articles

Incubation period: Usually 2–5 d, possibly longer

Period of communicability: Variable, until virulent bacilli are *no* longer present (identified by three negative cultures), usually 2 wk, but as long as 4 wk

Vary according to anatomic location of pseudomembrane

Nasal: Resembles common cold, serosanguineous mucopurulent nasal discharge without constitutional symptoms; may be frank epistaxis

Tonsillar/pharyngeal: Malaise; anorexia; sore throat, low-grade fever, pulse increased above expected for temperature within 24 h; smooth, adherent, white or gray membrane; lymphadenitis possibly pronounced (bull's neck); in severe cases, toxemia, septic shock,

Laryngeal: Fever, hoarseness, cough, with or without previous signs listed; potential airway obstruction, apprehensive dyspneic retractions, cyanosis

Treatment:

Antitoxin (usually intravenous), preceded by skin or conjunctival test to rule out sensitivity to horse serum

Antibiotics (*penicillin or erythromycin*)

Complete bed rest (prevention of myocarditis)

Tracheostomy for airway obstruction

Treatment of infected contacts and carriers

Complications:
Myocarditis (second week)
Neuritis and death within 6-10 d

⚠ Maintain *strict isolation* in hospital

Participate in sensitivity testing; have *epinephrine* available

Administer *antibiotics*; observe for signs of sensitivity to penicillin

Administer complete care to maintain bedrest

☞ Use suctioning as needed

Observe respirations for signs of obstruction

☞ Administer humidified oxygen if prescribed

ERYTHEMA INFECTIOSUM (FIFTH DISEASE)

Agent: Human parvovirus B19 (HPV)

Source: Infected persons

Transmission: Unknown; possibly respiratory secretions and blood

Incubation period: 4–14 d, may be as long as 20 d

Period of communicability: Uncertain but *before* onset of symptoms in most children; also for about 1 wk *after* onset of symptoms in children with aplastic crisis

Rash appears in three stages:

I—Erythema on face, chiefly on cheeks, "slapped face" appearance; disappears by 1–4 d

II—About 2 d after rash appears on face, maculopapular red spots appear, symmetrically distributed on upper and lower extremities; rash progresses from *proximal to distal* surfaces and may last a week or more

III—Rash subsides but reappears if skin is irritated or traumatized (sun, heat, cold, friction)

In children with aplastic crisis, rash is usually absent and prodromal illness includes: fever, myalgia, lethargy, nausea, vomiting, and abdominal pain

Treatment:

Symptomatic and supportive: *antipyretics, analgesics, antiinflammatory* drugs. Possible blood transfusion for transient aplastic anemia

Complications:
Aplastic crisis in children with hemolytic disease or immune deficiency

Arthritis (self-limited) and arthralgia (arthritis may become chronic)

Fetal death if mother infected during pregnancy, but no evidence of congenital anomalies

Myocarditis (rare)

Isolation of child not necessary, except hospitalized child (immunosuppressed or with aplastic crises) suspected of HPV infection is placed on respiratory

⚠ isolation and *standard precautions*

Pregnant women: need not be excluded from workplace where HPV infection is present; should *not* care for patients with aplastic crises; explain low risk of fetal death to those in contact with affected children

(continued)

TABLE 17.1 COMMUNICABLE DISEASES OF CHILDHOOD (continued)

Disease	◄ Assessment: Clinical Manifestations	Therapeutic Management/Complications ◄	Nursing Considerations
EXANTHEMA SUBITUM (ROSEOLA)			
Agent: Human herpes virus type 6 (HHV-6) **Source:** Unknown **Transmission:** Unknown (virtually limited to children between 6 months and 3 yr of age) **Incubation period:** 5-15d **Period of communicability:** Unknown	Persistent *high fever* for 3–4 d in child who appears well Precipitous drop in fever to normal with appearance of rash **Rash:** Discrete rose-pink macules or maculopapules appearing first on trunk, then spreading to neck, face, and extremities; nonpruritic, fades on pressure, lasts 1-2 d **Associated signs and symptoms:** Cervical/postauricular lymphadenopathy, injected pharynx, cough, coryza	**Treatment:** Nonspecific *Antipyretics* to control fever **Complications:** Encephalitis (rare) Febrile seizures (recurrent, possibly from latent infection of central nervous system that is reactivated by fever)	Teach parents measures for lowering temperature If child is prone to seizures, discuss appropriate precautions, possibility of recurrent febrile seizures.
MEASLES (RUBEOLA)			
Agent: Virus **Source:** Respiratory tract secretions, blood, and urine of infected person **Transmission:** Usually by *direct* contact with *droplets* of infected person **Incubation period:** 10–20 d **Period of communicability:** From 4 d *before* to 5 d *after* rash appears but mainly *during* prodromal (catarrhal) stage	**Prodromal (catarrhal) stage:** Fever and malaise, followed in 24 hours by coryza, cough, conjunctivitis, *Koplik spots* (small, irregular red spots with a minute, bluish white center first seen on buccal mucosa opposite molars 2 days *before* rash); symptoms gradually increase in severity until second day after rash appears, when they begin to subside **Rash:** Appears 3 to 4 days after onset of prodromal stage; begins as erythematous maculopapular eruption on face and gradually spreads downward; more severe in *earlier* sites (appears confluent) and less intense in *later* sites (appears discrete); after 3 to 4 d, assumes brownish appearance, and fine desquamation occurs over areas of extensive involvement **Constitutional signs and symptoms:** Anorexia, malaise, generalized lymphadenopathy	**Treatment:** *Vitamin A* supplementation **Supportive:** *bed rest* during febrile period; *antipyretics*, *antibiotics* to prevent secondary bacterial infection in children who are high-risk **Complications:** Bronchiolitis Encephalitis Obstructive laryngitis and laryngotracheitis Otitis media Pneumonia	*Isolation* until fifth day of rash; if hospitalized, institute *respiratory precautions* Maintain *bed rest* during prodromal stage; provide quiet activity **Fever:** Instruct parents to administer *antipyretics; avoid* chilling; if child is prone to *seizures*, institute appropriate precautions (fever spikes to 40°C [104°F] between fourth and fifth days) **Eye care:** Dim lights if photophobia present; clean eyelids with warm saline solution to remove secretions or crusts; keep child from rubbing eyes; examine cornea for signs of ulceration **Coryza/cough:** Use cool mist vaporizer, protect skin around nares with layer of petrolatum; encourage fluids and *soft, bland* foods **Skin care:** Keep skin clean; use tepid baths as necessary

(continued)

TABLE 17.1 COMMUNICABLE DISEASES OF CHILDHOOD *(continued)*

Disease	► Assessment: Clinical Manifestations	Therapeutic Management/Complications	► Nursing Considerations

MUMPS

Agent: Paramyxovirus

Source: Saliva of infected persons

Transmission: Direct contact with or droplet spread from an infected person

Incubation period: 14–21 d

Period of communicability: Most communicable immediately *before* and *after* swelling begins

Prodromal stage: Fever, headache, malaise, and anorexia for 24 h, followed by "earache" that is aggravated by chewing

Parotitis: By third day, parotid gland(s) (either unilateral or bilateral) enlarges and reaches maximum size in 1-3 d; accompanied by pain and tenderness

Other manifestations: Submaxillary and sublingual infection; orchitis, and meningoencephalitis

Treatment:

Symptomatic and supportive: *analgesics* for pain and *antipyretics* for fever; intravenous fluid may be necessary for child who refuses to drink, or vomits because of meningoencephalitis

Complications:
Arthritis
Epididymo-orchitis
Hepatitis
Myocarditis
Postinfectious encephalitis
Sensorineural deafness
Sterility

⚠ *Isolation:* respiratory precautions during period of communicability

Bed rest during prodromal phase, until no swelling

⬭ *Analgesics* for pain; if unwilling to chew, use elixir form

🍎 *Fluids* and *soft, bland* foods; *avoid* foods requiring chewing

☞ Hot or cold compresses to neck, whichever is more comforting

☞ *To relieve orchitis*, provide warmth, local support (tight-fitting underpants; stretch bathing suit)

PERTUSSIS (WHOOPING COUGH)

Agent: *Bordetella pertussis*

Source: Discharge from respiratory tract of infected persons

Transmission: Direct contact or droplet spread from infected person; indirect contact with freshly contaminated articles

Incubation period: 5 to 21 days, usually 10

Period of communicability: Greatest during catarrhal stage *before* onset of paroxysms, and may extend to fourth week *after* onset of paroxysms

Catarrhal stage: Begins with symptoms of upper respiratory tract infection, such as coryza, sneezing, lacrimation, cough, and low-grade fever; symptoms continue 1–2 wk, when dry, hacking cough becomes more severe

Paroxysmal stage: Cough most often occurs at *night* and consists of short, rapid coughs followed by sudden inspiration associated with a high-pitched crowing sound or "whoop"; during paroxysms: cheeks become flushed or cyanotic, eyes bulge, and tongue protrudes; paroxysm may continue until thick mucus plug is dislodged; vomiting frequently follows attack; stage generally lasts 4–6 wk, followed by convalescent stage

Treatment:

⬭ *Antimicrobial* therapy (e.g. *erythromycin*)

⬭ Administration of *pertussis-immune globulin*

Supportive treatment:
Hospitalization required for infants, children who are dehydrated, or those who have complications
Bed rest
Increased oxygen intake and humidity
Adequate fluids
Intubation possibly necessary

Complications:
Atelectasis
Convulsions
Hemorrhage (subarachnoid, subconjunctival, epistaxis)
Hernia
Otitis media
Pneumonia (usual cause of death)
Prolapsed rectum
Weight loss and dehydration

⚠ *Isolation* during catarrhal stage; if hospitalized, institute *respiratory precautions*

Maintain *bed rest* as long as fever present

Keep child occupied during day (increased interest in play associated with fewer paroxysms)

Reassure parents during frightening episodes of whooping cough

Provide restful environment and reduce factors that promote paroxysms (dust, smoke, sudden change in temperature, chilling, activity, excitement); keep room well-ventilated

Encourage fluids; offer *small* amount of *fluids* frequently; refeed child after vomiting

☞ Provide high humidity (humidifier or tent); suction gently but often to prevent choking on secretions

(continued)

TABLE 17.1 COMMUNICABLE DISEASES OF CHILDHOOD *(continued)*

Disease	◄ Assessment: Clinical Manifestations	Therapeutic Management/Complications ◄	Nursing Considerations
PERTUSSIS (WHOOPING COUGH) *(continued)*			
			Observe for signs of *airway obstruction* (increased restlessness, apprehension, retractions, cyanosis)
			Involve community health nurse if child cared for at home
POLIOMYELITIS			
Agent: Enteroviruses three types:	May be manifested in three different forms:	**Treatment:** No specific treatment, including *antimicrobials* or *gamma globulin*	Maintain *complete* bed rest
type 1—most frequent cause of paralysis, both epidemic and endemic;	**Abortive or inapparent**— Fever, uneasiness, sore throat, headache, anorexia, vomiting, abdominal pain; lasts a few hours to a few days	*Complete bed rest* during acute phase	Administer mild *sedatives* as necessary to relieve anxiety and promote rest
type 2—least frequently associated with paralysis;		☞ Assisted respiratory ventilation in case of respiratory paralysis	☞ Participate in *physiotherapy* procedures (use of moist hot packs and range-of-motion exercises)
type 3—second most frequently associated with paralysis	**Nonparalytic**—Same manifestations as **abortive** but more severe, with pain and stiffness in neck, back, and legs	Physical therapy for muscles following acute stage	*Position* child to maintain body alignment and prevent contractures or decubiti; use footboard
Source: Feces and oropharyngeal secretions of infected persons, especially young children	**Paralytic**—Initial course similar to **non-paralytic** type, followed by recovery and then signs of central nervous system paralysis	**Complications:** Hypertension Kidney stones from demineralization of bone during prolonged immobility Permanent paralysis Respiratory arrest	Encourage child to move; administer *analgesics* for maximum comfort during physical activity
Transmission: Direct contact with persons with apparent or inapparent active infection; spread is via *fecal-oral* and *pharyngeal-oropharyngeal* routes			⚡ Observe for *respiratory paralysis* (difficulty in talking, ineffective cough, inability to hold breath, shallow and rapid respirations); report such signs and symptoms to practitioner; have tracheostomy tray at bedside
Incubation period: Usually 7-14 d, with range of 5-35 d			
Period of communicability: Not exactly known; virus is present in throat and feces shortly *after* infection and *persists* for about 1 wk in throat and 4–6 wk in *feces*			

(continued)

TABLE 17.1 COMMUNICABLE DISEASES OF CHILDHOOD *(continued)*

Disease	▶ *Assessment: Clinical Manifestations*	*Therapeutic Management/Complications*	▶ *Nursing Considerations*
RUBELLA (GERMAN MEASLES)			
Agent: Rubella virus **Source:** Primarily nasopharyngeal secretions of person with apparent or inapparent infection; virus also present in blood, stool, and urine	**Prodromal stage:** Absent in children, present in adults and adolescents; consists of: low-grade fever, headache, malaise, anorexia, mild conjunctivitis, coryza, sore throat, cough, and lymphadenopathy; lasts for 1 to 5 days, subsides 1 day *after* appearance of rash	**Treatment:** *No treatment necessary* other than *antipyretics* for low-grade fever and *analgesics* for discomfort **Complications:** Rare (arthritis, encephalitis, or purpura); *most benign* of all childhood communicable diseases; **greatest danger is teratogenic effect on fetus**	Reassure parents of benign nature of illness in affected child Employ comfort measures as necessary *Isolate child from pregnant women*
Transmission: *Direct contact and spread via infected person, indirectly via articles freshly contaminated with nasopharyngeal secretions, feces, or urine* **Incubation period:** 14–21 d **Period of communicability:** 7 d *before*—about 5 d *after* appearance of rash	**Rash:** First appears on face and rapidly spreads downward to neck, arms, trunk, and legs; by end of first day: body is covered with a discrete, pinkish red maculo-papular exanthema; disappears in same order as it began, and is usually gone by third day **Constitutional signs and symptoms:** Occasionally low-grade fever, headache, malaise, and lymphadenopathy		

(continued)

TABLE 17.1 COMMUNICABLE DISEASES OF CHILDHOOD (continued)

Disease	Assessment: Clinical Manifestations	Therapeutic Management/Complications	Nursing Considerations
SCARLET FEVER			
Agent: Group A ß- hemolytic streptococci **Source:** Usually from nasopharygeal secretions of infected persons and carriers **Transmission:** *Direct* contact with infected person or droplet spread; *indirectly* by contact with contaminated articles, ingestion of *contaminated milk* or other food **Incubation period:** 2–4 d, with range of 1–7 d **Period of communicability:** During incubation period and clinical illness approximately 10 d; during first 2 wk of carrier phase, although may persist for months	**Prodromal stage:** Abrupt high fever, pulse increased out of proportion to fever; vomiting, headache, chills, malaise, abdominal pain **Enanthema:** Tonsils enlarged, edematous, reddened, and covered with patches of exudate; in severe cases appearance resembles membrane seen in diphtheria; pharynx is edematous and beefy red; during first 1–2 d: tongue is coated and papillae become red and swollen (*white strawberry tongue*); by 4–5 d: white coat sloughs off, leaving prominent papillae (*red strawberry tongue*); palate is covered with erythematous punctate lesions **Exanthema:** Rash appears within 12 h after prodromal signs; red pinhead-sized punctate lesions rapidly become generalized but are *absent* on face, which becomes flushed with striking *circumoral pallor*; rash is more intense in *folds of joints*; by end of 1 wk: desquamation begins (fine, sandpaper-like on torso; sheet-like sloughing on palms and soles), which may be complete by 3 wk or longer	**Treatment:** Treatment of choice is a full course of *penicillin (or erythromycin* in penicillin-sensitive children); fever should subside 24 h after beginning therapy *Antibiotic* therapy for newly diagnosed carriers (nose or throat cultures positive for streptococci) **Supportive measures:** bed rest during febrile phase; *analgesics* for sore throat **Complications:** Carditis Glomerulonephritis Otitis media Peritonsillar abscess Polyarthritis (uncommon) Sinusitis	Institute *respiratory precautions* until 24 h after initiation of treatment Ensure compliance with oral *antibiotic therapy (intramuscular benzathine penicillin G [Bicillin]* may be given if parents' reliability in giving oral drugs is questionable) Provide quiet activity during convalescent period Relieve discomfort of sore throat with *analgesics*, gargles, lozenges, antiseptic throat sprays (*Chloraseptic*), and inhalation of cool mist Encourage *fluids* during febrile phase; *avoid* irritating liquids (citrus juices) or rough foods; when child is able to eat, begin with *soft diet* Advise parents to consult practitioner if fever persists after beginning therapy Discuss procedures for preventing spread of infection

Source: Wong, D. *Whaley and Wong's Nursing Care of Infants and Children* (7th ed). St. Louis: Mosby.

⋈ B. Analysis/nursing diagnosis:
1. *Altered tissue perfusion* (liver) related to hepatic necrosis.
2. *Fluid volume deficit* related to increased loss of fluids secondary to vomiting and diaphoresis.
3. *Risk for injury* related to bleeding and clotting disorders.
4. *Anxiety* related to parental/child feelings of guilt, uncertainty as to outcome, and invasive nature of treatments.
5. *Knowledge deficit* regarding accident prevention.

⋈ C. Nursing care plan/implementation:
1. Goal: *promote excretion of acetaminophen and prevent permanent liver damage.*
   ☞ a. If possible, induce vomiting; save, bring to emergency department.
   ☞ b. Assist with gastric lavage, if appropriate.
   ⬭ c. Administer *activated charcoal.*
   ᜠ d. Assist with obtaining acetaminophen level 4 h after ingestion.
   e. Treatment must begin as soon as possible; therapy begun later than 10 h after ingestion has *no* value.
   ⬭ f. Administer antidote (*acetylcysteine*) per MD order. Usually administered via NG tube because of offensive odor. Given as one loading dose and 17 maintenance doses.
   g. Monitor hepatic functioning—assist with obtaining specimens and check results frequently; be aware that liver
   ᜠ enzymes will rise and peak within 3 days and then should rapidly return to normal.
2. Goal: *restore fluid and electrolyte balance.*
   ☞ a. Monitor vital signs and perform neurologic checks q2–4h and prn.
   ᜠ b. Monitor I&O, urine analysis, including specific gravity, and weight.
   c. Monitor IV fluids as ordered.
3. Goal: *prevent bleeding.*
   ᜠ a. Assist in monitoring child's prothrombin time; notify MD of significant changes.
   ᜠ b. Monitor urine and stool for occult blood.
   c. Observe for and report any petechiae or unusual bruising.
4. Goal: *control anxiety.*
   a. Allow parents to ventilate feelings.
   b. Support parents; be non-judgemental.
⌂ 5. Goal: **health teaching.** *Prevent another accidental poisoning* (see **Chapter 13**, nursing care plan, Goal **5** for **salicylate poisoning**).

⋈ D. Evaluation/outcome criteria:
1. Acetaminophen is successfully removed from child's body and normal liver functioning is re-established.
2. Fluid and electrolyte balance is restored and maintained.
3. No bleeding occurs.
4. Anxiety is controlled.
5. No further episodes of poisoning occur.

Infestations

I. Lice (Pediculosis)
   A. *Introduction*: In children, the most common form of lice is *Pediculosis capitis*, head lice. This parasite feeds on the scalp, and its saliva causes severe itching. Head lice are frequently associated with the sharing of combs and brushes, hats, and clothing; thus, they are more common in *girls*, especially those with long hair. Lice are also associated with *over-crowded* conditions and poor hair *hygiene*.

⋈ B. Assessment:
1. Severe itching of scalp.
2. Visible eggs/nits on shafts of hair.

⋈ C. Analysis/nursing diagnosis:
1. *Impaired skin integrity* related to infestation of scalp with lice and scratching caused by pruritus.
2. *Knowledge deficit* related to transmission and prevention of disease and treatment regimen.

⋈ D. Nursing care plan/implementation:
1. Goal: *eradicate lice infestation and restore skin integrity.*
   ⬭ a. *Apply permethrin (NIX or RID)*—rub in 4–5 min, then comb with fine-tooth comb to remove dead lice and nits (eggs). May need to be repeated if evidence of reinfestation is noted, or first treatment does not completely eradicate infestation.
   b. Wear gloves and cap to protect self.
   c. Inspect other family members; treat prn
   ⬭ with *permethrin.*
⌂ 2. Goal: **health teaching.** *Teach family preventitive measures to safeguard against reinfestation.*
   a. Wash all clothes and linens to kill any lice that may have fallen off the child's hair.
   b. Encourage short hair, if acceptable.
   c. *Teach preventive measures*: don't share comb, brushes, hats.

⋈ E. Evaluation/outcome criteria:
1. Skin integrity is restored.
2. Family knowledgeable regarding preventitive measures.

II. Pinworms (Enterobiasis)

A. *Introduction*: In children, the most common parasitic infestation is pinworms. Infestation usually occurs when the child places fingers (and the pinworm eggs) into the mouth. Breaking the *anus-to-mouth contamination cycle* can best be accomplished by good hygiene, especially handwashing before eating and after toileting. If one family member has pinworms, it is highly likely that other family members are also infested; therefore, treat the *entire* family to eradicate the parasite. Pinworms are easily eradicated with *antiparasitic* medications.

B. **Assessment:**
1. Intense perianal itching.
2. Visible pinworms in the stool.
3. Vague abdominal discomfort.
4. Anorexia and weight loss.

C. **Analysis/nursing diagnosis:**
1. *Risk for infection/injury* related to the anus-to-mouth contamination cycle of pinworm infestation, severe rectal itching.
2. *Knowledge deficit* related to transmission and prevention of disease and treatment regimen.

D. **Nursing care plan/implementation**:
1. Goal: *eradicate pinworm infestation.*
   a. Treat *all* family members simultaneously with an antiparasitic agent, e.g., *pyruvinium pamoate (Povan)* or *mebendazole.* Then repeat in 2 weeks to prevent reinfestation.
   b. Launder all underwear, bed linens, and towels in hot soapy water to kill eggs.
2. Goal: **health teaching.** T*each family preventitive measures to safeguard against reinfestation.*
   a. Teach family members the importance of good hygiene, especially handwashing before eating (or preparing food) and after toileting. Stress to children to keep their fingers out of their mouths.

E. **Evaluation/outcome criteria:**
1. Pinworms are eradicated.
2. Family knowledgeable regarding prevenatitive measures.

Other Special Needs of Children

Pediatric Surgery

I. In general, basic care principles for children are the same as those for adults having surgery.

II. *Exceptions*:
A. Children should be prepared according to their developmental level and learning ability.

B. Children *cannot* sign own surgical consent form; this must be done by parent or legal guardian.
C. Parents should be actively involved in the child's care.

III. **Table 17.2 p. 181** reviews *specific nursing care* for the *most common pediatric surgical procedures.*

Down Syndrome

I. *Introduction*: Down syndrome (*trisomy 21; mongolism*) is a chromosomal abnormality involving an extra *chromosome 21* and resulting in *47* chromosomes instead of the normal 46 chromosomes. As a consequence, the child usually presents with varying degrees of mental retardation, characteristic facial and physical features, and other congenital anomalies. Down syndrome is the most common chromosomal disorder, occurring in approximately 1/800-1000 live births. *Perinatal risk factors* include advanced maternal age, especially with the first pregnancy; paternal age is also thought to be a related factor.

II. **Assessment:**
A. *Physical characteristics*
1. Brachycephalic (small, round *head*) with oblique palpebral fissures ("Oriental" *eyes*) and *Brushfield* spots (speckling of *iris*), depressed *nasal* bridge (saddle nose) and small, low-set *ears*.
2. Mouth:
   a. Small oral cavity with protruding tongue causes difficulty sucking and swallowing.
   b. Delayed eruption/misalignment of teeth.
3. Hands:
   a. Clinodactyly (in-curved little finger).
   b. *Simian* crease (transverse palmar crease).
4. Muscles: hypotonic ("floppy baby") with hyperextensible joints.
5. Skin: dry, cracked.
B. *Genetic* studies reveal an extra chromosome 21 (trisomy 21).
C. *Intellectual characteristics*
1. Mental retardation—varies from severely retarded to low-average intelligence.
2. Most fall within "trainable" range: IQ of 36–51 (moderate mental retardation).
D. *Congenital anomalies/diseases*
1. 30–40% have congenital *heart* defects: mortality rates highest in those with Down syndrome and cyanotic heart disease.
2. *GI*: tracheoesophageal fistula, Hirschsprung's disease.
3. *Thyroid* dysfunction, especially hypothyroidism.
4. *Visual* defects: cataracts, strabismus.
5. *Hearing* loss.
6. Increased incidence of *leukemia.*

(*continued on p. 182*)

TABLE 17.2   PEDIATRIC SURGERY: NURSING CONSIDERATIONS

Surgical Procedure	✉ *Specific Nursing Care*
Appendectomy	Observe same principles of preoperative and postoperative care as for adult GI surgery. ■ NPO until bowel sounds return (24–48 h). ☞ ■ If appendix ruptured pre- or intraoperatively, place in *semi-Fowler's position* and implement wound precautions. ⊂⊃ ■ Administer *antibiotics* per MD order. ■ Monitor for signs and symptoms of peritonitis. Typical course—speedy recovery, with discharge in about 2-3 d; excellent *prognosis*.
Herniorrhaphy (umbilical/inguinal)	*Umbilical*: ↑ incidence in infants who are African-American. *Inguinal*: ↑ incidence in boys. **Preoperative**: monitor for possible complications of strangulation. **Postoperative**: routine GI surgery care. *Prognosis*—excellent; usually outpatient procedure with same day discharge.
Myringotomy (with tympanostomy) A myringotomy is a crescent shaped slit in the tympanic membrane. Tympanostomy tubes are for pressure equalization (supply air to middle ear). Two separate procedures but can also be done at the same time.	**Postoperative**: ■ *Position*—place with operated *ear down*, to allow for drainage. Expect moderate amount of purulent drainage initially. ■ Keep *external* ear canal clean and dry. 🏠 *Teach parents/discharge planning*: ■ Need to keep water out of ear—use special ear plugs when bathing or swimming. ■ Tubes will remain in place 3–7 mo and then fall out spontaneously with healing of ear drum.
Tonsillectomy (most frequently performed pediatric surgical procedure)	Preoperative: check bleeding and clotting times. **Postoperative**: ■ *Position*—place on abdomen or semi-prone with head turned to side to prevent aspiration. ■ *Observe for most frequent complication—hemorrhage* (frequent swallowing, emesis of bright red blood, shock). *Prevent bleeding*: ■ Do *not* suction—may cause bleeding. ■ Do *not* encourage coughing, clearing throat, or blowing nose—may aggravate operative site and cause bleeding. ■ Minimize crying. *Decrease pain*: ■ Offer ice collar to decrease pain and for vasoconstriction, but do *not* force. ⊂⊃ ■ *Acetaminophen* for pain (*no* aspirin). 🍎 *Nutrition*: ■ NPO initially, then *cool, clear fluids* such as cool water, crushed ice, flavored icepops, diluted (non-citrus) fruit juice. ■ **No: red fluids** (punch, jello, icepops), citrus juices, warm fluids (tea, broth), toast, milk/ice cream/pudding, carbonated sodas. Progress to *soft, bland*. 🏠 *Teach parents/discharge planning*: ■ Signs and symptoms of infection—call physician promptly. ■ 5–10 d postoperatively expect slight bleeding. 🍎 ■ Continue *soft, bland diet* as tolerated.

Source: ©Lagerquist, S. *Little, Brown's NCLEX-RN® Examination Review*. Boston: Little, Brown (out of print).

E. *Growth and development*
1. Slow growth, especially in height.
2. Delay in developmental milestones.

F. *Sexual development*
1. Delayed or incomplete.
2. Women—small number have had offspring (majority have had abnormality).
3. Men—infertile.

G. *Aging*
1. Premature aging, with shortened life expectancy.
2. Death usually before age 40—generally related to *respiratory* complication: repeated infections, pneumonia, lung disease.

▶ III. **Analysis/nursing diagnosis:**
A. *Risk for aspiration* related to hypotonia.
B. *Altered nutrition, less than body requirements*, related to hypotonia and/or congenital anomalies.
C. *Altered growth and development* related to Down syndrome.
D. *Knowledge deficit* related to Down syndrome.

▶ IV. **Nursing care plan/implementation:**
A. Goal: *prevent physical complications.*
☞ 1. Respiratory
   a. Use bulb syringe to clear nose, mouth.
   b. Use vaporizer.
   c. Make frequent *position* changes.
   d. *Avoid* contact with people with upper respiratory infections.
2. Aspiration
   a. *Small*, more *frequent* feedings.
   b. Burp well during/after infant feedings.
   c. Allow sufficient time to eat.
   d. *Position after meals*: head of bed *elevated, right side*—or on stomach, with head to side.
B. Goal: *meet nutritional needs.*
☞ 1. Suction (before meals) to clear airway.
2. Adapt feeding techniques to meet special needs of infant/child; e.g., use long, straight-handled spoon.
3. Monitor height and weight.
4. As child grows, monitor caloric intake (tends toward obesity).
5. Offer foods *high in bulk* to prevent constipation related to hypotonia.
C. Goal: *promote optimal growth and development.*
1. Encourage parents to enroll infant/toddler in early stimulation program and to follow through with suggested exercises at home.
2. Preschool/school-age: special education classes.
〰 3. Screen frequently, using DDST to monitor development.
4. Help parents focus on normal or positive aspects of infant/child.

5. Help parents work toward realistic goals with their child.
🏠 D. Goal: **health teaching.**
1. Explain that tongue-thrust behavior is normal and that food should be re-fed.
2. Before adolescence—counsel parents and child about delay in sexual development, decreased libido, marriage and family relations.
3. In severe cases, assist parents to deal with issue of placement/institutionalization.

▶ V. **Evaluation/outcome criteria:**
A. Physical complications are prevented.
B. Adequate nutrition is maintained.
C. Child attains optimal level of growth and development.
D. Parents have appropriate knowledge base regarding child with Down syndrome.

Child Abuse

Abuse takes several forms: *physical* (battering), *sexual*, and/or *emotional* abuse, as well as *neglect*. This section focuses on identification of the child who is a victim of violence and nursing care of children who are sexually abused.

I. **Victim of Physical Abuse**: signs of battering in children are listed in **Table 17.3 p. 183.**

II. **Sexual Abuse of Children**
▶ A. **Assessment**—characteristic behaviors:
1. *Relationship* of offender to victim: many filling paternal role (uncle, grandfather, cousin) with repeated, unquestioned access to the child.
2. Methods of *pressuring* victim into sexual activity: offering material goods, misrepresenting moral standards ("it's O.K."), exploiting need for human contact and warmth.
3. Method of pressuring victim to *secrecy* (to conceal the act) is inducing fear of: punishment, not being believed, rejection, being blamed for the activity, abandonment.
4. Disclosure of sexual activity via:
   a. Direct visual or verbal confrontation and *observation* by others.
   b. *Verbalization* of act by victim.
   c. *Visible clues*: excess money and candy, new clothes, pictures, notes.
   d. *Signs and symptoms*: bed-wetting, excessive bathing, tears, avoiding school, somatic distress (*GI and urinary tract pains*).
▶ B. **Analysis/nursing diagnosis:**
1. *Altered protection* related to inflicted pain.
2. *Personal identity disturbance* related to abuse as child and feeling guilty and responsible for being a victim.

TABLE 17.3 SUMMARY: CLUES TO THE IDENTIFICATION OF A CHILD WHO IS A VICTIM OF VIOLENCE

CLUES IN THE HISTORY

- Significant DELAY in seeking medical care
- Major DISCREPANCIES in the history:
  1. Discrepancy between different people's versions of the story
  2. Discrepancy between the history and the observed injuries
  3. Discrepancy between the history and the child's developmental capabilities
- History of multiple emergency room visits for various injuries
- A story that is VAGUE AND CONTRADICTORY

CLUES IN THE PHYSICAL EXAMINATION

- Child who seems apathetic and DOES NOT CRY despite his injuries
- Child who DOES NOT TURN TO PARENTS FOR COMFORT
- Child who is POORLY NOURISHED and POORLY CARED FOR
- The presence of MULTIPLE BRUISES and abrasions, especially around the trunk and buttocks
- The presence of OLD BRUISES IN ADDITION TO FRESH ONES
- The presence of SUSPICIOUS BURNS:
  1. Cigarette burns
  2. Scalds without splash marks or involving the buttocks, hands, or feet but sparing skin folds
- Injuries about the MOUTH
- RIB FRACTURES
- FRACTURES in an infant < 1 yr of age
- Pattern of injury DESCRIPTIVE OF OBJECT USED (e.g. belt buckle, wire hanger, etc.)
- Injury denotes TYPE OF ABUSE (e.g. whiplash from shaking; dislocation from twisting).

Adapted from Caroline N. *Emergency Care in the Streets* (5th ed). Boston: Little, Brown (out of print).

C. **Nursing care plan/implementation:**
1. Goal: *protect child from further trauma.*
   a. Establish safe environment and the termination of trauma.
   b. Encourage child to verbalize feelings about incident to dispel tension built up by secrecy.
   c. Ask child to draw a picture or use dolls and toys to show what happened.
   d. Observe for symptoms over a period of time:
      (1) *Phobic* reactions when seeing or hearing offender's name.
      (2) *Scholastic* pattern changes; usually declining.
      (3) *Sleep pattern changes*, recurrent dreams, nightmares.

2. Goal: *reestablish a sense of self in child.*
   a. Look for *silent reaction* to being an accessory to sex (that is, child keeping burden of the secret activity within self); help deal with unresolved issues.
   b. Establish therapeutic alliance with parent who is abusive, if possible or feasible.

3. Goal: **health teaching.**
   a. Teach child that his (her) body is private and to inform a responsible adult when someone violates privacy without consent.
   b. Teach adults in family to respond to victim with sensitivity, support, and concern.

D. **Evaluation/outcome criteria:**
1. Child's needs for affection, attention, personal recognition, or love met without sexual exploitation. Child experiences protective environment.
2. Child maintains a sense of self.

The Child Who is Dying

I. *Introduction*: There are many causes of death in children. Many diseases formerly associated with death in childhood (e.g. cystic fibrosis) are now chronic in nature with children surviving into their second and third decades. However, accidents, congenital anomalies and some disease processes (e.g. cancer) continue to be associated with childhood mortality.

II. **Assessment:**
A. Look for signs of impending death (see **Table 17.4 p. 184**).
B. Assess family's response to child's anticipated or actual death.
C. Assess family for signs and symptoms of grief and grieving.
D. Assess family's ability to cope with this situational crisis.
E. Assess what the child has been told or knows about prognosis and what the family would like the child to know.

III. **Analysis/nursing diagnosis:**
A. *Fear/anxiety* related to terminal prognosis, diagnostic procedures and treatments.
B. *Powerlessness* (child) related to dying process.
C. *Altered nutrition*, less than body requirements, related to anorexia.
D. *Anticipatory grieving* related to the probable death of a child or of family.

IV. **Nursing care plan/implementation:**
A. Goal: *reduce anxiety experienced by child and family.*
1. Limit interventions to symptomatic support and treatment only; discuss other interventions with family and MD.

TABLE 17.4 PHYSICAL SIGNS OF APPROACHING DEATH

Spurts of energy followed by lethargy

Sleep needs increase

Loss of sensation and movement in the lower extremities, progressing toward the upper body

Sensation of heat, although body feels cool

Loss of senses:

Tactile sensation decreases

Sensitive to light

Hearing is *last* sense to fail

Confusion, loss of consciousness, slurred speech

Muscle weakness

Loss of bowel and bladder control

Urine output decreases

Decreased appetite/thirst

Difficulty swallowing

Skin: pale, gray-blue color, cool to touch

Change in respiratory pattern:

Cheyne-Stokes respirations (waxing and waning of depth of breathing with regular periods of apnea)

"Death rattle" (noisy chest sounds from accumulation of pulmonary and pharyngeal secretions)

Weak, slow pulse; decreased blood pressure

Adapted from Wong D. Nursing Care of Infants and Children (7th ed.) St. Louis: Mosby.

2. Explain all diagnostic procedures and treatments to the child and family.

3. Be scrupulously honest in all interactions with family and child; stress the utmost importance of honesty in all interpersonal relationships, especially at this time.

4. Answer as honestly and completely as possible any questions that the child may ask.

5. Keep the parents as involved in the child's care as they are able and willing to be.

6. Remain with the child or have a responsible adult remain with the child at all times; do *not* leave the child unattended.

7. Assume a nonjudgmental attitude toward the behavior of the child and family.

B. Goal: *provide adequate emotional and physical support for child during the terminal phase of a disease.*

1. Emotional support:

a. Continue to talk to the child, even if the child is unresponsive or appears comatose.

b. Position the nurse or family members in such a way that the child can easily see the person who is speaking.

c. Speak in a normal tone of voice; do *not* whisper.

d. Do *not* talk about the child in the child's presence, even if the child appears to be comatose.

e. If child is able to respond, ask "yes" or "no" questions to help conserve energy. Provide choices.

f. If child appears to be awake, help orient the child to time and place.

g. Play soothing music for the child.

h. Encourage parents to remain close to the child and to hold and cuddle the child.

i. Do *not* repeat vital signs routinely; this unnecessarily disturbs the child.

2. Physical support:

a. Administer medications per MD order to provide 24-h pain relief.

b. *Avoid* excessive stimulation with noise or light, but also *avoid* dim lights.

c. Assist child to *change position* frequently or change the child's position if child is unable to do so.

d. *Avoid* pressure on reddened or irritated bony prominences; maintain anatomically correct body alignment.

e. Use pillows and other supportive equipment to support the child in a position of maximal comfort.

f. Provide toileting assistance as necessary and administer perineal care if child is incontinent.

g. Provide comfort measures (soothing massage) but *avoid* routine care unless necessary.

C. Goal: *provide adequate nutrition.*

1. Offer foods and fluids that the child *prefers*.

2. Encourage *small, frequent* meals and snacks.

3. Feed slowly in an *upright* position to avoid aspiration.

4. *Avoid* foods with strong or offensive odors.

5. Make the environment as conducive as possible for meals; encourage family members to eat with the child.

6. Suggest foods that are *easy to chew* and *swallow*, such as soups or custard.

7. Administer *antiemetic* per MD order.

8. Provide good oral hygiene both before and after meals.

D. Goal: *provide support for the family* (see also **Table 17.5 p. 185**).

1. Remain open and available to all family members; enter the child's room often and spend time with the family.

2. Encourage the family to express their feelings concerning the child's illness, dying, and death.

3. Discuss the need for family members to care for their own needs as well as the child's; encourage family members to eat and sleep.

4. Provide for the physical comfort and emotional needs of the family.

TABLE 17.5 GUIDELINES: SUPPORTING GRIEVING FAMILIES

GENERAL

Stay with the family; sit quietly if they prefer not to talk; cry with them if desired.

Accept the family's grief reactions; *avoid* judgmental statements (e.g., "You should be feeling better by now").

Avoid offering rationalizations for the child's death (e.g., "You should be glad your child isn't suffering anymore").

Avoid artificial consolation (e.g., "I know how you feel," or "You are still young enough to have another baby").

Deal openly with feelings such as guilt, anger, and loss of self-esteem.

Focus on feelings by using a "feeling" word in the statement (e.g., "You're still feeling all the pain of losing a child").

Provide for participation in care (if desired).

Extend visiting hours and number of visitors.

Identify/appoint one "spokesperson" on staff to keep family updated and avoid misinformation.

Refer the family to an appropriate self-help group or for professional help if needed.

AT THE TIME OF DEATH

Reassure the family that everything possible is being done for the child, if they wish lifesaving interventions.

Do everything possible to ensure the child's comfort, especially relieving pain.

Provide the child and family the opportunity to review special experiences or memories in their lives.

Express personal feelings of loss and/or frustrations (e.g., "We will miss him so much," or "We tried everything; we feel so sorry that we couldn't save him").

Provide information that the family requests and be honest.

Respect the emotional needs of family members, such as siblings, who may need brief respites from the child who is dying.

Make every effort to arrange for family members, especially parents, to be with the child at the moment of death, if they wish to be present.

Allow the family to stay with the child who died for as long as they wish and to rock, hold, or bathe the child.

Provide practical help when possible, such as collecting the child's belongings.

Arrange for spiritual support, such as clergy; pray with the family if no one else can stay with them.

AFTER THE DEATH

Attend the funeral or visitation if there was a special closeness with the family.

Initiate and maintain contact (e.g., sending cards, telephoning, inviting them back to the unit, or making a home visit).

Refer to the child who died by name; discuss shared memories with the family.

Discourage the use of drugs or alcohol as a method of escaping grief.

Encourage all family members to communicate their feelings rather than remaining silent to avoid upsetting another member.

Emphasize that grieving is a painful process that often takes years to resolve.

"Family" refers to all significant persons involved in the child's life, such as parents, siblings, grandparents, or other close relatives or friends.

Adapted from Wong D. *Nursing Care of Infants and Children* (7th ed). St. Louis: Mosby.

5. Involve family in important decisions regarding the child's treatment; serve as advocate for the child and family.
6. Refer family to clergyperson for additional support.

▶ **V. Evaluation/outcome criteria:**
   A. Child and family appear as calm and anxiety-free as possible.
   B. Child will feel in control (powerful) despite terminal prognosis.
   C. Child is able to take in at least a minimal amount of foods or fluids.
   D. Family members remain present and involved with child's care through death.

⬭ Guidelines for Administering Medications to Infants and Children

I. **Developmental considerations**
   A. Be honest. Do *not* bribe or threaten child to obtain cooperation.
   B. Administer medication in the least traumatic manner possible.
   C. Describe any sensations child may expect to experience, e.g., "pinch" of needle during IM.
   D. Explain how child can "help" nurse, e.g., "Lie as still as you can." Enlist parental assistance (if available).
   E. Tell child that it is OK to cry; provide privacy.
   F. Offer support, praise, and encouragement during and after giving medication.

G. Allow child opportunity for age-appropriate therapeutic play to work through feelings and experiences, to clarify any misconceptions, and to teach child more effective coping strategies.

II. Safety considerations

A. Be absolutely sure dose is both safe (check recommended mg/kg) and accurate (have another nurse check your calculations). *Remember*: dose should generally be smaller than adult dose.

B. Check identification band or ask parent or another nurse for child's first and last name.

C. Restrain child to avoid injury while giving medication; a second person is often required to help hold child.

III. Oral medications

A. Use syringe without needle to draw up medication.

B. *Position*: upright or semireclining.

C. Place tip of syringe along the side of infant's tongue, and give medication slowly, in small amounts, allowing infant to swallow. Medicine cups can be used for older infants and children. **Never** pinch infant or child's nostrils to force him or her to open mouth.

D. When giving tablets or capsules (that are **not** enteric-coated), crush and mix into smallest possible amount of food or liquid to ensure that child takes entire dose. Do *not* mix with essential food or liquid (e.g., milk); select an optional food, such as applesauce.

IV. Ophthalmic installations

A. *Position*: supine or sitting with head extended.

B. For eye *drops*: hold dropper 1–2 cm above middle of conjunctival sac.

C. For eye *ointment*: squeeze 2 cm of ointment from tube onto conjunctival sac.

D. After giving drops or ointment, encourage child to keep eyes closed briefly to maximize contact with eyes. Child should be asked to look in all directions (with eyes closed) to enhance even distribution of medication.

E. Whenever possible, administer eye ointments at nap or bed time, because of possible blurred vision. Administer eye drops *prior* to eye ointment if they are ordered for the same time.

V. Otic installations

A. *Position*: head to side so that *affected* ear is *uppermost*.

B. For child **under** 3 yr: pull pinna gently **down** and back.

C. For child **over** 3 yr: pull pinna gently **up** and back.

D. After administering ear drops, encourage child to remain with *head to side* with *affected* ear *uppermost*, to maximize contact with entire external canal to reach eardrum. Gentle massage of area in front of ear facilitates entry of ear drops into canal.

E. If ear drops are kept in refrigerator, allow to warm to room temperature before instilling.

VI. Dermatologic installations

A. *Remember*: young child's skin is more permeable, therefore there is increased risk for medication absorption and resultant systemic effects; monitor for systemic effects.

B. Apply thin layer of cream or ointment and confine it to portions of skin where it is essential.

VII. Rectal medication

A. Prepare child emotionally and physically; rectal route is invasive and embarrassing, particularly for children.

B. *Position*: *side-lying* with *upper leg flexed*.

C. Lubricate rounded end of suppository and insert past anal sphincter with gloved fingertip (wear gloves when inserting rectal medication).

D. Remove fingertip and hold child's buttocks gently together until child no longer strains or indicates urge to expel medication.

VIII. Intramuscular medication

A. Because the infant or child is much smaller physically than an adult, the nurse should select a shorter needle, generally $5/8$ inch (infant) to 1 inch (child).

B. Preferred injection sites are on the *thigh*: vastus lateralis—lateral aspect; on thigh: dorsogluteal and ventrogluteal (if walking for 1 year). The *deltoid* muscle, though small, provides easy access and can be used in children with adequate muscle mass.

C. **Avoid** posterior gluteal muscle in children under age 4 yr.

D. Because of vast differences in size, muscle mass, and subcutaneous tissue, it is especially important to note bony prominences as landmarks for intramuscular injections.

E. Have a second adult present to help restrain the child.

F. Once the nurse has told the child he or she is to receive an injection, the procedure should be carried out as quickly and skillfully as possible.

COMMONLY PRESCRIBED MEDICATIONS

Medication	Administration	Use/Action	▶ Nursing Consideration
Antidote Acetylcysteine/ *Mucomyst*	• Oral and inhalation • Calculate to child's weight in kilograms • Administer in provided dropper or calibrated syringe • **NEVER** use household measuring spoon • Should be mixed in a carbonated beverage (has "rotten eggs" [sulfa] odor)	Used in treatment of acetaminophen overdose/ingestion Increases hepatic glutathione, which inactivates toxic metabolites in acetaminophen	• Dilute in 1:4 ratio to mask odor/taste • Begin therapy within 24 hours of ingestion • Obtain serum level 4 hours after reported ingestion to ensure peak level of drug has been reached
Antihelmintics Mebendazole/*Vermox* Pyrantel Pamoate/ *Antiminth*	• Oral • Calculate to child's weight in kilograms • Administer in provided dropper or calibrated syringe • **NEVER** use household measuring spoon	Used in treatment of pinworms and other parasitic infections Causes release of acetylcholine and inhibits cholinesterase, paralyzing the parasites Inhibits glucose uptake which depletes glycogen storage necessary for parasites' reproduction	• Infected child should sleep alone • Clean toilet daily with disinfectant • Increase fruit juice consumption (aids in worm's expulsion by eliminating accumulation in intestinal mucosa)
Antihistamines/ **Antipruritics** Diphenhydramine/ *Benadryl* Hydroxyzine/*Atarax*	• Oral, parenteral and topical • Calculate to child's weight in kilograms • Administer in provided dropper or calibrated syringe • **NEVER** use household measuring spoon	Used in common communicable diseases of childhood to suppress pruritis (itching) Blocks histamine release Decreases allergic response	• *Avoid* use in children with seizure disorders (depresses subcortical levels of central nervous system) • Provide for age-appropriate safety measures since medication causes drowsiness
Corticosteroids/ **Glucocorticoids** Hydrocortisone Cream/*Cortaid*	• Topical • Apply lotion or cream sparingly to affected area • Cleanse area first to prevent cumulative depot effect • Do **not** cover with occlusive dressing unless directed by pediatrician	Used in treatment of eczema Suppresses inflammatory response	• *Avoid* over-usage because repeated application promotes capillary fragility and "thinning" of skin • *Avoid* contact with mucus membranes
Emetics Ipecac/*Syrup of Ipecac*	• Oral • Calculate to child's age • Administer in provided dropper or calibrated syringe • **NEVER** use household measuring spoon	Used in treatment of specific overdoses/ingestions of poisonous substances Irritates gastric mucosa and stimulates medullary chemoreceptor trigger zone to induce vomiting	• Use *Ipecac Syrup*—**NOT** fluid extract (which is 14 times more potent and can cause death) • Use with caution in children with cardiac disorders (medication can cause tachycardia, cardiotoxicity) • Do *not* give with milk (delays action of *Ipecac*)

(continued)

COMMONLY PRESCRIBED MEDICATIONS *(continued)*

Medication	Administration	Use/Action	Nursing Consideration
Pediculicides Permethrin/*NIX* Pyrethrins/*RID*	• Topical • Shampoo according to instructions on bottle • Leave on for 10 minutes, then rinse with water and comb hair with fine-tooth comb • Repeat in 7–10 days	Used in treatment of head lice Kills parasites by affecting nervous system and inducing paralysis	• Evaluate all family members for possible infestation • Thorough cleaning of all infested areas • Assess for allergy to chrysanthemums (also contain permethrin) before initial application

Study and Memory Aids

Otitis Media—Complications

The sudden cessation of pain in a child with otitis media usually means that the ear drum has *ruptured*.
The nurse should check the auditory canal for drainage of purulent material, which should be gently cleansed away.

Eczema—Prevention

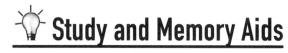
The most common offending allergen in eczema is *cow's milk*; infants should be kept on formula or breast milk for *1 yr* to prevent this problem.

Eczema—Care

The child with eczema should have only *cotton* clothing, bed linens, towels, and toys, e.g., cotton terrycloth doll.

Eczema—Prognosis

Half of children with eczema go into permanent, spontaneous remission; the other half of children with eczema develop other allergic manifestations such as *hay fever or asthma*.

Communicable Disease—Prevention

Immunizations can prevent most childhood communicable diseases.

Poisoning—Treatment

Syrup of ipecac is used to induce vomiting in children who have ingested a poison if vomiting is indicated.
Acetaminophen poisoning can cause potentially fatal *liver* damage; it is treated with the antidote *acetylcysteine*.

Lice Infestations—Treatment

Lice is treated with permethrin (*NIX* or *RID*), followed by use of a fine-toothed comb.

Pinworm Infestations—Treatment

Pinworms are treated with pyruvinium pamoate or mebendazole.

Tonsillectomy—Complications: Postoperative Hemorrhage. Signs and Symptoms:

1. Frequent swallowing
2. Emesis of bright red blood
3. Shock

Down Syndrome (the most common chromosomal abnormality)—Signs and Symptoms Include:

1. Small, round head
2. "Oriental" eyes
3. Brushfield spots
4. Saddle nose
5. Small, low-set ears
6. Simian crease

Most common cause of death with Down syndrome: respiratory complications.

Children's Concept of Death

Infants	Unaware of death May sense stress in caregivers
Toddlers	No real understanding of death Death is "something that makes parents worry"
Preschoolers	Death is reversible or temporary Dead people still breathe, eat, sleep Magical thinking may bring dead person back
School-age	More realistic understanding of death Death is irreversible Death is personified as grim reaper or boogeyman
Adolescents	Realistic understanding of death

Questions

1. When caring for a child who has recently undergone tonsillectomy, the nurse should be aware that the child should be discouraged from:
   1. Talking.
   2. Blowing the nose.
   3. Eating flavored ice pops.
   4. Taking pain medication.

2. The MD has recommended frequent baths for hydration for a child with eczema. Following each bath, the nurse should:

1. Apply a light coating of emollient to the child's skin while it is still wet.
2. Dry the skin thoroughly and apply baby powder.
3. Dry the skin thoroughly and leave it exposed to the air.
4. Apply a dilute solution of 1 part hydrogen peroxide mixed with 9 parts normal saline.

3. While caring for a child with otitis media, the nurse has heard numerous complaints about the severe pain the child is experiencing. However, the parent calls the nurse to report that suddenly the child has no pain at all. What action should the nurse advice the parent to take at this time?

1. Continue giving the ordered antibiotic.
2. Check the child's temperature.
3. Look at the ear for any drainage.
4. Bring the child to the clinic for further evaluation immediately.

4. Which statement is most therapeutic for the nurse to offer to the family of a child who has just died?

1. "You should feel relieved that at least your child is not suffering now."
2. "I know how sad you must be feeling now."
3. "We did everything we could. I'm very sorry we could not save your child."
4. "At least you are young enough to try to have another baby."

5. The nurse should be aware that preschoolers typically think of death as:

1. Something that makes their parents worried or sad.
2. Going away to a place where the dead person still breathes, eats, and sleeps.
3. The grim reaper, the devil, or a boogeyman.
4. The irreversible end of life as it is generally known.

6. A preschooler has head lice and must have her head shampooed with a pediculicide that must remain on the scalp and hair for several minutes. How could the nurse best gain this child's cooperation during the necessary treatment?

1. Offer the child a reward for good behavior during the treatment.
2. Inform the child that her parents will be notified if she fails to cooperate during the treatment.
3. Allow the child to apply her own shampoo.
4. Make a game of the treatment, such as "Beauty Parlor."

7. In assessing for parasites, the nurse should recognize that a classic behavior associated with the young child who has pinworms is:

1. Complaints of intense perianal itching.
2. General irritability.
3. Poor sleep pattern.
4. Short attention span.

8. The nurse instructs the parents of a child with pinworms of the need for a specimen, which is collected by:

1. Venipuncture.
2. Stool culture and sensitivity.
3. Transparent tape test.
4. Urine specimen.

9. Which procedure, performed by parents of an infant with infantile eczema, would lead the nurse to realize that additional health teaching is necessary?

1. Frequent colloid baths.
2. Topical steroid applications to affected areas.
3. Avoidance of wool clothing.
4. Applications of alcohol to crusted areas.

10. When assessing a child who is preverbal for otitis media, the nurse should anticipate that the child will:

1. Have difficulty swallowing.
2. Rub the affected side of the head on the mattress.
3. Have a runny nose.
4. Have vomiting and diarrhea.

11. The nurse's health care teaching to assist parents in preventing otitis media should include instructions to:

1. Finish the entire prescription of antibiotics.
2. Administer acetaminophen to reduce ear pain.
3. Apply warm compresses to the affected ear.
4. Refrain from putting the child to bed with a bottle of milk.

12. In which type of poisonings should the nurse question orders to induce vomiting?

1. Aspirin.
2. Acetaminophen.
3. Iron tablets.
4. Drain cleanser.

13. A 10-year-old child takes an overdose of acetaminophen. The nurse prepares to administer the antidote acetylcysteine to the child, but the child refuses to take the medication because it smells like "rotten eggs." The nurse's first action should be to:

1. Notify the pediatrician regarding the child's refusal to take the medication.
2. Instruct the child to pinch the nose to avoid smelling the medication as he swallows it.
3. Mix the medication in a carbonated beverage and attempt to readminister it to the child.
4. Telephone the pediatrician to request another antidote.

14. When caring for a child who has had a tonsillectomy, the nurse's priority observation should be for:

1. "Coffee ground " emesis.
2. Frequent swallowing.
3. Complaints of sore throat.
4. A slight increase in temperature.

15. When planning activities for a school-age child with Down syndrome, the nurse should:
    1. Speak loudly and clearly to help the child understand what is going to happen.
    2. Involve the parents but not the child who is cognitively impaired.
    3. Gear the activities to the child's developmental, not chronologic, age.
    4. Anticipate that the child will not willingly engage in planned activities.

Answers/Rationale

1. (2) Following a tonsillectomy, the child should be discouraged from coughing frequently, clearing the throat, or blowing the nose, which could irritate the operative site and cause bleeding. The child *can* certainly speak in a normal tone of voice (1). The child *should* be offered cool, clear liquids or ice pops (3) that are not red (to avoid any confusion about possible hemorrhage). The child's throat will be very sore after surgery and pain medication ordered by the MD *should* be given (4). **IMP, APP, 1, PhI, Reduction of risk potential**

2. (1) When a child with eczema is treated with frequent baths for hydration, the nurse should apply an emollient preparation to moist, damp skin. The skin should *not* be dried thoroughly (2, 3) because the purpose of the bath is hydration of the skin. Powder (2) further dries skin. Applying peroxide (4) would be painful and *not* therapeutic after a bath. **IMP, COM, 1, PhI, Basic care and comfort**

3. (3) The child whose ear drum has ruptured frequently presents with a sudden cessation of pain, perhaps accompanied by a decrease in fever. The caregiver should look at the external auditory canal and note the presence (or possible absence) of any purulent drainage, which would need to be gently cleansed away. The child should obviously finish all medication the MD has ordered, but in this case continuing the antibiotic (1) would be inadequate; the nurse needs to know whether the eardrum has ruptured. The child's temperature should continue to be monitored (2), and it may take a while for fever to drop; the nurse needs to know whether the eardrum has ruptured. There is no reason to hurry the child to the clinic (4) because this is *not an emergency*, although the child will need long-term followup for possible hearing loss. **EV, ANL, 2, PhI, Reduction of risk potential**

4. (3) At the time of death, it is appropriate for the nurse to express personal feelings of loss or frustration through this kind of statement. It is *not* appropriate or therapeutic for the nurse to offer rationalizations regarding the child's death (1) or to offer trite, artificial consolation (2, 4). **IMP, APP, 7, PsI, Psychosocial integrity**

5. (2) Preschoolers have usually heard the word "death" and often view it as a leaving or departure of a person from this world to another in which the dead person carries on all the usual living activities such as breathing, eating, and sleeping. *Toddlers* conceptualize death as something that primarily affects their parents' mood (1). *School-age* children typically personify death (3), and *adolescents* have a realistic understanding of death (4). **AN, APP, 5, PsI, Psychosocial integrity**

6. (4) Preschoolers enjoy games that mimic adult behaviors or occupations, so the child would be most receptive to the idea of playing "Beauty Parlor." Depending on the pediculicide used, the treatment may have to be repeated in 7-10 days to kill hatching nymphs; therefore, offers of rewards (1) can become costly and may not capture the child's cooperation. Rewards are never a totally appropriate means of gaining a child's cooperation. Threatening the child with informing her parents (2) regarding poor behavior only further stresses a child who is already traumatized. Since pediculicides are irritating if they come in contact with the child's eyes, the child should not be allowed to independently apply the shampoo (3). **IMP, APP, 7, HPM, Health promotion and maintenance**

7. (1) Intense perianal itching is the principal symptom of pinworm infection in a young child. The itching is due to the movement of the pinworms on skin and mucous membrane surfaces. General irritability (2), poor sleep pattern (3), and short attention span (4) are not usual behaviors associated with pinworms in a young child; these behaviors may be cues in a *toddler*, who cannot describe the perianal itching that is being experienced. **AS, COM, 1, PhI, Physiological adaptation**

8. (3) The transparent tape test involves placing a loop of the tape (sticky side out) against the child's perianal area and examining the tape under a microscope. The test should be performed as soon as the child awakens (pinworms migrate to the perianal area seeking warmth as the internal body temperature cools during sleep) and before evidence is lost via a bowel movement or bath. Venipuncture

---

Key to Codes

Nursing process: AS, assessment; **AN**, analysis; **PL**, planning; **IMP**, implementation; **EV**, evaluation. (See **Appendix L** for explanation of nursing process steps.)

Cognitive level: RE/KN, recall/knowledge; **COM**, comprehension; **APP**, application; **ANL**, analysis; **EVL**, evaluation; **SYN**, synthesis. (See **Appendix L** for explanation.)

Category of human function: 1, protective; **2**, sensory-perceptual; **3**, comfort, rest, activity, and mobility; **4**, nutrition; **5**, growth and development; **6**, fluid-gas transport; **7**, psychosocial-cultural; **8**, elimination. (See **Appendix N** for explanation.)

Client need: SECE, safe, effective care environment; **HPM**, health promotion and maintenance; **PsI**, psychosocial integrity; **PhI**, physiological integrity. (See **Appendix O** for explanation.)

Client subneed: See **Appendix O** for explanation.

(1), stool specimen (2), and urine specimen (4) are *not* appropriate collection techniques for a pinworm sample. **IMP, COM, 1, PhI, Reduction of risk potential**

9. (4) Drying agents, such as alcohol, must be avoided because they may intensify the itching associated with infantile eczema. Frequent colloid baths (1), such as cornstarch added to bath water; topical steroid applications (2) to decrease inflammation; and avoidance of wool clothing (3), which can potentiate itching, *are* appropriate treatment modalities in the management of infantile eczema. **EV, APP, 1, PhI, Pharmacological and parenteral therapies**

10. (2) Children who are preverbal rub the affected ear or shake their heads from side to side. Older children will verbalize complaints of ear pain or ache. Pain is caused by pressure on surrounding structures and is the *priority* assessment associated with otitis media. Difficulty swallowing (1), a runny nose/rhinorrhea (3), and vomiting and diarrhea (4) are *secondary* assessment criteria associated with otitis media. **AS, ANL, 1, PhI, Physiological adaptation**

11. (4) Instructions to refrain from putting the child to bed with a bottle of milk is a *preventive* nursing intervention for otitis media. This action prevents fluid from draining via the eustachian tube to the middle ear during swallowing. Instructions to finish the antibiotics (1), reduce the pain (2), and apply warm compresses to the affected ear (3) *are* appropriate nursing interventions *during* the course of the active infection. **IMP, ANL, 1, HPM, Health promotion and maintenance**

12. (4) Corrosives, such as toilet and drain cleansers, cause damage when they initially enter the esophagus and again when they are passed through the esophagus in the form of vomitus. Therefore, vomiting would be contraindicated. Water is usually given orally to dilute and neutralize the corrosive substance. As long as the child is alert and able to swallow, vomiting would not be harmful in toxic ingestions of aspirin (1), acetaminophen (2), and iron (3). **IMP, COM, 1, SECE, Management of care**

13. (3) Mixing acetylcysteine in a carbonated beverage helps decrease the objectionable smell of the medication and makes it more palatable. Should this intervention fail, the offensive medication may have to be administered via a nasogastric tube. The physician should be notified of the child's refusal to take the medication (1) only if the child continues to refuse to cooperate in spite of being offered the carbonated beverage mixture. Pinching off the nose (2) is *insufficient* to avoid the odor of the medication. Acetylcysteine is the *only* available antidote for acetaminophen poisoning (4). **IMP, ANL, 1, PhI, Pharmacological and parenteral therapies**

14. (2) Hemorrhage from the surgical site is a priority concern following a tonsillectomy; excessive swallowing indicates that blood is trickling down the child's throat. Tachycardia, pallor, and excessive swallowing are critical postoperative assessments for a child who has undergone a tonsillectomy. Dark brown or "coffee ground" emesis (1) indicates a vomitus of *old blood*, which is *anticipated* postoperatively. Bright red blood is a cause for concern. A sore throat (3) is *expected* and can usually be controlled with oral acetaminophen and codeine. A slight increase in temperature (4) is *normal* in most postoperative tonsillectomy clients. These children will receive acetaminophen and antibiotics for the fever. **AS, ANL, 1, PhI, Physiological adaptation**

15. (3) Activities must be directed toward what the child can do developmentally. The child with Down syndrome is not hearing-impaired, so the nurse does *not* need to speak loudly (1) to be understood. The interaction with the child must instead be on a level that the child is capable of understanding. Most children with Down syndrome are "moderately retarded," and are capable of being involved in planning their activities (2). Children with Down syndrome tend to be "easy" children who participate willingly (4), and who do *not* present difficulties to their caregivers. **PL, APP, 5, HPM, Health promotion and maintenance**

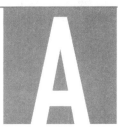

Common Acronyms and Abbreviations

This list provides a review of **over 200 need-to-know acronyms and abbreviations** used in charting, verbal communication/directives, and study guides.

a	Before (*ante*)
Ab	Antibody; abortion
Abd	Abdomen; abdominal
ABG	Arterial blood gas
ac	Before meals (*ante cibum*)
ADH	Antidiuretic hormone
ADHD	Attention deficit hyperactivity disorder
ad lib	As much as desired (*ad libitum*)
ADLs	Activities of daily living
AFB	Acid-fast bacillus
Afib	Atrial fibrillation
Aflutter	Atrial flutter
AG	Antigen
AIDS	Acquired immunodeficiency syndrome
A-K (AKA)	Above-the-knee amputation
ALL	Acute lymphocytic (lymphoblastic) leukemia
AMA	Against medical advice
A&O x 3	Alert, oriented to person, place, time
AP	Anteroposterior; alkaline phosphatase
APSGN	Acute post streptoccoal glomerulonephritis
ARC	AIDS-related complex
ARF	Acute renal failure
ASA	Acetylsalicylic acid (aspirin)
ASAP	As soon as possible
ASD	Atrial septal defect
AV	Atrioventricular; arteriovenous; aortic valve
AVB	Atrioventricular block
AVM	Arteriovenous malformation
bid	Twice daily (*bis in die*)
BKA	Below-the-knee amputation
BM	Bowel movement/bone marrow
BMR	Basal metabolic rate
BP	Blood pressure
BPM	Beats per minute
BUN	Blood urea nitrogen
c	With (*cum*)
CA	Carcinoma; cancer
CBC	Complete blood count
CCU	Cardiac (intensive) care unit
CF	Cystic fibrosis
CHD	Congenital heart disease
CHF	Congestive heart failure (see HF)
CMV	Cytomegalovirus
CNA	Certified Nursing Assistant
CNS	Central nervous system; coagulase-negative staphylococcus

CNS	Clinical nurse specialist
C/O	Complains of
COA	Coarctation of aorta
COPD	Chronic obstructive pulmonary disease
CP	Cerebral palsy
CPK	Creatine phosphokinase (now *creatine kinase* [CK])
CPR	Cardiopulmonary resuscitation
CRF	Chronic renal failure; cardiac risk factors
CRP	C-reactive protein
C&S	Culture & sensitivity
CSF	Cerebrospinal fluid
CVA	Cerebrovascular accident (now *stroke*, *brain attack*); costovertebral angle
CVP	Central venous pressure
Δ	Change (Greek letter delta)
D&D	Dehydration & diarrhea
Dig	Digitalis
DM	Diabetes mellitus (also called **DBM**)
DOB	Date of birth
DOE	Dyspnea on exertion
DPT	Diphtheria, pertussis, and tetanus
DRG	Diagnosis-related group
DTR	Deep tendon reflex
D_5W	5% dextrose in water
Dx	Diagnosis
ECG	Electrocardiogram
Echo	Echocardiogram
ED	Emergency department
EEG	Electroencephalogram
EKG	Electrocardiogram (common version)
EMG	Electromyogram
EMT	Emergency medical technician
ENT	Ear, nose, and throat
ER	Emergency room (now called *Emergency department*)
ESR	Erythrocyte sedimentation rate
ETOH	Alcohol (ethanol)
FBS	Fasting blood sugar
FEV_1	Forced expiratory volume in 1 second
FRC	Functional residual capacity
FTT	Failure to thrive
FUO	Fever of unknown origin
FVC	Forced vital capacity
g	Gram
GB	Gallbladder
GC	Gonococcus; gonorrhea
GI	Gastrointestinal

GTT	Glucose tolerance test
gtt(s)	Drop(s) (*guttae*)
GU	Genitourinary
HBV	Hepatitis B virus
HCG	Human chorionic gonadotropin
Hct	Hematocrit
HEENT	Head, eyes, ears, nose, throat
HF	Heart failure
HgbA$_{1c}$	Glycosylated hemoglobin
HIV	Human immunodeficiency virus
HMO	Health maintenance organization
HOB	Head of bed
HR	Heart rate
Hx	History
ICP	Intracranial pressure
ICU	Intensive care unit
I&D	Incision and drainage
IDDM	Insulin-dependent diabetes mellitus
Ig	Immunoglobulin
IM	Intramuscular
INH	Isoniazid
I&O	Intake and output
IPPB	Intermittent positive pressure breathing
IQ	Intelligence quotient
IV	Intravenous
IVC	Inferior vena cava
IVP	Intravenous pyelogram; intravenous push
JIA	Juvenile idiopathic arthritis
KD	Kawasaki's disease
KUB	Kidneys, ureters, bladder (flat/upright abdominal x-ray)
L&B	Laryngoscopy & bronchoscopy
L-C-P	Legg-Calvé-Perthes disease
LFTs	Liver function tests
LGIs	Lower GI series
LLL	Left lower (lung) lobe
LLQ	Left lower quadrant
LOC	Loss of consciousness; level of consciousness
LPN/LVN	Licensed practical nurse; licensed vocational nurse
LUL	Left upper (lung) lobe
LUQ	Left upper quadrant
MAP	Mean arterial pressure
MCL	Midclavicular line
Med	Medication
MMR	Measles, mumps, rubella
MOM	Milk of magnesia
Mono	Mononucleosis
MR	Mitral regurgitation; mental retardation
MRI	Magnetic resonance imaging
MS	Mental status; mitral stenosis; multiple sclerosis; morphine sulfate

NA	Not applicable
NG	Nasogastric
NIDDM	Non-insulin-dependent diabetes mellitus
NL	Normal
NOC	Night (nocturnal)
NPH	Neutral-protamine-hagedorn (intermediate-acting insulin)
NPO	Nothing by mouth (*nil per os*)
NS	Normal saline
NSAID	Nonsteroidal anti-inflammatory drug
NSR	Normal sinus rhythm
N/V	Nausea, vomiting
NVD	Nausea, vomiting, diarrhea
O$_2$	Oxygen
OM	Otitis media
OOB	Out of bed; out of breath
O&P	Ova and parasites
OR	Operating room
P	Para; pulse
p	Post (after)
PA	Posterior-anterior; physician's assistant; pulmonary artery
PAO$_2$	Alveolar oxygen pressure
PaO$_2$	Arterial partial pressure of oxygen
PAS	Para-aminosalicylic acid
PAT	Paroxysmal atrial tachycardia
pc	After meals (*post cibum*)
PCA	Patient-controlled analgesia (pump); patient care assistant
PCP	*Pneumocystis carinii* pneumonia; phencyclidine
PDA	Patent ductus arteriosus
PEEP	Positive end-expiratory pressure
PERRL(A)	Pupils equally round and reactive to light (and accommodation)
pH	Hydrogen ion concentration
PICU	Pediatric intensive care unit
PKU	Phenylketonuria
PMI	Point of maximum impulse
PO	By mouth (*per os*)
PPD	Purified protein derivative (TB skin test); percussion and postural drainage
PPO	Preferred provider organization
prn	When necessary (*pro re nata*)
Pt	Patient
PT	Prothrombin time; physical therapy
PTA	Prior to admission
PTT	Partial thromboplastin time
PVC	Premature ventricular contraction
q	Each, every (*quaque*)
qid	Four times a day (*quarter in die*)
R	Respirations
RA	Rheumatoid arthritis; right atrium
RBC	Red blood cell
RDS	Respiratory disease syndrome
RHD	Rheumatic heart disease
RLL	Right lower (lung) lobe

RLQ	Right lower quadrant		**TGV**	Transposition of great vessels
RML	Right middle (lung) lobe		**tid**	Three times a day (*ter in die*)
R/O	Rule out		**TKO**	To keep open
ROM	Range of motion		**TLC**	Total lung capacity; tender loving care
ROS	Review of systems		**TOF**	Tetralogy of Fallot
RUL	Right upper (lung) lobe		**TPN**	Total parenteral nutrition
RUQ	Right upper quadrant		**TPR**	Temperature, pulse, respirations
Rx	Prescription; therapy		**TSH**	Thyroid-stimulating hormone
			TV	Total volume; tidal volume
s	Without (*sine*)		**Tx**	Treatment
S_1	First heart sound			
S_2	Second heart sound		**UA**	Urinalysis
S_3	Third heart sound		**UGI**	Upper gastrointestinal series
S_4	Fourth heart sound		**UQ**	Upper quadrant
SBE	Subacute bacterial endocarditis		**URI**	Upper respiratory infection
SGA	Small for gestational age		**UTI**	Urinary tract infection
SIADH	Syndrome of inappropriate antidiuretic hormone		**UV**	Ultraviolet
SICU	Surgical intensive care unit			
SIDS	Sudden infant death syndrome		**VC**	Vital capacity
SL	Sublingually		**VCUG**	Voiding cystourethogram
SLE	Systemic lupus erythematosus		**Vfib (VF)**	Ventricular fibrillation
SOB	Short(ness) of breath		**VS**	Vital signs
SR	Sinus rhythm		**VSD**	Ventricular septal defect
S/S	Signs, symptoms			
Stat	Immediately (*statim*)		**WBC**	White blood count; white blood cells
STD	Sexually transmitted disease		**WNL**	Within normal limits
Sx	Symptoms		**w/o**	Without
T	Temperature			
T&A	Tonsillectomy and adenoidectomy			
TB	Tuberculosis			

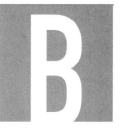

Quick Guide to Common Clinical Signs

Many clinical signs have been named for the physicians who first described them or the phenomena they resemble. The following is a list of **25 of the most common clinical signs**, for use as a quick reference as you review.

Babinski reflex   dorsiflexion of the big toe after stimulation of the lateral sole; normal 6 months of age; associated with *corticospinal tract lesions.*

Barlow test   *developmental hip dysplasia* is present if the femoral head moves into or out of the back of the acetabulum when pressure is applied from the front.

Blumberg's sign   transient pain in the abdomen after approximated fingers pressed gently into abdominal wall are suddenly withdrawn—rebound tenderness; associated with *peritoneal inflammation.*

Brudzinski's sign   flexion of the hip and knee induced by flexion of the neck; associated with *meningeal irritation.*

Brushfield spots   speckling of the iris; associated with *Down syndrome.*

Cheyne-Stokes respiration   rhythmic cycles of deep and shallow respiration, often with apneic periods; associated with *central nervous system respiratory center dysfunction.*

Chvostek's sign   facial muscle spasm induced by tapping on the facial nerve branches; associated with *hypocalcemia.*

Coppernail's sign   ecchymoses on the perineum, scrotum, or labia; associated with *fracture of the pelvis.*

Cullen's sign   bluish discoloration of the umbilicus; associated with *acute pancreatitis* or *hemoperitoneum,* especially *rupture of fallopian tube in ectopic pregnancy.*

Doll's eye sign   dissociation between the movements of the head and eyes: as the head is raised, the eyes are lowered, and as the head is lowered, the eyes are raised; associated with global-diffuse disorders of the *cerebrum;* also seen in normal newborns.

Fluid wave   transmission across the abdomen of a wave induced by snapping the abdomen; associated with *ascites.*

Goldstein's sign   wide distance between the great toe and the adjoining toe; associated with *cretinism and trisomy* 21.

Harlequin sign   in the newborn infant, reddening of the lower half of the laterally recumbent body and blanching of the upper half, due to a *temporary vasomotor disturbance.*

Kehr's sign   severe pain in the left upper quadrant, radiating to the top of the shoulder; associated with *splenic rupture.*

Kernig's sign   inability to extend leg when sitting or lying with the thigh flexed on the abdomen; associated with *meningeal irritation.*

Knie's sign   unequal dilatation of the pupils; associated with *Graves's disease.*

Kussmaul's respiration   paroxysmal air hunger; associated with acidosis, especially *diabetic ketoacidosis.*

McBurney's sign   tenderness at McBurney's point (located two-thirds of the distance from the umbilicus to the anterior-superior iliac spine); associated with *appendicitis.*

Ortolani's (click) sign   "click" sound sometimes heard if *hip dysplasia* is present; on assessment, head of femur can be felt (or heard as a click) to slip forward in acetabulum and slip back when pressure is released and legs returned to their original position.

Osler's sign   small painful erythematous swellings in the skin of the hands and feet; associated with *bacterial endocarditis.*

Psoas sign   pain induced by hyperextension of the right thigh while lying on the left side; associated with *appendicitis.*

Setting-sun sign   downward deviation of the eyes so that each iris appears to "set" beneath the lower lid, with white sclera exposed between it and the upper lid; associated with *increased intracranial pressure* or irritation of the *brainstem;* sometimes seen in normal infants.

Simian crease   transverse palmar crease; associated with *Down syndrome.*

Trendelenburg sign   when the child bears weight on the affected hip, the pelvis tilts downward on the unaffected side instead of upward; associated with *developmental dysplasia of the hip.*

Williamson's sign   markedly diminished blood pressure in the leg as compared with that in the arm on the same side; associated with *pneumothorax* and *pleural effusions.*

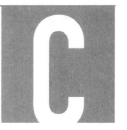
For a quick review, use this index to locate **55 selected diagnostic tests and procedures** covered in this book as they relate to specific conditions.

Test/Procedure	Condition/Situation	Page(s)
Arthrography	Developmental dysplasia of the hip (DDH)	153
Barium enema	Intussusception	69, 73, 79
Barlow test	DDH	153
Biopsy	Brain tumors	109
Blood tests:		
Acetaminophen levels	Poisoning	171, 179, 187
Aso titer	Acute poststreptococcal glomerulonephritis (APSGN)	88, 90
	Rheumatic fever (RF)	59
C-reactive protein	RF	59
Clotting	Acetaminophen poisoning	171, 179
Digoxin level, serum	Congenital heart disease (CHD)	62, 63
Enzymes (liver)	Acetaminophen poisoning	171, 179
Glucose, blood	Diabetes	76, 77
	Hypoglycemia	77
Hepatic function	Acetaminophen poisoning	171, 179
Latex fixation	Juvenile idiopathic arthritis (JIA)	130, 134
Lead levels, serum	Lead poisoning	118
Phenytoin levels, serum	Seizures (bacterial meningitis)	122
Rheumatoid factor	JIA	130, 134
Salicylate level, serum	Salicylate poisoning	119
Bone marrow aspiration	Ewing sarcoma	107
	Leukemia	111
Cardiac catheterization	CHD	58, 63
Cardiopneumogram	Apnea of infancy	45
CT scan	Bone tumors	107
	Brain tumors	109
	DDH	153
	Hydrocephalus	150
	Osteomyelitis	127
Cerebral angiography	Brain tumors	109
Cerebrospinal tap	Guillain-Barré syndrome (GBS)	142
Culture and sensitivity	Antibiotic medication	128, 133
Culture, throat	RF	59
	Scarlet fever	178
ECG	CHD	58
	Kawasaki's disease	61
	RF	59

Test/Procedure	Condition/Situation	Page(s)
Echocardiogram	CHD	58
	Kawasaki's disease	61
EEG	Seizures	117
EMG	Duchenne muscular dystrophy	141
	GBS	142
Glucose tolerance	Diabetes	76, 77
Gluten challenge	Celiac disease	74
Hemoglobin electrophoresis	Sickle cell anemia (SCA)	96
IVP	Wilms' tumor	109
Jejunal biopsy	Celiac disease	74
MRI	Brain tumors	109
	Legg-Calvé-Perthes disease	128
	Osteomyelitis	127
	Scoliosis	131
	Seizures	117
Muscle biopsy	Duchenne muscular dystrophy	141
Ortolani test	DDH	153, 160
Peak expiratory flow rate	Asthma	44
Pneumocardiogram	Apnea of infancy	45
Polysomnography	Apnea of infancy	45
Pulmonary function tests	Chemotherapy agents (e.g. bleomycin)	110
Scoliometer	Scoliosis	131
Sickledex	SCA	96
Spinal tap (lumbar puncture)	Bacterial meningitis	116
	Brain tumors	109
Stool:		
Culture	Acute gastric enteritis (AGE)	71
	Celiac disease	74
	Cystic fibrosis	40
Occult blood	Acetaminophen poisoning	179
	Hormones	110
	Reye syndrome	121
Pinworms	Infestation (pinworms)	180
Sweat test	Cystic fibrosis	40, 51
Trendelenburg sign	DDH	153
Ultrasound	Clubfoot	152
	DDH	153
Upper GI series	Pyloric stenosis	70
Urine:		
Blood	APSGN	88
	Salicylate poisoning	119
Culture	Urinary tract infections	89, 90
Protein	APSGN	88
Specific gravity	Acetaminophen poisoning	179
	AGE	71

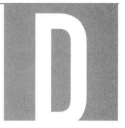 Laboratory Values

Use this chart as a quick overview of lab values: both normal and conditions that result in *high* or *low* values. Terms in **bold** identify **common** occurrences in **children and adolescents**.

Test	Normal Values	Possible Significance	
		Increases	*Decreases*
HEMATOLOGY			
Aspartate aminotransferase (AST)—*formerly* called serum glutamic oxaloacetic transaminase (SGOT)	*Men*: 10-40 U/L *Women*: 9-25 U/L **Newborns**: 2-3 times higher	**Reye syndrome**, myocardial infarction, cardiac surgery, hepatitis, cirrhosis, trauma, **severe burns**, progressive muscular dystrophy, infectious mononucleosis, **acute renal failure**.	Uremia, chronic dialysis, ketoacidosis.
Bleeding time—indication of hemostatic efficiency	1-9 min	Hemorrhagic purpura, **acute leukemia**, aplastic anemia, DIC, oral anticoagulant therapy.	
Hematocrit—volume of packed red blood cells per 100 mL of blood	*Men*: 45% (38-54%) *Women*: 40% (36-47%) **Children**: same as adult after age 8-13 yr	**Dehydration**, polycythemia, **congenital heart disease**.	**Anemia, hemorrhage, leukemia, dietary deficiencies**.
Hemoglobin—oxygen-combining protein	*Men*: 14-18 g/dL *Women*: 12-16 g/dL **Children**: same as adult by age 8-13 yr	See hematocrit.	See hematocrit.
Partial thromboplastin time (PTT)—tests coagulation mechanism; stage I deficiencies	*APTT*: 30-40 secs *PTT*: 60-70 secs **Newborn**: higher	**Deficiency** of factors VIII, IX, X, XI, XII; **anticoagulant therapy**.	Extensive cancer, DIC.
Platelets—thrombocytes	150,000-400,000/mm³ **Newborn**: lower	Polycythemia, postsplenectomy, **anemia**.	**Leukemia**, aplastic anemia, cirrhosis, multiple myeloma, **chemotherapy**.
Prothrombin time—tests extrinsic clotting; stages **II** and **III**	11-15 sec **Newborn**: higher	**Anticoagulant** therapy, DIC, hepatic disease, **malabsorption**.	**Digitalis** therapy, diuretic reaction, **vitamin K therapy**.
Red blood cell count—number of circulating erythrocytes per cubic millimeter (mm³) of whole blood	*Men*: 4.5–6.2 million/mm³ *Women*: 4.0–5.5 million/mm³ **Newborn**: *high*; lower by 1 yr **Children**: same as adult by age 8-13 yr	Polycythemia vera, anoxia, **dehydration**.	**Leukemia, hemorrhage, anemias, Hodgkin's disease**.
Sedimentation rate—speed at which red blood cells settle in uncoagulated blood	*Men*: 0-15 mm/h *Women*: 0-20 mm/h **Newborn/children**: slower	Acute bacterial infection, cancer, **infectious disease**, numerous inflammatory states.	Polycythemia vera, **sickle cell anemia**.

Test	Normal Values	Possible Significance	
		Increases	Decreases
White blood cell count—number of leukocytes in 1 mm³	5000-10,000 mm³ **Newborn**: *extremely high*	**Leukemia, bacterial** infection, severe sepsis.	Viral infection, overwhelming bacterial infection, **lupus erythematosus**, antineoplastic **chemotherapy.**
White blood cell differential—enumeration of individual leukocyte distribution			
Neutrophils	55-70%	**Bacterial infection**, tumor, **inflammation**, stress, drug reaction, trauma, metabolic disorders.	**Acute viral** infection, **anorexia nervosa**, radiation therapy, drug-induced, alcoholic ingestion.
Eosinophils	1-4%	Allergic disorder, **parasitic** infestation, **eosinophilic leukemia.**	Acute or chronic stress; excess ACTH, cortisone, or epinephrine; endocrine disorder.
Basophils	0-1%	Myeloproliferative disease, **leukemia.**	**Anaphylactic** reaction, hyperthyroidism, radiation therapy, **infections.**
Lymphocytes	20-40%	**Chronic lymphocytic leukemia**, infectious mononucleosis, chronic bacterial infection, **viral infection.**	**Leukemia**, systemic **lupus erythematosus**, immune deficiency disorders.
BLOOD CHEMISTRY **Alkaline phosphatase (ALP)**	30-85 U/mL **Infants, children**: 1.6-2.6 times adult level **Puberty**: 6-7 times adult level	Hyperparathyroidism, Paget's disease, cancer with bone metastasis, obstructive jaundice, cirrhosis, infectious hepatitis, **rickets.**	Malnutrition, scurvy, **celiac disease**, chronic nephritis, **hypothyroidism, cystic fibrosis.**
Amylase	53-123 U/L **Children**: 25-125 U/L **Newborn**: 5-65 or absent	Acute pancreatitis, **mumps**, duodenal ulcer, pancreatic cancer, perforated bowel, **renal failure.**	Advanced chronic pancreatitis, chronic alcoholism.
Bilirubin, serum	*Direct*: 0.1-0.3 mg/dL *Indirect*: 0.2-0.8 mg/dL *Total*: 0.1-1.0 mg/dL *Newborn*: higher until age 1 mo	Massive hemolysis, low-grade hemolytic disease, cirrhosis, obstructive liver disease, hepatitis, biliary obstruction, **erythroblastosis fetalis.**	
Calcium, serum	9-10.5 mg/dL, or 4.5-5.6 mg/dL, ionized **Newborn**: lower **Children**: slightly higher	Hyperparathyroidism, multiple myeloma, bone metastasis, bone fracture, thiazide-diuretic reaction, milk-alkali syndrome.	Hypoparathyroidism, **renal failure**, pregnancy, massive transfusion.
Carbon dioxide	24-30 mEq/L **Infants/children**: lower	Emphysema, **salicylate toxicity, vomiting.**	Starvation, **diarrhea.**

		Possible Significance	
Test	*Normal Values*	*Increases*	*Decreases*
Chloride, serum	90-110 mEq/L	Hyperventilation, diabetes insipidus, uremia.	Heart failure, **pyloric obstruction,** hypoventilation, **vomiting,** chronic respiratory acidosis.
Cholesterol (total serum)	<200 mg/dL **Children:** lower	Hypercholesterolemia, hyperlipidemia, myocardial infarction, uncontrolled diabetes mellitus, high cholesterol diet, atherosclerosis, stress, **glomerulonephritis** (nephrotic stage), familial.	**Malnutrition,** cholesterol-lowering medication, **anemia,** liver disease, hyperthyroidism.
Creatinine, serum	*Men:* 0.6-1.2 mg/dL *Women:* 0.5-1.1 mg/dL **Children:** lower	Chronic **glomerulonephritis,** nephritis, **heart failure,** muscle disease.	Debilitation.
Creatine kinase (CK) (Creatine phosphokinase [CPK])	*Men:* 12-70 U/mL (55-170 U/L) *Women:* 10-55 U/mL (30-135 U/L) **Newborn:** higher	Acute myocardial infarction, acute stroke, **convulsions,** surgery, **muscular dystrophy,** hypokalemia, **birth trauma.**	
Isoenzymes: CPK-MM/CK-MM:	100%	**Muscular dystrophy,** delirium tremens, surgery, hypokalemia, crush injuries, **hypothyroidism.**	
CPK-MB/CK-MB	0%	Acute myocardial infarction, cardiac defibrillation, myocarditis, cardiac ischemia.	
CPK-BB/CK-BB	0%	Pulmonary infarction, brain surgery, stroke, pulmonary embolism, **seizures,** intestinal ischemia.	
Fibrinogen, serum	0.2-0.4 g/100 dL or 200-400 mg/dL **Newborn:** lower	**Pneumonia,** acute infection, **nephrosis,** rheumatoid arthritis.	Cirrhosis, toxic liver necrosis, **anemia,** obstetric complications, DIC, advanced carcinoma.
Glucose (fasting)	80-120 mg/dL **Newborn/children:** lower	Acute stress, Cushing's syndrome, hyperthyroidism, acute or chronic pancreatitis, **diabetes mellitus, hyperglycemia.**	Addison's disease, liver disease, reactive **hypoglycemia,** pituitary hypofunction.
Glycosylated hemoglobin (HbA$_1$c)	4.0-7.0%	**Newly diagnosed or poorly controlled diabetes mellitus.**	
Iron-binding capacity (total)	25-420 mcg/L	**Lead poisoning,** hepatic necrosis.	**Iron deficiency anemia,** chronic blood loss.

| | | Possible Significance | |
| | | Increases | Decreases |
Test	Normal Values		
Lactic dehydrogenase (LDH)	*Adult*: 40-90 U/L **Newborn:** very *high* **Children:** 60-170 U/L LDH-1: 17-27% LDH-2: 27-37% LDH-3: 18-25% LDH-4: 3-8% LDH-5: 0-5%	Myocardial infarction, hemolytic and macrolytic anemias, **leukemia**, shock, trauma, **non-Hodgkin's lymphoma**, PCP.	
Phosphorus, inorganic, serum	3.0-4.5 mg/dL **Newborn:** highest **Adolescents:** decline	Chronic glomerular disease, hypoparathyroidism, milk-alkali syndrome, sarcoidosis.	Hyperparathyroidism, **rickets**, osteomalacia, renal tubular necrosis, **malabsorption** syndrome, vitamin D deficiency.
Potassium, serum	3.5-5.0 mEq/L **Newborn:** slightly higher	**Diabetic ketosis, renal failure**, Addison's disease, excessive intake.	Thiazide diuretics, Cushing's syndrome, cirrhosis with ascites, hyperaldosteronism, steroid therapy, malignant hypertension, poor dietary habits, chronic diarrhea, diaphoresis, renal tubular necrosis, **malabsorption syndrome, vomiting.**
Protein, serum (albumin/globulin)	*Total*: 6.4-8.3 g/dL **Children:** slightly lower *Albumin*: 3.5-5.0 g/dL *Globulin*: 2.3-3.5 g/dL	**Dehydration**, multiple myeloma.	Chronic liver disease, myeloproliferative disease, **burns.**
Sodium, serum	138-144 mEq/L	Increased intake, either orally or IV; Cushing's, **excessive sweating**, diabetes insipidus.	Addison's disease, sodium-losing nephropathy, **vomiting, diarrhea**, fistulas, tube drainage, **burns**, renal insufficiency with acidosis, starvation with acidosis, paracentesis, thoracentesis, ascites, **heart failure, SIADH.**
T_3 uptake	24-34%	**Hyperthyroidism**, thyroxine-binding globulin (TBG) deficiency.	**Hypothyroidism**, pregnancy, TBG excess.
Thyroxine	5-12 mcg/dL	**Hyperthyroidism.**	**Hypothyroidism, renal failure.**
Serum glutamic oxaloacetic transaminase (SGOT)— *see* AST			
Urea nitrogen, serum (BUN)	10-20 mg/dL **Newborn/infant:** lower	**Acute or chronic renal failure**, heart failure, obstructive uropathy, **dehydration.**	Cirrhosis, malnutrition.
Uric acid, serum	*Men*: 2.1-8.5 mg/dL *Women*: 2.0-6.6 mg/dL **Children:** lower until puberty	Gout, **chronic renal failure, starvation**, diuretic therapy.	

Test	Normal Values	Possible Significance	
		Increases	*Decreases*
BLOOD GASES			
Bicarbonate (HCO_3)	21-28 mEq/L **Newborn/Children**: lower	Metabolic alkalosis.	Metabolic acidosis
pH, serum	7.35-7.45 **Newborn**: lower	Metabolic alkalosis—alkali ingestion, respiratory alkalosis-hyperventilation.	Metabolic acidosis—ketoacidosis, shock, respiratory acidosis-alveolar hypoventilation.
Oxygen pressure (PO_2), whole blood, arterial	80-100 mm Hg **Newborn**: lower	Oxygen administration in the absence of severe lung disease.	Chronic obstructive lung disease, severe pneumonia, pulmonary embolism, pulmonary edema, respiratory muscle disease.
Carbon dioxide pressure (PCO_2), whole blood, arterial	35-45 mm Hg	Primary respiratory acidosis, loss of H+ through nasogastric suctioning or **vomiting**.	Primary respiratory alkalosis.
IMMUNODIAGNOSTIC STUDIES			
Carcinoembryonic antigen	<3 ng/mL	Cancer of: colon, lung, metastatic breast, pancreas, stomach, prostate, ovary, bladder, limbs; also neuroblastoma, **leukemias**, osteogenic carcinoma. Elevated in noncancer conditions such as: hepatic cirrhosis, uremia, pancreatitis, colorectal polyposis, or peptic ulcer disease, ulcerative colitis, and regional enteritis.	
URINALYSIS			
pH	4.8-8.0	Metabolic alkalosis.	Metabolic acidosis.
Specific gravity	1.010-1.030 **Children**: lower until age 2 yr	**Dehydration**, pituitary tumor, hypotension.	Distal renal tubular disease, polycystic kidney disease, diabetes insipidus, overhydration.
Glucose	Negative	Diabetes mellitus.	
Protein	Negative	**Nephrosis, glomerulonephritis, lupus erythematosus.**	
Casts	Negative	**Nephrosis, glomerulonephritis, lupus erythematosus, infection.**	
Red blood cells	Negative	Renal calculi, hemorrhagic cystitis, tumors of the kidney.	
White blood cells	Negative **Newborn**: extremely high	Inflammation of the kidneys, ureters, or bladder.	

		Possible Significance	
Test	*Normal Values*	*Increases*	*Decreases*
Color	Normal yellow	*Abnormal*: red to reddish brown—**hematuria**; brown to brownish gray—**bilirubinuria** or urobilinuria; tea-colored—possible obstructive jaundice.	*Almost colorless*: chronic kidney disease, diabetes insipidus, **diabetes mellitus**.
Sodium	40-220 mEq/L/24 h	Salt-wasting renal disease, SIADH, **dehydration**.	Heart failure, primary aldosteronism.
Chloride	110-250 mEq/L/24 h	Chronic obstructive lung disease, **dehydration**, **salicylate toxicity**.	Gastric suction, HF, emphysema.
Potassium	25-120 mEq/L/24 h **Newborn**: slightly higher	Diuretic therapy.	**Renal failure.**
Creatinine clearance	90-139 mL/min		**Renal disease.**
Hydroxycorticosteroids	2-10 mg/24 h	Cushing's disease.	Addison's disease.
Ketosteroids	*Men*: 7-25 mg/24 h *Women*: 4-15 mg/24 h **Newborn**: low	Hirsutism, adrenal hyperplasia.	Thyrotoxicosis, Addison's disease.
Catecholamines (VMA)	*Epinephrine*: 0.5-20.0 mcg/ 24 h *Norepinephrine*: 15-80 mcg/ 24 h	Pheochromocytoma, severe anxiety, numerous medications.	

URINE TESTS

Schilling test	Excretion of 8-40% or more of test dose should appear in urine.		Gastrointestinal malabsorption, **pernicious anemia**.

Index to: Selected Pediatric Emergencies

 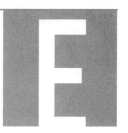

For a quick review, use this index to locate content on **20 pediatric emergencies** that are covered in this book.

Index to: Nursing Treatments (Hands-On Care, Skills, Activities and Procedures)

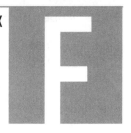

Use this index as a **quick checklist of 53 skills and procedures** (with page references to selected conditions mentioned in this book) that nurses need to know or be able to perform in giving direct client care.

Procedure	Condition/Situation	Page(s)
Head circumference, monitor	Hydrocephalus	150, 151
	Spina bifida	148
Heat application	Juvenile idiopathic arthritis (JIA)	131
	SCA	98
(Heimlich's) Foreign body airway obstruction maneuver	Airway obstruction	48
Humidifier/mist vaporizer, cool	Asthma	45
	Croup	42
	Down syndrome	182
	LTB	42
	Pediatric respiratory conditions	43
	Pertussis	175
	Rubeola	174
	Scarlet fever	178
Hyperalimentation	Hirschsprung's	72
Hypothermia blanket	Kawasaki's disease	61
	Respiratory infections (LTB, croup, epiglottitis)	43
	Salicylate poisoning	120
Incentive spirometer	Cystic fibrosis	41
Inhaler, use of	Anti-asthmatic medication	45
Intravenous fluids	Acetaminophen poisoning	179
	AGE	69, 71
	Appendicitis	75
	Bacterial meningitis	116
	Hirschsprung's	72
	Intussusception	73
	Kawasaki's disease	61
	Mumps	175
	Osteomyelitis	128
	Pyloric stenosis	70
	Respiratory infections (LTB, etc.)	43
	Reye syndrome	121
	Salicylate poisoning	115, 119
	Sickle cell anemia	97
	TEF	156
Isolation	Diphtheria	173
	Mumps	175
	Rubella	177
	Rubeola	174
	Varicella	172
Isolation, respiratory	Bacterial meningitis	116
	Fifth disease	173
	Pertussis	175
	Rubeola	174
	Scarlet fever	178
Isolation, reverse (protective)	Leukemia	106
Isolette care	Bone tumors	108
	Myelomeningocele (spina bifida)	148
Medication (IM) administration	Hemophilia	99
	Lead poisoning	115, 118
Myelomeningocele apron	Myelomeningocele (spina bifida)	148
Neurologic checks	Acetaminophen poisoning	179
	Hydrocephalus	150, 151
	Reye syndrome	121

Procedure	Condition/Situation	Page(s)
Oral hygiene, special	Child who is dying	184
	Kawasaki's disease	61
	Leukemia	106
Oxygen	Apnea	45
	Asthma	45
	Brain tumors	109
	C.F.	43
	C.P.	140
	Congenital heart disease	57
	Diphtheria	173
	Iron deficiency anemia	96
	Pediatric respiratory infections	43
	RF	60
	Sickle cell anemia	98
	TEF	156
Pavlik harness	DDH	129, 147, 154
Perineal care	AGE	72
	Child who is dying	184
Physiotherapy	Polio	176
Postural drainage	C.F.	40, 41
	Pediatric respiratory infections	43
Pressure, application of	Hemophilia	99
Range-of-motion exercises	C.P.	141
	DMD	141
	GBS	142
	Hemophilia	99
	Juvenile I.A.	134
Restraints	Bacterial meningitis	116
	Cleft lip/palate	57
	RF	60
Seizure precautions	Bacterial meningitis	116
	Brain tumors	109
	C.P.	140
	Kawasaki's disease	61
	Lead poisoning	119
	Reye syndrome	121
	Roseola	174
	Rubeola	174
Skin care	APSGN	89
	Bone tumors	108
	Eczema	170-171
	Kawasaki's disease	61
	Leukemia	106
	Nephrosis	86
	Rubeola	174
	Suture line—pyloric stenosis	60
	Varicella	172
Soaks, cool	Eczema	170
Soaks, warm	Juvenile I.A.	131
	Lead poisoning	115, 119
	Mumps	175
	Salicylate poisoning	120
Splints	Club foot	129
	DMD	141
	Juvenile I.A.	129, 130, 131
	Osteomyelitis	129

Procedure	Condition/Situation	Page(s)
Standard precautions	AGE	71
	Bacterial meningitis	116
	Bone tumors	108
	C.F.	40
	Communicable diseases	169, 171, 172, 173
	Congenital heart disease	57
	Eczema	171
	Leukemia	106
	Myelomeningocele (spina bifida)	148
	Sickle cell anemia	98
Suction	Apnea of infancy	45
	Brain tumors	109
	C.F.	40
	Diphtheria	173
	Down syndrome	182
	Respiratory infections	43
Temperature, rectal	Kawasaki's disease	61
Traction	Developmental hip dysplasia	129
	Legg-Calvé-Perthes	128, 134
	Scoliosis	129
Vomiting, induced	Poisonings, ingestions	119, 169, 171, 179
Wound care	Osteomyelitis	128
	Ruptured appendix/appendicitis	75, 81

☞ Index to: Tubes

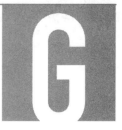
For a quick reference as you study or review, use this index for a quick review of **hands-on care** related to **15 different tubes** that are featured in the pediatric conditions covered in this book.

Type	Condition/Situation	Page(s)
Chest tubes	TEF	156
Colonic irrigations	Hirschsprung's	72
CVP	Osteomyelitis	128
	Reye syndrome	121
Endotracheal tube	Pediatric respiratory infections (epiglottitis)	42
	TEF (tracheoesophageal fistula)	156
	Reye syndrome	121
Enema	Hirschsprung's	72
Foley catheter	Reye syndrome	121
Gastric lavage	Acetaminophen poisoning	179
	Salicylate poisoning	119
Gastrostomy tube	TEF	156
Gavage feeding	CHD (congenital heart disease)	57
N.G. tube	Hirschsprung's	72
	Reye syndrome	121
	Salicylate poisoning	119
	TEF	156
Respirator	GBS (Guillain-Barré syndrome)	142
Suction	Apnea of infancy	45
	CHD	57
	C.P. (cerebral palsy)	140
	Cystic fibrosis	40
	Down syndrome	182
	GBS	142
	Pediatric respiratory infections	43
	Pertussis	175
	TEF	156
Tracheostomy	Diphtheria	173
	GBS	142, 143
Urinary drainage apparatus	Hypospadias	159
Ventilation, mechanical	Reye syndrome	121
	TEF	156

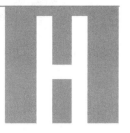

☞ Index to: Positioning the Client

For a quick reference as you study or review, use this index to locate **27 positions of choice** (or contraindications) for various conditions.

Position	Selected Condition/Situation	Page(s)
Avoid prone	Apnea of infancy	45, 51
	Cleft lip	157
Bed rest	APSGN	89
	Diphtheria	173
	Kawasaki's disease	61
	Legg-Calvé-Perthes	129
	Mumps	175
	Nephrosis	86
	Osteomyelitis	129
	Polio	176
	Rheumatic fever	60
	Rubeola	174
	Scarlet fever	178
	Sickle cell crisis	98
	Whooping cough	175
Body alignment	GBS	142
	Polio	176
Ear affected, uppermost	Giving otic meds	186
Ear, operative-down	Myringotomy	181
Extremities, elevate	Kawasaki's disease	61
Flat	Hydrocephalus, postshunt	151, 160
	Juvenile I.A.	131
Fowler's, high-, semi-	Cyanotic heart defects	57
	Hirschsprung's (pre-op)	72
	Iron deficiency anemia	96
	Pediatric respiratory infections	43
	Pyloric stenosis	70, 79
	Ruptured appendix	181
Fowler's, low-	Appendicitis	75
Head of bed, elevated	Bacterial meningitis	115, 116, 122
	Down syndrome	182
	Reye syndrome	121
	TEF	156, 160
Hips, abducted	Myelomeningocele (spina bifida)	148
Immobilized	Hemophilia	99
	Osteomyelitis	127, 128, 129
Joints extended	JIA	131
Knee-chest (squatting)	Cyanotic heart defects	56, 57
Lung-expansion, maximum	GBS	142
Neck, hyperextended	Cyanotic heart defects	57
Orthopneic	Asthma	44

Position	*Selected Condition/Situation*	*Page(s)*
Prone	Cleft palate	157
	JIA	131
	Myelomeningocele (pre-op) (spina bifida)	148, 160
Prone, semi	Down syndrome	182
	T&A (post-op)	181
Right side	Down syndrome	182
	Pyloric stenosis	70, 79
Side-lying	Bacterial meningitis	116, 122
	Giving rectal meds	186
	Myelomeningocele (post-op)	148
	Opisthotonus	115, 116, 122
Sit up, lean forward	Hemophilia, epistaxis	99
Supine	Apnea of infancy	45
	Giving ophthalmic meds	186
Turn, position frequently	APSGN	89
	Bone cancer	108
	Child who is dying	184
	Cystic fibrosis	40
	Down syndrome	182
	GBS	142
	Hydrocephalus	151
	Nephrosis	86
Unoperative side	Shunt procedure (post-op), hydrocephalus	151
Upright	Child who is dying	184
	Giving oral meds	186

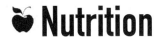

Nutrition

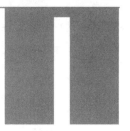

This table lists age-related desirable weights, heights, and energy needs useful in determining recommended daily intake of calories.

Median Heights and Weights and Recommended Energy Intake

Category	Age (yr) or condition	Weight (kg)	(lb)	Height (cm)	(in)	REE[a] (kcal/day)	Multiples of REE	Average energy allowance (kcal)[b] Per kg	Per day[c]
Infants	0.0-0.5	6	13	60	24	320		108	650
	0.5-1.0	9	20	71	28	500		98	850
Children	1-3	13	29	90	35	740		102	1300
	4-6	20	44	112	44	950		90	1800
	7-10	28	62	132	52	1130		70	2000
Men	11-14	45	99	157	62	1440	1.70	55	2500
	15-18	66	145	176	69	1760	1.67	45	3000
	19-24	72	160	177	70	1780	1.67	40	2900
	25-50	79	174	176	70	1800	1.60	37	2900
	51+	77	170	173	68	1530	1.50	30	2300
Women	11-14	46	101	157	62	1310	1.67	47	2200
	15-18	55	120	163	64	1370	1.60	40	2200
	19-24	58	128	164	65	1350	1.60	38	2200
	25-50	63	138	163	64	1380	1.55	36	2200
	51+	65	143	160	63	1280	1.50	30	1900
									+0
									+300
									+300
									+500
									+500

From Food and Nutrition Board, National Research Council: *Recommended dietary allowances*, ed 10, Washington, DC, National Academy of Sciences.

[a]Resting energy expenditure.

[b]In the range of light to moderate activity, the coefficient of variation is ± 20%.

[c]Figure is rounded.

The data in this table have been assembled from the observed median heights and weights of children together with desirable weights for adults for the mean heights of men (70 inches) and women (64 inches) between the ages of 18 and 34 years as surveyed in the United States population (HEW/NCHS data). The energy allowances for the young adults are for men and women doing light work. The allowances for the two older age-groups represent mean energy needs over these age spans, allowing for a 2% decrease in basal (resting) metabolic rate per decade and a reduction in activity of 200 kcal/day for men and women between 51 and 75 years of age, 500 kcal for men over 75, and 400 kcal for women over 75. The customary range of daily energy output is shown for adults and is based on a variation in energy needs of ± 400 kcal at any one age, emphasizing the wide range of energy intakes appropriate for any group of people. Energy allowances for children through age 18 are based on medium energy intakes of children these ages followed in longitudinal growth studies.

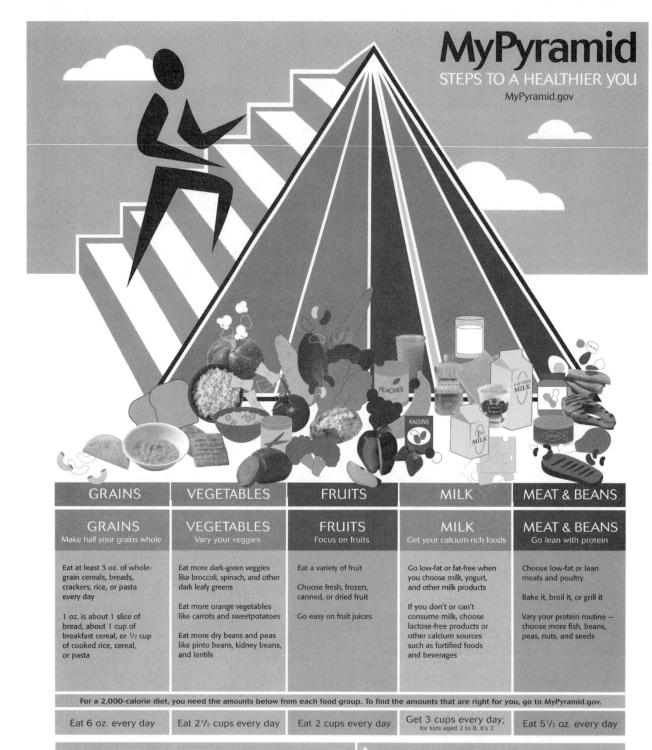

MyPyramid
STEPS TO A HEALTHIER YOU
MyPyramid.gov

GRAINS	VEGETABLES	FRUITS	MILK	MEAT & BEANS
GRAINS Make half your grains whole	**VEGETABLES** Vary your veggies	**FRUITS** Focus on fruits	**MILK** Get your calcium-rich foods	**MEAT & BEANS** Go lean with protein
Eat at least 3 oz. of whole-grain cereals, breads, crackers, rice, or pasta every day 1 oz. is about 1 slice of bread, about 1 cup of breakfast cereal, or ½ cup of cooked rice, cereal, or pasta	Eat more dark-green veggies like broccoli, spinach, and other dark leafy greens Eat more orange vegetables like carrots and sweetpotatoes Eat more dry beans and peas like pinto beans, kidney beans, and lentils	Eat a variety of fruit Choose fresh, frozen, canned, or dried fruit Go easy on fruit juices	Go low-fat or fat-free when you choose milk, yogurt, and other milk products If you don't or can't consume milk, choose lactose-free products or other calcium sources such as fortified foods and beverages	Choose low-fat or lean meats and poultry Bake it, broil it, or grill it Vary your protein routine — choose more fish, beans, peas, nuts, and seeds

For a 2,000-calorie diet, you need the amounts below from each food group. To find the amounts that are right for you, go to MyPyramid.gov.

Eat 6 oz. every day	Eat 2½ cups every day	Eat 2 cups every day	Get 3 cups every day; for kids aged 2 to 8, it's 2	Eat 5½ oz. every day

Find your balance between food and physical activity
- Be sure to stay within your daily calorie needs.
- Be physically active for at least 30 minutes most days of the week.
- About 60 minutes a day of physical activity may be needed to prevent weight gain.
- For sustaining weight loss, at least 60 to 90 minutes a day of physical activity may be required.
- Children and teenagers should be physically active for 60 minutes every day, or most days.

Know the limits on fats, sugars, and salt (sodium)
- Make most of your fat sources from fish, nuts, and vegetable oils.
- Limit solid fats like butter, stick margarine, shortening, and lard, as well as foods that contain these.
- Check the Nutrition Facts label to keep saturated fats, trans fats, and sodium low.
- Choose food and beverages low in added sugars. Added sugars contribute calories with few, if any, nutrients.

MyPyramid.gov
STEPS TO A HEALTHIER YOU

U.S. Department of Agriculture
Center for Nutrition Policy and Promotion
April 2005
CNPP-15

USDA is an equal opportunity provider and employer.

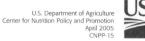

🍎 Index to: Diets

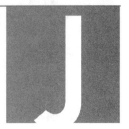
For a quick review, use this index to locate pages where **25 special dietary considerations** are covered in this book as they relate to specific conditions/situations.

Type	Selected Condition/Situation	Page(s)
Bland	Kawasaki's disease	61
	Mumps	175
	Rubeola	174
	Tonsillectomy (post-op)	181
Bulk, *high*	Down syndrome	182
Calorie, *high*	Cerebral palsy	140
	Cystic fibrosis	40
	Leukemia	106
Calorie, *low*	Osteomyelitis	128, 134
Diabetic	Diabetes	78
Elimination/hypoallergenic	Eczema	171
Fluids, cool	Febrile seizures	117
	Kawasaki's disease	61
	Tonsillectomy	181
Fluids, extra	Leukemia	106
	Myelomeningocele (spina bifida)	148
	Osteomyelitis	128, 134
	Sickle cell anemia	97
Fluids, extra, push	Communicable diseases	169, 171
	Cystic fibrosis	40
	Kawasaki's disease	61
	Leukemia	106
	Mumps	175
	Scarlet fever	178
	UTI	90
Fluid restrictions	APSGN	89
Gluten-free	Celiac disease	69, 74, 75
Iron, *high*	Anemia, Fe^+ deficiency	96
	CHD (congenital heart disease)	57
	Leukemia	106
Lactose-free	Eczema	171
Liquids, clear	Bacterial meningitis	116
	Bronchiolitis	42
	Cleft lip/palate, post-op	158
	Pyloric stenosis	70
	Respiratory infections	44
	TEF, post-op	156
NPO	Appendix, ruptured; postop	75, 181
	Bacterial meningitis	116
	Hydrocephalus	151
	Pyloric stenosis	70
	Respiratory infections	43
	Salicylate poisoning	119

Type	Selected Condition/Situation	Page(s)
	TEF	156
	Tonsillectomy	181
Oral rehydration therapy	AGE	69, 71
Potassium, *high*	CHD	57
	Kawasaki's disease	62
Potassium, *low*	APSGN (with oliguria)	89
Protein, *high*	Cystic fibrosis	40
	Leukemia	106
	Nephrosis	86, 87
	Osteomyelitis	128, 134
Protein (restricted)	APSGN (with azotemia)	89
Residue, *low*	Hirschsprung's	72
Small, frequent feedings	Apnea of infancy	46
	APSGN	89
	Down syndrome	182
	Child who is dying	184
	Hydrocephalus (post op)	151
	Leukemia	106
	Osteomyelitis	128
Sodium, increased	Cystic fibrosis	40
Sodium, *low*	APSGN	89
	CHD	57
	Nephrosis	86, 87
	Rheumatic fever	60
Soft	Child who is dying	184
	Mumps	175
	Rubeola	174
	Scarlet fever	178
	Tonsillectomy	181

AVOID:		
Carbonated sodas	Tonsillectomy	181
Citrus juices	Scarlet fever	178
	Tonsillectomy	181
Dairy products	Eczema	171
	Respiratory infections	44, 51
	Tonsillectomy	181
Foods requiring chewing	Child who is dying	184
	Mumps	175
Foods with strong odors	Child who is dying	184
Raw fruits, vegetables	Leukemia	106
Red fluids	Tonsillectomy	181
Spicy foods	Kawasaki's disease	61
Toast	Tonsillectomy	181
Tyramine foods, high in	Alkylating agents	110
Warm fluids (tea, broth)	Tonsillectomy	181

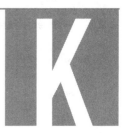
For a quick review of essential information related to **health care teaching and home health care,** use this index to locate what you need to know to provide **basic home care teaching** in 35 conditions/situations.

NCLEX-RN® Test Plan: 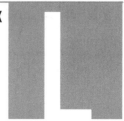 Nursing Process/Cognitive Level: Definitions/Descriptions

The phases of the nursing process include:

I. Assessment: Establishing a database.

A. *Gather objective and subjective information relative to the client:*
   1. Collect information from the client, significant others and/or health care team members; current and prior health records; and other pertinent resources.
   2. Utilize assessment skills appropriate to client's condition.
   3. Recognize *symptoms* and significant findings.
   4. Determine client's ability to assume self-care of daily health needs.
   5. Determine health team member's ability to provide care.
   6. Assess *environment* of client.
   7. Identify own or staff reactions to client, significant others and/or health care team members.

B. *Confirm data:*
   1. *Verify* observation or perception by obtaining additional information.
   2. *Question* prescriptions and decisions by other health care team members when indicated.
   3. *Observe* condition of client directly when indicated.
   4. *Validate* that an appropriate client assessment has been made.

C. *Communicate information gained in assessment:*
   1. Document assessment findings thoroughly and accurately.
   2. Report assessment findings to relevant members of the health care team.

II. Analysis: Identifying actual or potential health care needs and/or problems based on assessment.

A. *Interpret data:*
   1. Validate data.
   2. Organize related data.
   3. Determine *need for additional* data.
   4. Determine client's unique needs and/or problems.

B. *Formulate client's nursing diagnoses:*
   1. Determine significant relationship between data and client needs and/or problems.
   2. Utilize *standard taxonomy* for formulating nursing diagnoses.

C. *Communicate results of analysis:*
   1. *Document client's nursing diagnoses.*
   2. Report results of analysis to relevant members of the health care team.

III. Planning: Setting goals for meeting client's needs and designing strategies to achieve these goals.

A. *Prioritize nursing diagnoses:*
   1. Involve client, significant others and/or health care team members when establishing nursing diagnoses.
   2. *Establish priorities among nursing* diagnoses.
   3. Anticipate needs and/or problems on the basis of established priorities.

B. *Determine goals of care:*
   1. Involve client, significant others and/or health care team members in setting goals.
   2. *Establish priorities among goals.*
   3. Anticipate needs and/or problems on the basis of established priorities.

C. *Formulate outcome criteria for goals of care:*
   1. Involve client, significant others and/or health care team members in formulating outcome criteria for goals of care.
   2. *Establish priorities among outcome criteria* for goals of care.
   3. Anticipate needs and/or problems on the basis of established priorities.

D. *Develop plan of care and modify as necessary:*
   1. Involve the client, significant others and/or health care team members in designing strategies.
   2. *Individualize* the plan of care based on such information as *age, gender, culture, ethnicity and religion.*
   3. Plan for client's safety, comfort and maintenance of optimal functioning.
   4. Select nursing interventions for delivery of client's care.
   5. Select *appropriate teaching approaches.*

E. *Collaborate with other health care team members when planning delivery of client's care:*
   1. Identify health or social resources available to the client and/or significant others.
   2. Select appropriate health care team members when planning assignments.
   3. Coordinate care provided by health care team members.

Source: Adapted from: National Council of State Boards of Nursing. *NCLEX-RN® Test Plan*.

F. *Communicate plan of care:*
1. Document plan of care thoroughly and accurately.
2. Report plan of care to relevant members of the health care team.
3. Review plan of care with client.

IV. **Implementation: Initiating and completing actions necessary to accomplish the defined goals.**
A. *Organize and manage client's care:*
1. Implement a plan of care.
2. Arrange for a client care conference.
B. *Counsel and teach client, significant others and/or health care team members:*
1. Assist client, significant others and/or health care team members to recognize and manage stress.
2. Facilitate client relationships with significant others and health care team members.
3. *Teach* correct principles, procedures and techniques for maintenance and promotion of health.
4. Provide client with health status information.
5. Refer client, significant others and/or health care team members to appropriate *resources.*
C. *Provide care to achieve established goals of care:*
1. Use *safe and appropriate techniques* when administering client care.
2. Use precautionary and *preventive* interventions in providing care to client.
3. *Prepare client for surgery, delivery* or other *procedures.*
4. Institute *interventions* to compensate for adverse responses.
5. *Initiate life-saving interventions* for emergency situations.
6. Provide an *environment* conducive to attainment of goals of care.
7. Adjust care in accord with client's expressed or implied needs, problems and/or preferences.
8. Stimulate and motivate client to achieve self-care and independence.
9. Encourage client to follow a treatment regime.
10. Assist client to maintain optimal functioning.
D. *Supervise and coordinate the delivery of client's care provided by nursing personnel:*
1. *Delegate* nursing interventions to appropriate nursing personnel.

2. Monitor and follow up on delegated interventions.
3. Manage health care team members' reactions to factors influencing therapeutic relationships with clients.
E. *Communicate nursing interventions:*
1. Record actual client responses, nursing interventions and other information relevant to implementation of care.
2. Provide complete, accurate reports on assigned client(s) to relevant members of the health care team.

V. **Evaluation: Determining the extent to which goals have been achieved and interventions have been successful.**
A. *Compare actual outcomes with expected outcomes of care:*
1. Evaluate responses (*expected* and *unexpected*) in order to determine the degree of success of nursing interventions.
2. Determine impact of therapeutic interventions on the client and significant others.
3. Determine need for modifying the plan of care.
4. Identify factors that may interfere with the client's ability to implement the plan of care.
B. *Evaluate the client's ability to implement self-care:*
1. Verify that *tests or measurements are performed* correctly by the client and/or other caregivers.
2. Ascertain client's and/or others' *understanding* of information given.
C. *Evaluate health care team members' ability to implement client care:*
1. Determine *impact of teaching* on health care team members.
2. Identify factors that might alter health care team members' response to teaching.
D. *Communicate evaluation findings:*
1. Document client's response to therapy, care and/or teaching.
2. Report client's response to therapy, care and/or teaching to relevant members of the health care team.
3. Report and document others' responses to teaching.
4. Document other caregivers' responses to teaching.

Notes:

1. Throughout the outline in this book, the stages of the *Nursing Process* are referred to as: **assessment, analysis/nursing diagnosis, nursing care plan/implementation, and evaluation/outcome criteria.**

2. The practice questions in this book are coded as to phase of the *Nursing Process* being tested; the codes are found following the answer/rationale for each question.

*Key to **Nursing Process** Codes:*

AS	Assessment
AN	Analysis
PL	Planning
IMP	Implementation
EV	Evaluation

For an **index to questions relating to each phase of the Nursing Process/Cognitive Level,** see **Appendix M.**

The phases of the *Cognitive Level* include:

A. **Recall/Knowledge:** Rote remembering of significant facts or terms; to define, to name and to list.

B. **Comprehension:** To understand; to restate; to reorganize; to translate; to find an illustration or example; to interpret by explanation or summary; to determine implications, consequences and effects.

C. **Application:** The use of abstractions in particular or concrete situations. They may be in the form of general ideas, rules, procedures, or general methods. The abstractions may also be technical principles, ideas, and theories that need to be remembered and applied, using a concept or principle in a new situation.

D. **Analysis:** The breakdown of the whole into constituent parts or elements so that a rank priority of ideas can emerge and relationships between ideas can be made clear.

E. **Synthesis:** Putting ideas together to form a new whole.

F. **Evaluation:** Judging material using criteria.

*Key to **Cognitive Level** Codes:*

RE/KN	Recall/Knowledge
COM	Comprehension
ANL	Analysis
APP	Application
SYN	Synthesis
EVL	Evaluation

For an **index to questions relating to each phase of the cognitive level,** see **Appendix M.**

Index to: Questions Related to
Nursing Process/Cognitive Level

 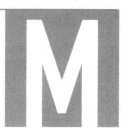

Use this index to locate **practice questions** in each **phase of the nursing process and cognitive level** throughout the book.

Please refer to the following pages for the complete table.

NURSING PROCESS / COGNITIVE LEVEL

Chapter	Assessment (AS) Question #:	Analysis (AN) Question #:	Planning (PL) Question #:	Implementation (IMP) Question #:	Evaluation (EV) Question #:	Recall/Know. (RE/KN) Question #:	Comprehension (COM) Question #:	Application (APP) Question #:	Analysis (ANL) Question #:	Evaluation (EVL) Question #:	Synthesis (SYN) Question #:
1—Clinical Assessment		1		3, 4, 5, 6	2, 7, 8		1, 2, 8	3, 4, 7	5, 6		
2—Growth and Development: Infant				1, 2, 3, 6	4, 5, 7, 8			1, 4, 5, 6, 8	2, 3, 7		
3—Growth and Development: Toddler	7		3, 4, 5	1, 2, 6	8		1	2, 3, 4, 5, 6, 8	7		
4—Growth and Development: Preschooler	3, 5		2	1, 4, 6	7, 8		6, 8	1, 2, 3, 4	5, 7		
5—Growth and Development: School-Aged	3	8	4	1, 2, 5, 6, 7			2, 5, 6	1, 3, 4, 7, 8			
6—Growth and Development: Adolescent		5	1	2, 4, 6, 7, 8	3		6	1, 2, 4, 7, 8	3, 5		
7—Respiratory Disorders	6, 15	8	7, 9, 11, 13	1, 2, 3, 4, 5, 12, 16, 17	10, 14, 18		1, 17	3, 4, 5, 6, 9, 11, 12, 13, 15, 18	2, 7, 8, 10, 14, 16		
8—Cardiovascular Disorders	4, 23	1, 6, 14, 17, 22, 24	9, 13	2, 5, 7, 10, 11, 15, 16, 18, 19, 20	3, 8, 12, 21		4	2, 3, 9, 10, 12, 13, 14, 15, 16, 19, 20, 21, 24	1, 5, 6, 7, 8, 11, 17, 18, 22, 23		
9—Gastrointestinal Disorders	1, 6, 10, 13	4, 12, 14, 22	7, 18	3, 5, 9, 11, 17, 19, 20, 21	2, 8, 15, 16		1, 13	4, 9, 11, 12, 15, 16, 19, 21, 22	2, 3, 5, 6, 7, 8, 10, 14, 17, 18, 20		
10—Genitourinary Disorders	1, 13	5		2, 3, 6, 7	4, 8, 9, 10, 11, 12, 14, 15		1	3, 10, 11, 12, 13, 14, 15	2, 4, 5, 6, 7, 8, 9		
11—Hematologic Disorders			7	1, 3, 6, 8, 9, 10, 11	2, 4, 5			11	1, 2, 3, 4, 5, 6, 7, 8, 9, 10		

(continued)

NURSING PROCESS / COGNITIVE LEVEL

Chapter	Assessment (AS) Question #:	Analysis (AN) Question #:	Planning (PL) Question #:	Implementation (IMP) Question #:	Evaluation (EV) Question #:	Recall/Know. (RE/KN) Question #:	Comprehension (COM) Question #:	Application (APP) Question #:	Analysis (ANL) Question #:	Evaluation (EVL) Question #:	Synthesis (SYN) Question #:
12—Neoplastic Disorders	1, 2, 3, 16, 17, 19	9, 10, 11	5	4, 6, 7, 8, 12, 13, 18	14, 15		6, 8, 11, 12, 19	2, 3, 7, 10, 13, 14, 15	1, 4, 5, 9, 16, 17, 18		
13—Central Nervous System Disorders	4		5, 10	1, 2, 3, 6, 7, 8, 9			1, 3, 5, 9	2, 6, 7, 8, 10	4		
14—Musculoskeletal Disorders	6, 7, 10	3, 8, 11, 13, 15, 16	1, 4	2, 5, 12, 14, 17, 18	9		6, 8	2, 5, 9, 11, 13, 14, 17	1, 3, 4, 7, 10, 12, 15, 16, 18		
15—Neuromuscular Disorders	1	7, 9	2, 12	3, 4, 6, 8, 11	5, 10		1, 7, 8, 10	3, 4, 6, 11	2, 5, 9, 12		
16—Problems of the Newborn (Birth Defects)	35	5, 7, 8, 34	1, 2, 4, 13, 14, 15, 18, 19, 29, 30	3, 6, 9, 10, 11, 12, 16, 17, 20, 21, 22, 23, 25, 26, 27, 28, 31, 32, 36, 37	24, 33, 38		10, 16, 32	1, 2, 4, 9, 12, 14, 17, 22, 23, 24, 26, 27, 28, 29, 30, 31, 33, 34, 36, 37, 38	3, 5, 6, 7, 8, 11, 13, 15, 18, 19, 20, 21, 25, 35		
17—Nursing Care for Children's Unique Needs	7, 10, 14	5	15	1, 2, 4, 6, 8, 11, 12, 13	3, 9		2, 7, 8, 12	1, 4, 5, 6, 9, 15	3, 10, 11, 13, 14		

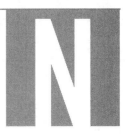

Definitions and Index to: Questions Related to Categories of Human Functions

This index lists *practice questions* for you to use in reviewing *categories of human functions* (which are *detailed* examples of what subtopics are covered by the four *broad* client needs categories).

The eight categories of human functions include:

Protective Functions   client's ability to maintain defenses and prevent physical and chemical trauma, injury, and threats to health status (e.g., communicable diseases, abuse, safety hazards, poisoning, skin disorders, and pre- and post-operative complications).

Sensory-Perceptual Functions   client's ability to perceive, interpret, and respond to sensory and cognitive stimuli (e.g., auditory, visual, verbal impairments, brain tumors, aphasia, sensory deprivation or overload, body image, reality orientation, learning disabilities).

Comfort, Rest, Activity, and Mobility Functions   client's ability to maintain mobility, desirable level of activity, adequate sleep, rest, and comfort (e.g., pain, sleep disturbances, joint impairment).

Nutrition   client's ability to maintain the intake and processing of essential nutrients (e.g., obesity, gastric and metabolic disorders that primarily affect the nutritional status).

Growth and Development   client's ability to maintain maturational processes throughout the life span (e.g., child bearing, child rearing, maturational crisis, changes in aging, psychosocial development).

Fluid-Gas Transport Functions   client's ability to maintain fluid-gas transport (e.g., fluid volume deficit/overload, acid-base balance, CPR, anemias, cardiopulmonary diseases).

Psychosocial-Cultural Functions   client's ability to function in intrapersonal/interpersonal relationships (e.g., grieving, death/dying, psychotic behaviors, self concept, therapeutic communication, ethical-legal aspects, community resources, situational crises, substance abuse).

Elimination Functions   client's ability to maintain functions related to relieving the body of waste products (e.g., conditions of GI and/or GU systems).

Chapter	Protective Functions (1) Question #:	Sensory-Perceptual Functions (2) Question #:	Comfort, Rest, Activity, and Mobility Functions (3) Question #:	Nutrition (4) Question #:	Growth and Development (5) Question #:	Fluid-Gas Transport Functions (6) Question #:	Psychosocial-Cultural Functions (7) Question #:	Eliminations Functions (8) Question #:
1—Clinical Assessment of the Child	1				2, 4, 5	7, 8	3	6
2—Growth and Development of the Infant					1, 2, 3, 4, 5, 6, 7	8		
3—Growth and Development of the Toddler					1, 2, 3, 4, 5, 6, 7, 8			
4—Growth and Development of the Preschooler				2	1, 3, 4, 5, 6, 7, 8			
5—Growth and Development of the School-Aged Child					1, 2, 3, 4, 5, 6, 7, 8			
6—Growth and Development of the Adolescent	7, 8				1, 2, 3, 6		4, 5	
7—Respiratory Disorders	5					1, 2, 3, 4, 6, 7, 9, 10, 11, 12, 13, 14, 15, 16, 17, 18	8	
8—Cardiovascular Disorders	1, 3, 4, 5, 7, 9, 20				10	8, 11, 12, 13, 14, 15, 17, 18, 19, 21, 22, 23, 24	2, 6, 16	
9—Gastrointestinal Disorders				1, 2, 3, 4, 5, 20	11, 22		21	6, 7, 8, 9, 10, 12, 13, 14, 15, 16, 17, 18, 19
10—Genitourinary Disorders	5, 9		6		2	3, 4, 7, 8, 9		1, 10, 11, 12, 13, 14, 15

Chapter	Protective Functions (1) Question #:	Sensory-Perceptual Functions (2) Question #:	Comfort, Rest, Activity, and Mobility Functions (3) Question #:	Nutrition (4) Question #:	Growth and Development (5) Question #:	Fluid-Gas Transport Functions (6) Question #:	Psychosocial-Cultural Functions (7) Question #:	Eliminations Functions (8) Question #:
11—Hematologic Disorders					11	1, 2, 3, 4, 5, 7, 8, 9	6, 10	
12—Neoplastic Disorders	4,6, 7, 8, 9, 12, 13, 14, 15, 18		1, 10, 11			2, 16, 17, 19		3, 5
13—Central Nervous System Disorders	1, 2, 3, 5	6, 7, 8, 9				4	10	
14—Musculoskeletal Disorders	15	10	1, 2, 3, 4, 5, 6, 7, 8, 9, 12, 16, 17, 18		11, 13, 14			
15—Neuromuscular Disorders	10, 12	11	1, 2, 4, 7, 8	5		9	3, 6	
16—Problems of the Newborn (Birth Defects)	2, 4, 8, 13, 14, 17, 18, 19, 26, 34, 36		3, 5, 6, 7, 9, 10, 11, 37	15, 16, 22, 23, 25, 27, 28, 35	20, 21, 24, 31, 32, 33, 38		12	1, 29, 30
17—Nursing Care for Children's Unique Needs	1, 2, 7, 8, 9, 10, 11, 12, 13, 14	3			5, 15		4, 6	

Definitions and Index to: Questions Related to CLIENT NEEDS/*Client Subneeds*

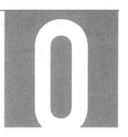

To *practice questions* in each of the 4 categories of **client needs** and *6 client subneeds* that are tested on NCLEX-RN®, refer to the questions listed on the following pages:

CLIENT NEEDS/*Client Subneeds:*

1. SAFE, EFFECTIVE CARE ENVIRONMENT
Management of Care
Safety and Infection Control

2. HEALTH PROMOTION AND MAINTENANCE—has no *client subneeds.*

3. PSYCHOSOCIAL INTEGRITY— has no *client subneeds.*

4. PHYSIOLOGICAL INTEGRITY
Basic Care and Comfort
Pharmacological and Parenteral Therapies
Reduction of Risk Potential
Physiological Adaptation

The four broad categories of **CLIENT NEEDS** include:

SAFE, EFFECTIVE CARE ENVIRONMENT—coordinated care, environmental safety, safe and effective treatment and procedures (e.g., client rights, confidentiality, principles of teaching/learning, control of infectious agents).

HEALTH PROMOTION AND MAINTENANCE—normal growth and development from birth to death, self-care and support systems, prevention and early treatment of disease (e.g., newborn care, normal perinatal care, family planning, human sexuality, parenting, end-of-life process, lifestyle choices, immunity).

PSYCHOSOCIAL INTEGRITY—psychosocial adaptation, coping (e.g., behavioral norms, chemical dependency, communication skills, family systems, mental health concepts, psychodynamics of behavior, psychopathology, treatment modalities).

PHYSIOLOGICAL INTEGRITY—physiological adaptation, reduction of risk potential, provision of basic care (e.g., drug administration, emergencies, nutritional therapies).

The six categories of *client subneeds* include:

1. *Management of Care*—staff development, collaboration, supervision of multidisciplinary health team; delegation; client rights; prioritization, ethical and legal responsibilities; referrals.

2. *Safety and Infection Control*—protecting clients, family/significant others and health care personnel from health and environmental hazards; e.g., disaster planning, home safety, medical and surgical asepsis, use of restraint/safety devices, safe use of equipment, standard precautions.

3. *Basic Care and Comfort*—performing routine nursing activities of daily living.

4. *Pharmacological and Parenteral Therapies*—expected and unexpected effects, chemotherapy; blood products; pain management; calculations; TPN, IV; central venous access devices.

5. *Reduction of Risk Potential*—monitoring, and reducing likelihood of complications related to existing conditions, treatments or procedures.

6. *Physiological Adaptation*—meeting acute, chronic or life-threatening physical health conditions

Chapter	CLIENT NEED: SAFE, EFFECTIVE CARE ENVIRONMENT (SECE) Client Subneed: Management of Care — Question #:	Client Subneed: Safety/Infection Control — Question #:	CLIENT NEED: HEALTH PROMOTION/ MAINTENANCE (HPM) — Question #:	CLIENT NEED: PSYCHOSOCIAL INTEGRITY (PsI)	CLIENT NEED: PHYSIOLOGICAL INTEGRITY (PhI) Client Subneed: Basic Care/Comfort — Question #:	Client Subneed: Pharmacological/Parenteral Therapies — Question #:	Client Subneed: Reduction of Risk Potential — Question #:	Client Subneed: Physiological Adaptation — Question #:
1—Clinical Assessment of the Child	5		1, 2, 6	3, 4			8	7
2—Growth and Development: Infant			1, 2, 3, 5, 6, 7, 8	4				
3—Growth and Development: Toddler		8	1, 6, 7	2, 3, 4, 5				
4—Growth and Development: Preschooler			1, 2, 3, 4, 6, 7, 8	5				
5—Growth and Development: School-Aged			1, 2, 3, 4, 5, 6, 8	7				
6—Growth and Development: Adolescent			1, 6, 7, 8	2, 3, 4, 5				
7—Respiratory Disorders	18	12	8, 9			3, 5	2, 4, 10, 11, 13, 14, 17	1, 6, 7, 15, 16
8—Cardiovascular Disorders	5		9	2, 6, 10		3, 12, 13, 15, 20, 21, 24	7, 8, 11, 14, 17, 22, 23	1, 4, 16, 18, 19
9—Gastrointestinal Disorders	12		11	3, 21, 22	5, 6, 7, 16, 19		8, 9, 10	1, 2, 4, 13, 14, 15, 17, 18, 20
10—Genitourinary Disorders	11		5, 7		6, 13	14	3, 8, 9, 15	1, 2, 4, 10, 12
11—Hematologic Disorders		7, 9	2, 3, 4, 5, 6, 10, 11					1, 8
12—Neoplastic Disorders	6, 14	18	4, 5, 8			10, 11	3, 7, 9, 17, 19	1, 2, 12, 13, 15, 16
13—Central Nervous System Disorders		2, 7		10		3, 8, 9	1, 6	4, 5 (continued)

Chapter	CLIENT NEED: SAFE, EFFECTIVE CARE ENVIRONMENT (SECE)		CLIENT NEED: HEALTH PROMOTION/ MAINTENANCE (HPM)	CLIENT NEED: PSYCHOSOCIAL INTEGRITY (PsI)	CLIENT NEED: PHYSIOLOGICAL INTEGRITY (PhI)			
	Client Subneed: Management of Care	Client Subneed: Safety/Infection Control			Client Subneed: Basic Care/Comfort	Client Subneed: Pharmacological/Parenteral Therapies	Client Subneed: Reduction of Risk Potential	Client Subneed: Physiological Adaptation
	Question #:	Question #:	Question #:		Question #:	Question #:	Question #:	Question #:
14—Musculo-skeletal Disorders	16	12	11, 14	6, 8, 13	3, 4, 5, 7, 9, 17		10	1, 2, 15, 18
15—Neuromuscular Disorders			2, 3, 7, 10	6	4, 5, 8		11, 12	1, 9
16—Problems of the Newborn (Birth Defects)		3	2, 6, 10, 20, 24, 29, 31, 38	9, 12, 32	16, 17, 22, 23, 28, 30		8, 11, 13, 14, 15, 18, 19, 25, 26, 27, 35, 36, 37	1, 4, 5, 7, 21, 33, 34
17—Nursing Care for Children's Unique Needs	12		6, 11, 15	4, 5	2	9, 13	1, 3, 8	7, 10, 14

Resources

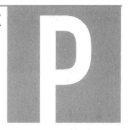

These are selected **sources of information and services.** Every effort has been made to provide current names and addresses; however addresses do change frequently.

Health and Welfare Agencies/Associations

American Burn Association
www.ameriburn.org

Shriner's Burn Institute
University of Cincinnati
www.med.uc.edu/departments/surgery/research/shriners.cfm

American Cancer Society
www.cancer.org

American Diabetes Association
www.diabetes.org

American Foundation for the Blind
www.afb.org

Asthma and Allergy Foundation of America
www.aafa.org

Centers for Disease Control and Prevention
Department of Health and Human Services
U.S. Public Health Service
www.cdc.gov

Concern for Dying
http://grief.netfirms.com/dying.html

Cystic Fibrosis Foundation
www.cff.org/home

Epilepsy Foundation of America
www.epilepsyfoundation.org

Guide for Infant Survival (Sudden Infant Death Syndrome)
www.5mcc.com/Assets/SUMMARY/TP0886.html

Leukemia Society of America
www.mdleukemia.org

National Association to Control Epilepsy
www.epilepsyfoundation.org

Sickle Cell Disease Association of America, Inc.
www.sicklecelldisease.org

National Cancer Institute
www.cancer.gov

National Hemophilia Foundation
www.hemophilia.org

National Institute of Allergy and Infectious Diseases
www.niaid.nih.gov/default.htm

National SIDS Alliance (Sudden Infant Death Syndrome)
www.sidsalliance.org

National Society to Prevent Blindness
www.eyeinfo.org/national.html

Office for Individuals with Disabilities
www.mdtap.org/oidcontent

The Phoenix Society for Burn Survivors, Inc.
www.phoenix-society.org/about.htm

National Scoliosis Foundation
http://scoliosis.org

United Cerebral Palsy Association (UCPA)
www.ucpahi.org

Professional Organizations/Associations

American Academy of Ambulatory Care Nursing
www.aaacn.org

American Academy of Nurse Practitioners
www.aanp.org

The American Assembly for Men in Nursing
www.aamn.org

American Holistic Nurses' Association
www.ahna.org

Association of Nurses in AIDS Care
www.hivpositive.com/f-Awards/ANAC/ANAC.html

Association of Pediatric Oncology Nursing
www.apon.org

Association of Rehabilitation Nurses
www.rehabnurse.org

Emergency Nurses Association
www.ena.org

National Association of Hispanic Nurses
www.thehispanicnurses.org

National Association of Home Care (NAHC)
www.nahc.org

National Association of Pediatric Nurse Associates and
   Practitioners
www.napnap.org

National Black Nurses Association, Inc.
www.nbna.org

North American Nursing Diagnosis Association
www.nanda.org

Oncology Nursing Society
www.ons.org

Transcultural Nursing Society
Department of Nursing Madonna College
www.tcns.org

Patient Education Materials

Abbott Laboratories
www.abbott.com

Cystic Fibrosis Foundation
www.cff.org

Juvenile Diabetes Foundation International
www.jdrf.org

Eli Lilly and Company
Educational Resources Program
www.lilly.com

March of Dimes Birth Defects Foundation
www.cehn.org/cehn/resourceguide/mod.html

National Hydrocephalus Foundation
www.nhfonline.org

National Safety Council
www.nsc.org

National Scoliosis Foundation
http://scoliosis.org

National Tay-Sachs and Allied Diseases Association
www.ntsad.org

Nutrition Education Association
www.nal.usda.gov/fnic

Phoenix Society for Burn Survivors, Inc.
www.phoenix-society.org

Schering Corporation
www.sch-plough.com

Spina Bifida Association of America
www.sbaa.org

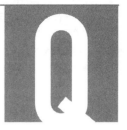
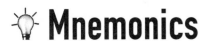 Mnemonics

Appendicitis—Assessment: PAINS
Pain (RLQ)
Anorexia
Increased temperature and WBC (15,000–20,000)
Nausea/vomiting
Signs: Psoas, McBurney's

*Appendicitis—Complications: 4 P's
Perforation
Peritonitis
Periappendiceal abscess
Pyelothrombophlebitis

Cleft Lip—Nursing Care Plan (postoperative): "CLEFT LIP"
Crying, minimize
Logan bow
Elbow restraints
Feed with Breck feeder
Tent, croup

Liquid (sterile water), rinse after feeding
Impaired feeding (no sucking)
Position—*never* on abdomen

Congenital Heart Disease—Assessment: HEARTS
Heart sounds (murmur)
Eating problem (poor sucking)
Assess weight (slow gain), growth (slow)
↑**R**espirations (also pulse); ↑ Respiratory infections →
    hypoxia
Tires easily
Septal defects: ASD, VSD

Developmental Dysplasia of the Hip—Assessment: ASSESS
Asymmetric gluteal and thigh folds (on affected side)
Signs: Barlow, Ortolani (newborn); Trendelenberg
    (older child)
Shortening of leg (on affected side)
Evaluate: abduction limitation, delayed walking
Spine, knee flexion, with hips abducted, cause "click"
Scan (CT) and ultrasound in young infants

Diabetes—Symptoms: 3 P's
Polyphagia
Polydipsia
Polyuria

Eardrops—administering: UP/DOWN

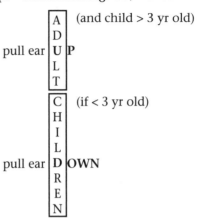

pull ear — ADULT — P   (and child > 3 yr old)

pull ear — CHILDREN — DOWN   (if < 3 yr old)

(Acyanotic) Heart Defects—Assessment: ABC's^2
Always Ⓛ → Ⓡ shunt
Blood loss (epistaxis)
Cerebral symptoms: headaches
Systemic pressure > pulmonary pressure
Syncope

(Cyanotic) Heart Defects—Assessment: ABC^2's
Always Ⓡ → Ⓛ shunt
Breathing difficulties ("Tet" spells)
Clubbing, **C**yanosis
Squatting relieves hypoxia

(Cyanotic) Heart Defects—Types: 3 T's
Transposition of the great vessels
Tetralogy of Fallot
Truncus arteriosus

Kawasaki's Disease—Assessment: LOTS of FEVER
Lymphadenopathy (cervical)
Oral inflammation (lips: cracked, dry; tongue: strawberry-
    color; mouth: erythema of oropharynx)
Thrombocytosis
Skin: erythema (palms, soles); desquamation, starting at
    fingertips
                        (of)
Fever ≥ 5 days
Eyes (bilateral conjunctivitis)
Vasculitis (coronary artery)
Edema
Rash (erythematous; polymorphous)

LTB—Assessment: R^{2}ES^{2}T
Retractions; **R**estlessness
Evening onset of "crowing" sounds
Stridors (inspiratory); **S**low onset
Temperature (elevated)

*Adapted from Rogers, P. *Medical Student's Guide to Top Board Scores*. Boston. Little, Brown.

Nephrotic Syndrome—Assessment: NAPLES
Nutrition (protein malnutrition)
Albumin (hypoalbuminemia)
Proteinuria
Lipidemia
Edema
Sequelae/complications: hypercoagulation; ↑ bacterial
    infections

Reye Syndrome—Clinical Features: $A^1V^3C^3R^3$
Aspirin ingestion
Viral infection (**V**aricella, influenzae → **V**omiting
    protracted)
Confusion → **C**ombativeness → **C**oma (acute metabolic
    encephalopathy)
Reflexes (brainstem) are lost → **R**igidity (decerebrate) →
    Respiratory failure

Reye Syndrome—Lab Values: ↑ LAB
Liver function tests (↑ ALT, AST, LDH)
Ammonia (>300: poor prognosis)
Bleeding times (↑ PT, PTT)

**Reye Syndrome—Supportive Treatment
(↓ sign/symtoms): Control GRAPH**
↓ Cerebral edema
↓ GI symptoms (vomiting)
↓ Respiratory failure
↓ Ammonia levels
↓ PT/PTT time
↓ Hypoglycemia

Sickle Cell Anemia—Clinical Assessment: $A^2S^3I^2C^3KLE^3$
Avascular necrosis (extreme pain!); **A**plastic crisis
Sickling of cells; **S**plenic sequestration; **S**hock
    (hypovolemia)
Infections (*H. influenza*, pneumococcus; osteomyelitis
    with *Staph. aureas* and *salmonella*); **I**schemia
Chronic hemolytic anemia; **C**risis (vaso-occlusive);
    Capillary stasis
Kidney damage (hematuria; ↓ urine concentration)
Leg ulcers
Electrophoresis of hemoglobin; ↓ **E**rythropoeisis
    (i.e. ↑ RBC destruction); **E**lectrolyte imbalances

**Sickle Cell Anemia—Prevention of Vaso-occlusive Crisis:
A^4HOPE**
Avoid precipitating factors: **A**ltitude (high), **A**irplane
    travel, **A**ctivity (strenuous)
Hydration (↑ fluids due to ↑ vomit and diarrhea)
Oxygenation (O_2)
Prophylactic penicillin and vaccination
Electrolyte imbalance

Stool—Assessment: ACCT
Amount
Color
Consistency
Timing

**Tetralogy of Fallot—Assessment of Cardiac Abnormalities:
HOPS**
Hypertrophy of ® ventricle
Over-riding aorta
Pulmonary stenosis
Septal defect (e.g., VSD)

Tracheoesophageal Fistula—Assessment: 3 C's
Coughing
Choking
Cyanosis

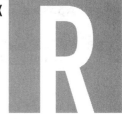

Crossword Puzzle:
Cardiopulmonary Failure
(Pediatrics)*

Clues (Answers on **page 248**)

Across

1. 0.5 to 1 gm/kg for hypoglycemia.
7. 0.5 mg of epinephrine (1:10,000) = _____ cc.
10. Measure of acid/base status.
11. Indicated for hypotension and/or poor perfusion.
12. Draw up this amount of atropine for a 5 kg infant.
13. Bradycardia rate.
14. A measure of skin perfusion.
19. First-line catecholamine.
20. State of poor oxygenation.
22. A crystalloid solution (abbr.)
25. Cardiopulmonary resuscitation + interventions for foreign body airway obstruction (FBAO) (abbr).
26. Dose (mg) of lidocaine for a 7 kg child.
27. Milliequivalent dose of sodium bicarbonate for a 10 kg child.
28. Basic life support for cardiopulmonary arrest (abbr).
29. Route of medication administration associated with many hazards (abbr).
30. Purpose of chest compressions.
31. Very rapid heart rate (abbr).
34. Crystalloid solution of choice (abbr).
35. Interventions for respiratory distress (2 words).
40. Do this before intervening.
41. Alternative route for certain medications when IV is not available.
42. For basic life support, check infant pulse here.
44. Treatment for ventricular fibrillation.
46. Provide abdominal _____s for FBAO in children.
47. Clinical state with decreased delivery of oxygen and metabolic substrates to the tissues.
49. Watch the _____ rise to assess ventilations.
50. To achieve vascular access.
55. Maneuver to open airway with suspected cervical injury.
56. Solutions used in volume expansion.
59. Hazard associated with assisted ventilation at high pressures.
60. Late and inconsistent sign of respiratory distress.
62. Check responsiveness to assess its perfusion.
64. Indicated for bradycardia, accompanied by poor perfusion or hypotension.
66. Slow rate = _____cardia.
69. Systematic, standardized approach to pediatric cardiopulmonary failure (acronym).
70. Large leg vein for central line.
71. Look for increased work of breathing as child tries to _____ .
74. 70 + (2X age in years) is lower limit for—(abbr).
76. End result of progressive deterioration in respiratory and circulatory function (2 words).

78. Prepare _____ cc of epinephrine (1:10,000) for a 20 kg child.
81. "Straight line"; no pulse.
84. Minimum dose of atropine is _____ cc = 0.1 mg.
86. Clear the airway.
87. To confirm endotracheal tube (ETT) placement.
88. Remember to provide support and information to these or significant others.

Down

2. Indicated for ventricular trachycardia or fibrillation.
3. Give back _____ and chest thrusts for infant FBAO.
4. ETT size for a one-year-old child.
5. Place infant's head in this position to open airway.
6. For basic life support, person one to eight years of age.
8. Safe and effective alternative route to vascular access.
9. Early sign of respiratory distress in infants.
10. Maintain to keep airway open.
15. Mottling, pallor, and slow capillary refill indicate poor _____ .
16. Assess _____ for rate and depth.
17. Provide bag-mask _____ for respiratory failure.
18. Used to treat hypoxemia.
19. Obtained with cardiac monitor to detect dysrhythmias (abbr).
21. Test to assess ventilation and acid-base balance (abbr).
23. Provide one breath every three _____ for an infant or child (abbr).
24. 1-2-3 steps in rapid cardiopulmonary assessment.
28. Heart rate X stroke volume.
32. Blood pressure may be maintained by increasing heart rate and _____ (2 words).
33. Newborns increase cardiac output by increasing heart _____ .
36. Administered during resuscitation to achieve therapeutic goals.
37. Decreased perfusion here is an early sign of shock.
38. Device applied to face to deliver oxygen and provide ventilation.
39. Gastric _____ , a possible side effect of assisted ventilation.
43. Indicates increased work of breathing.
45. Increased respiratory rate.
48. Ranges from pale to cyanotic.
51. Narcotic antagonist.
52. Sign of brain hypoperfusion.
53. Maintain to avoid hypothermia.
54. Late sign of cardiac decompensation.
56. Weak _____ , irritability in a baby may be early signs of shock.
57. pH less than 7.35.
58. Continuous infusion of medication.
60. 20 _____/kg fluid bolus for volume expansion.

*Galuska, L.A. *Solve the puzzle of pediatric and cardiopulmonary failure.* MCN, 20, 334, 336.

61. ETT size for an eight-year-old child.
63. _____ trauma, side effect of excessive ventilatory pressures.
65. Provided to family members.
66. Device used to ventilate child without ETT (abbr).
67. A must after each intervention.
68. Urine output < 1 cc/kg/hr is a sign of _____ renal perfusion.
71. Check a child's pulse here.
72. Use suction and positioning to maintain patency.
73. Tube placed in the trachea (abbr).
75. _____ D50 to make D25.
77. Insert to relieve gastric distension.
79. Flaring and retractions = increased _____ of breathing.
80. For basic life support, an infant is younger than_____ year.
82. Ranges from awake and alert to unresponsive (abbr).
83. Airway used in unconscious child.
85. Positive _____-expiratory pressure = PEEP.

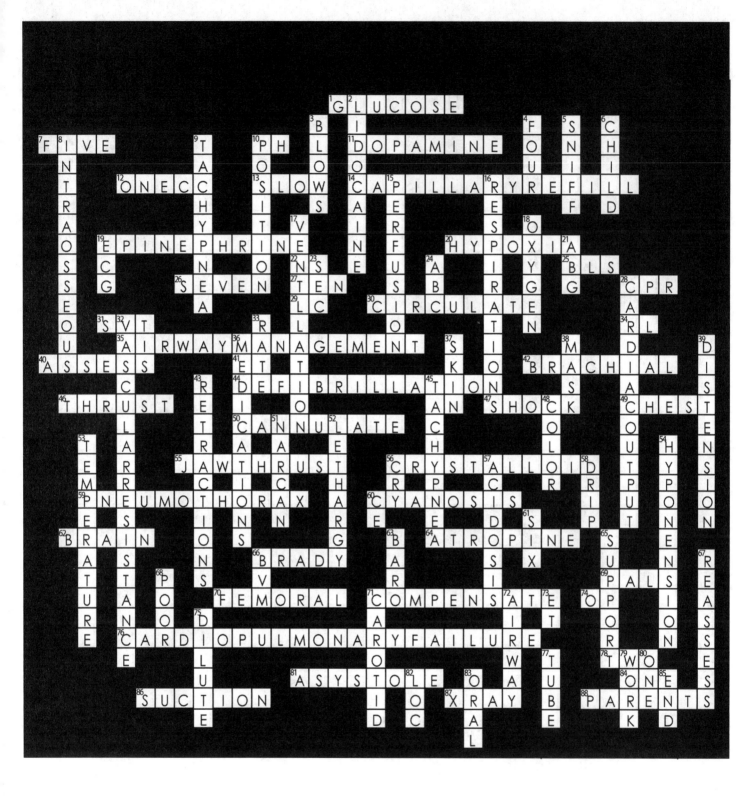

BIBLIOGRAPHY

Baker LK and Anderson B. *Plans of Care for Specialty Practice Series: Pediatrics*. Albany: Delmar.

Ball J. and Bindler R. *Pediatric Nursing: Caring for Children*. Norwalk, CT: Appleton and Lange.

Betz C., Hunsberger M., and Wright S. *Family-Centered Nursing Care of Children* (2nd ed). Philadelphia: WB Saunders.

Boynton RW, et al. *Manual of Pediatrics Nursing* (3rd ed). Philadelphia: JB Lippincott.

Castiglia PT and Harbin RE. *Child Health Care: Process and Practice*. Philadelphia: JB Lippincott.

Gulanick M., Gradishar D., and Puzas MK. *Ambulatory Pediatric Nursing: Plans of Care for Specialty Practice*. Albany: Delmar.

Hickey P. Pediatric collaborative practice: A cardiovascular program. *Nurs Clin North Am* 30:2.

Instant Nursing Assessment Series: Pediatrics Albany: Delmar.

Jackson DB and Saunders R. *Child Health Nursing: A Comprehensive Approach to the Care of Children and Their Families*. Philadelphia: JB Lippincott.

Olds SB, London ML, and Ladewig PW. *Maternal-Newborn Nursing: A Family Centered Approach* (5th ed). Menlo Park: Addison-Wesley.

Pilliteri A. *Maternal and Child Health Nursing: Care of the Childbearing and Childrearing Family* (2nd ed). Philadelphia: JB Lippincott.

Pilliteri A. *Pocket Companion for Maternal and Child Health Nursing*. Philadelphia: JB Lippincott.

Rapid Nursing Intervention Series: Pediatrics. Albany: Delmar.

Skale N. *Manual of Pediatric Nursing Procedures*. Philadelphia: JB Lippincott.

Wong DL. *Clinical Manual of Pediatric Nursing*. St. Louis: Mosby.

Wong DL. *Whaley and Wong's Nursing Care of Infants and Children*. St. Louis: Mosby.

INDEX

DATE DUE

PRINTED IN U.S.A.